Kinesiology and Sports Science

Kinesiology and Sports Science

Edited by Tilly Martin

SYRAWOOD
PUBLISHING HOUSE

New York

Published by Syrawood Publishing House,
750 Third Avenue, 9th Floor,
New York, NY 10017, USA
www.syrawoodpublishinghouse.com

Kinesiology and Sports Science
Edited by Tilly Martin

International Standard Book Number: 978-1-64740-253-2 (Hardback)

Cataloging-in-Publication Data

Kinesiology and sports science / edited by Tilly Martin.
    p. cm.
Includes bibliographical references and index.
ISBN 978-1-64740-253-2
1. Kinesiology. 2. Sports sciences. 3. Sports. I. Martin, Tilly.
QP303 .K56 2022
612.7--dc23

TABLE OF CONTENTS

Permissions

List of Contributors

Index

PREFACE

The scientific study of human body movement is known as kinesiology. It primarily addresses the physiological, biomechanical and psychological dynamic principles and mechanisms of movement. Human kinesiology have applications in the area of biomechanics, orthopedics and sports psychology. Kinesiology involves various principles of neuroplasticity, adaptation through exercise, motor redundancy, etc. It primarily applies the sciences of biomechanics, anatomy, physiology, psychology and neuroscience to study movements. The discipline of sports science studies how the human body works during exercise and how health is promoted through sports and physical activities. The study of sports science includes areas like physiology, psychology, anatomy, biomechanics and biokinetics. This book studies, analyzes and upholds the pillars of kinesiology and sports science and their utmost significance in modern times. It traces the progress of these fields and highlights some of their key concepts and applications. This book aims to serve as a resource guide for students and experts.

This book is a comprehensive compilation of works of different researchers from varied parts of the world. It includes valuable experiences of the researchers with the sole objective of providing the readers (learners) with a proper knowledge of the concerned field. This book will be beneficial in evoking inspiration and enhancing the knowledge of the interested readers.

In the end, I would like to extend my heartiest thanks to the authors who worked with great determination on their chapters. I also appreciate the publisher's support in the course of the book. I would also like to deeply acknowledge my family who stood by me as a source of inspiration during the project.

Editor

The Effect of Elevation on Volumetric Measurements of the Lower Extremity

Cordial M. Gillette[1]*, Scott T. Doberstein[2], Danielle L. DeSerano[3], Eric J. Linnell[4]

[1]*Exercise and Sport Science, University of Wisconsin – La Crosse, 1725 State Street, 148 Mitchell Hall, La Crosse, Wisconsin, 54601, USA*
[2]*Exercise and Sport Science, University of Wisconsin – La Crosse, 1725 State Street, 144 Mitchell Hall, La Crosse, Wisconsin, 54601, USA*
[3]*UW-Health Sports Medicine, 621 Research Drive, Madison, Wisconsin, 53711, USA*
[4]*Athletics, University of Wisconsin – Madison, 1440 Monroe Street, Madison, Wisconsin, 53711, USA*

Corresponding Author: Cordial M. Gillette, E-mail: cgillette@uwlax.edu

ARTICLE INFO

Conflicts of interest: None
Funding: None

ABSTRACT

Background: The empirical evidence for the use of RICE (rest, ice, compression, elevation) has been questioned regarding its clinical effectiveness. The component of RICE that has the least literature regarding its effectiveness is elevation. **Objective:** The objective of this study was to determine if various positions of elevation result in volumetric changes of the lower extremity. **Methodology:** A randomized crossover design was used to determine the effects of the four following conditions on volumetric changes of the lower extremity: seated at the end of a table (seated), lying supine (flat), lying supine with the foot elevated 12 inches off the table (elevated), and lying prone with the knees bent to 90 degrees (prone). The conditions were randomized using a Latin Square. Each subject completed all conditions with at least 24 hours between each session. Pre and post volumetric measurements were taken using a volumetric tank. The subject was placed in one of the four described testing positions for 30 minutes. The change in weight of the displaced water was the main outcome measure. The data was analyzed using an ANOVA of the pre and post measurements with a Bonferroni post hoc analysis. The level of significance was set at $P<.05$ for all analyses. **Results:** The only statistically significant difference was between the gravity dependent position (seated) and all other positions ($p<.001$). There was no significant difference between lying supine (flat), on a bolster (elevated), or prone with the knees flexed to 90 degrees (prone). **Conclusions:** From these results, the extent of elevation does not appear to have an effect on changes in low leg volume. Elevation above the heart did not significantly improve reduction in limb volume, but removing the limb from a gravity dependent position might be beneficial.

Key words: Swelling, Injury, Edema, Treatment

INTRODUCTION

For many decades, the use of rest, ice, compression, and elevation (RICE) has been the main-stay and a widely accepted treatment for acute musculoskeletal injuries. The proposed mechanisms for assisting in the healing process are to limit the various unwanted cellular changes that occur with injury and thus decrease the amount and extent of tissue damage. In theory, this would lead to quicker healing and a faster return to normal function and activity levels. However, RICE has been questioned regarding its clinical effectiveness based on the limited evidence available to date (van den Bekerom et al., 2012). Of all the components of RICE, ice has been researched the most extensively and thus clinicians practice injury management based on very good evidence related to its use for acute injuries (Jutte, Merrick, Ingersoll, & Edwards, 2001; Merrick, Jutte, & Smith, 2003; Merrick, Knight, Ingersoll, & Potteiger, 1993; Merrick, Rankin, Andres, & Hinman, 1999; Otte, Merrick, Ingersoll, & Cordova, 2002; Prentice, 2009a). Greenwood and Gillette (2017), however, showed that cold water immersion increases metabolic rate in humans and therefore is more beneficial for exercise recovery than treatment of acute injuries. Even though it is very common for injuries to be elevated during acute treatment and makes sense theoretically, the empirical evidence supporting its use is lacking, so much so that some clinicians question using this part of the RICE protocol at all. Several questions regarding the use of elevation include is there a most beneficial degree of elevation or is elevation even necessary?

Elevation is utilized based on theories that it will eliminate the effects of gravity, augment venous return (Hirai & Iwata, 2004), assist lymphatic drainage of blood and other fluids (Prentice, 2009b, 2009c, 2011, 2013), and decrease capillary hydrostatic pressure (Knight, 1995; Warren, Hardiman, & Woolf, 1992). There is limited and conflicting evidence on the effects of venous return and lymphatic drainage in regards to elevation (Elkins, Herrick, Grindlay, Mann, & De Forest, 1953; Hirai & Iwata, 2004; Warren et al., 1992). The leading theory for the use of elevation is to decrease capillary hydrostatic pressure thereby decreasing the loss of fluid across the capillary (Merrick et al., 1993) and potentially limit fluid accumulation in the extremity. While there is evidence of changes in capillary hydrostatic pressures and significant changes in the volume of lower legs after 4 hours (Hargens, 1983), the window of opportunity for limiting secondary injury lies within the first 30 minutes following acute injury (Merrick & McBrier, 2010) and there is currently no evidence for volume changes due to elevation over a 30 minute time period. Therefore, there is a need to examine volume changes in the lower extremity over a 30 minute time period and determine if limb position affects volumetric changes. To determine changes in limb volume due to elevation, the effects of multiple positions must first be determined in a non-edematous limb. The objective of this study was to determine if various positions of elevation result in volumetric changes of the lower extremity of non-injured individuals in a 30 minute window. The hypothesis was positions of elevation would cause greater decreases in volumetric measurements than a non-elevated or gravity dependent position.

METHODOLOGY

Participants

The subjects included 21 healthy, college-aged student volunteers (9 males, 12 females) ages 19 – 22 with an average age of 21.05 (males – 21.00; females - 21.09) and no previous (6 month) history of low leg injury. The average height, weight, and BMI were 174.18 cm (males – 176.16 cm; females – 172.20 cm), 74.11 kg (males – 77.4 kg; females – 70.82 kg), and 24.36 (males – 24.82; females – 23.91), respectively.

Study Design

A randomized crossover design was used to determine the effects of the four following conditions on volumetric changes of the lower extremity: seated at the end of a table (seated, Figure 1), lying supine (flat, Figure 2), lying supine with the foot elevated 12 inches off the table (elevated, Figure 3), and lying prone with the knees bent to 90 degrees (prone, Figure 4). The conditions were randomized using a Latin Square. Each subject completed all conditions with at least 24 hours between each condition session.

Volumetric Measurements

Pre and post volumetric measurements were taken using a volumetric tank. The volumetric tank had been modified to position the overflow spout parallel to the floor. The beginning weight of the volumetric tank and water was 9000 g (Figure 5) using a Mettler Toledo XS32000L Precision Balance (Columbus, OH). The volumetric tank was transferred

to the floor without loss of water and the collection container was placed under the spout. The subject was seated in a chair to allow proper positioning of the foot in the tank. Before placing the subject's right foot in the volumetric tank, it was wiped with a wet towel to avoid absorption of any water through the skin and air bubbles from accumulating on the skin. The subject's foot and ankle were submersed in the vol-

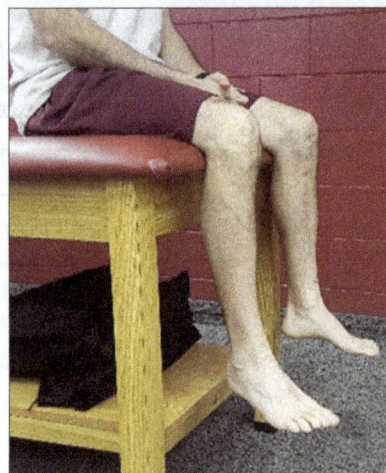

Figure 1. Seated

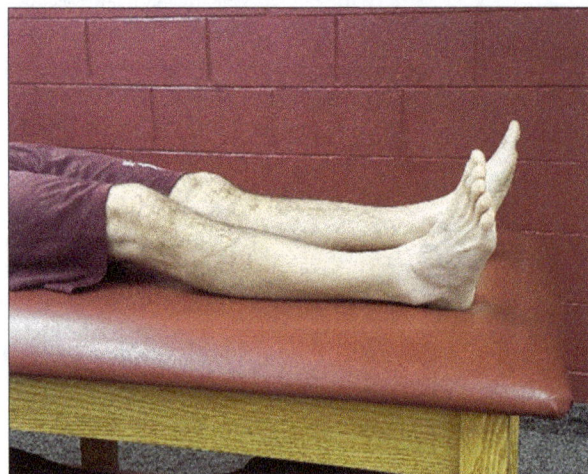

Figure 2. Lying Supine

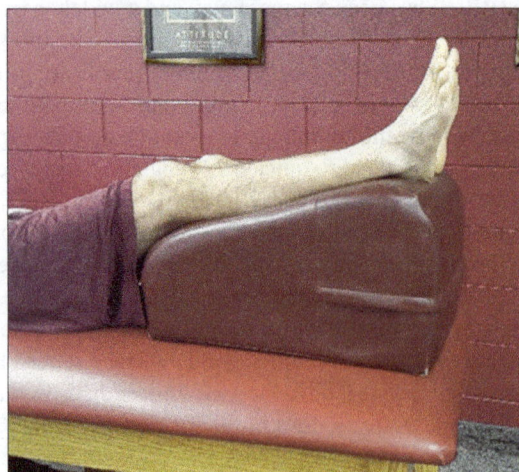

Figure 3. Elevated 12 inches

umetric tank and they were instructed to place the MP joint of their great toe and medial malleolus against the side wall and their heel and low leg against the back wall of the tank. The subject remained seated with their foot in the tank while the water was collected in the container until dripping from the spout ceased (Figure 6). The collection container and displaced water were again weighed (Figure 7). This measurement was taken before and after each condition.

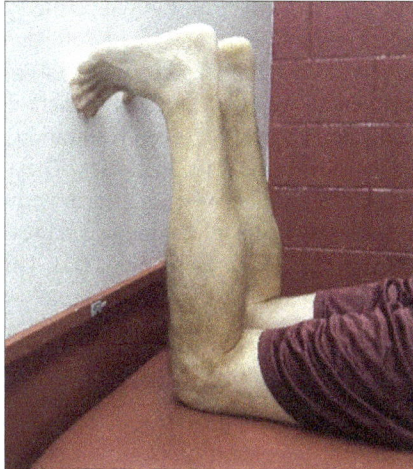

Figure 4. Prone with knees at 90 degrees

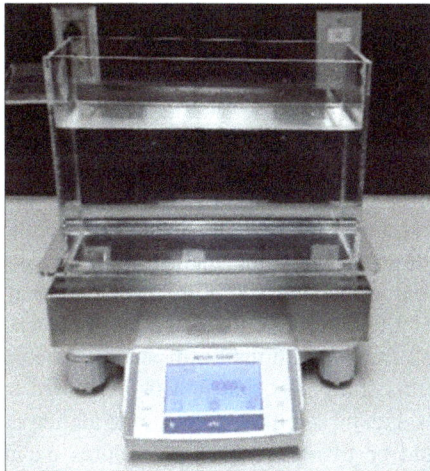

Figure 5. Beginning volume

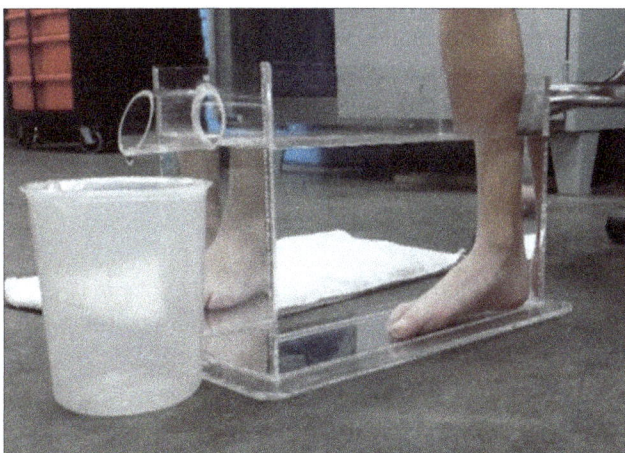

Figure 6. Foot placed in tank for collection

Testing Positions

After the initial volumetric measurement was taken, the subject was placed in one of the four testing positions as described above. They remained in this position for 30 minutes and were instructed to avoid movement (i.e. dorsiflexion/plantarflexion, toe flexion/extension, etc.) throughout the 30 minutes. Upon completion of the intervention, the post volumetric measurement was taken utilizing the above described procedures.

Statistical Analysis

The change in weight of the displaced water was the main outcome measure. The data was normally distributed. The data was analyzed using a paired samples t-test of the pre and post measurements as well as an ANOVA of the mean change in pre and post measurements with a Bonferroni post hoc analysis. The level of significance was set at $P<.05$ for all analyses. Statistical analysis was performed with SPSS version 23.

RESULTS

The paired samples t-test indicated significant changes in volume from pre to post-test volumetric measurements for all positions except for the seated position (seated, p =.087; supine, p =.001; elevated 12 inches, p =.004; prone, p =.002). The seated, gravity-dependent position was the only position which caused a mean increase in volume; all other positions demonstrated decreases in volume, including the neutral position. The ANOVA revealed the difference was significant between the gravity dependent position (seated) and all other positions (seated, p =.003; elevated 12 inches, p =.037, prone at 90, p =.004). There was no significant difference between lying supine (flat), with the foot elevated 12 inches while in a supine position (elevated), p = 1.00, or prone with the knees flexed to 90 degrees (prone), p = 1.00; nor was there a difference between the elevated position and prone, p =.611. The volumetric changes based on positioning are presented in Table 1.

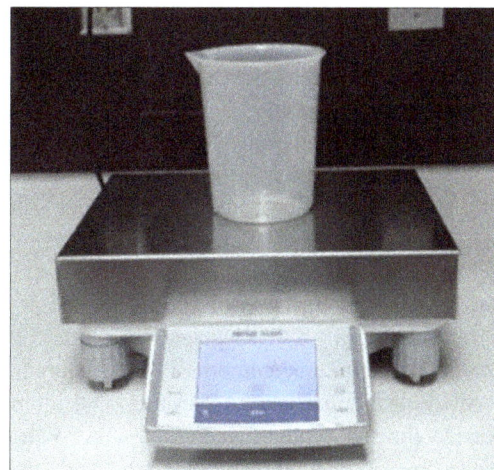

Figure 7. Displaced water

Table 1. Volumetric changes in the low leg

Position	Mean±SD		Mean change in volume±standard error
	Pre-test	Post-test	
Seated	510.4±148.2	522.1±152.7	11.7±6.47
Supine (flat)	518.7±159.5	504.3±160.1	−14.3±3.58*
Elevated 12 inches	511.5±164.3	502.2±164.4	−9.3±2.83*
Prone at 90	525.9±168.7	509.6±162.9	−16.3±4.46*

*Denotes significant change compared to baseline (p<0.05).

DISCUSSION

The results of this study indicate elevated positions did not have a greater decrease in limb volume than a neutral or gravity dependent positon. The recommended extent of elevation, based on expert opinion is 15 to 25 centimeters (6-10 inches) above the heart (Knight, 1995). It is reasonable to state that elevation above the heart is not necessary for removing edema, while removing the limb from a gravity dependent position might be beneficial. Several texts (Prentice, 2009a, 2009c, 2011, 2013) indicate the higher the elevation, the greater effect; however, Warren et al.(1992) assessed volume changes in human calves during 45 and 90 degrees of elevation using strain gauge plethysmography and found the higher angle produced slower exsanguination with greater venous return when the lower leg was elevated to 45. Therefore, a greater degree of elevation may not promote greater results in preventing or removing edema. In our study, the 90 degree position (prone) did demonstrate the greatest change in volume, but it was not significant.

These results are comparable to those found by Tsang et al.(2000) in which significant changes in limb volume were found after 30 minutes of elevation in healthy individuals. At 90 degrees of elevation in a supine position, their study showed a volumetric decrease of 15.3 mL immediately post treatment while we found volumetric decreases of 16.3 mL in a prone position with the knee bent to 90 degrees. Their study also showed a continued decrease in limb volume of 9.8 mL 60 minutes after returning to a gravity dependent position. They reported that elevation does decrease volume due to increases in venous flow and lymphatic absorption of interstitial fluid; however, only one position was studied. We did not look at results other than immediately following the intervention; therefore, the duration of the effect of removing gravity cannot be concluded from our study, but perhaps repeating this study with varying degrees of elevation may be useful given the findings of Warren et al.(1992). A follow-up study by Tsang et al. (2003) looked at the effects of returning to a gravity-dependent position following elevation and intermittent compression on injured ankles and revealed elevation alone, or elevation and intermittent compression did not produce decreased ankle volume for an extended period of time. While they did find significant decreases in volume immediately post treatment, the effects were negated when the limb returned to a gravity-dependent position, yet 60 minutes in a gravity-dependent position did not increase the volume beyond baseline measurements. Our results were also consistent with Sims (1986) who examined ankle volume changes in healthy, uninjured ankles in an elevated position compared to a gravity dependent position. He found a 14 – 17 mL decrease in volume in an elevated position compared to a 16 to 18 ml increase in a gravity dependent position. Sims (Sims, 1986) attributed changes in position to gravity's effect on the lymphatic system. The question still remains if there are greater effects on venous return or lymphatic flow. Hirai and Iwata (2004) investigated peak femoral venous velocity and calf muscle volume before and during limb elevation, deep respiration, calf compression and various types of leg exercises. They found that while elevation did promote venous return, active exercise utilizing ankle plantar and dorsiflexion was more effective to promote venous return (Hirai & Iwata, 2004). This supports the use of early, pain-free range of motion exercises following acute injury.

CONCLUSION

From these results, the extent of elevation does not appear to have an effect on changes in low leg volume. This study was conducted on healthy individuals and more information is needed to determine if these effects would occur in an individual with swelling. Given these results, elevation is not harmful to the patient, yet its benefit is not clearly evident.

A limitation of all the studies conducted on elevation thus far is that we have examined volume changes on either healthy subjects or post-acute injury. An attempt to determine the effects of elevation on the formation of edema in acute lateral ankle sprains was made by Hageman (2006), but no injuries meeting the inclusion criteria occurred or were brought to the attention of the investigator. It is, therefore, difficult to determine the potential of elevation to prevent edema from accumulating in an injured limb. A limitation of this study was that it was conducted on healthy individuals with no swelling. A recommendation for a future study would be to repeat these procedures on individuals with swelling or simulated swelling. In conclusion, further evidence must be sought to elucidate the significance of elevation. If our treatment goal is to limit secondary injury and prevent edema formation, yet treatments in a gravity dependent position, such as ice immersion, may be more useful to limit secondary injury through tissue temperature decrease, the question remains if there is enough evidence to keep elevation as a main-stay in acute injury management.

REFERENCES

Elkins, E. C., Herrick, J. F., Grindlay, J. H., Mann, F. C., & De Forest, R. E. (1953). Effect of various procedures on the flow of lymph. *Archives of Physical Medicine and Rehabilitation, 34*(1), 31-39.

Greenwood, A., & Gillette, C. (2017). Effect of cold water immersion on metabolic rate in humans. *International Journal of Kinesiology and Sports Science, 5*(2), 1 - 6.

doi: doi:10.7575/aiac.ijkss.v.5n.2p.1

Hargens, A. R. (1983). Fluid shifts in vascular and extra-vascular spaces during and after simulated weightlessness. *Medicine & Science in Sports & Exercise, 15*(5), 421-427.

Hirai, M., & Iwata, H. (2004). A comparison of physical methods for prophylaxis of deep vein thrombosis on augmentation of venous flow velocity and reduction of calf volume. *Phlebology, 19*(2), 72-76. doi:10.1258/026835504323080344

Jutte, L. S., Merrick, M. A., Ingersoll, C. D., & Edwards, J. E. (2001). The relationship between intramuscular temperature, skin temperature, and adipose thickness during cryotherapy and rewarming. *Archives of Physical Medicine and Rehabilitation, 82*(6), 845-850. doi: http://dx. doi.org/10.1053/apmr.2001.23195

Knight, K. (1995). Cryotherapy in sport injury management. Champaign, IL: Human Kinetics.

Merrick, M. A., Jutte, L. S., & Smith, M. E. (2003). Cold modalities with different thermodynamic properties produce different surface and intramuscular temperatures. *Journal of Athletic Training, 38*(1), 28-33.

Merrick, M. A., Knight, K. L., Ingersoll, C. D., & Potteiger, J. A. (1993). The effects of ice and compression wraps on intramuscular temperatures at various depths. *Journal of Athletic Training, 28*(3), 236-245.

Merrick, M. A., & McBrier, N. M. (2010). Progression of secondary injury after musculoskeletal trauma—A window of opportunity? *Journal of Sport Rehabilitation, 19*, 380-388.

Merrick, M. A., Rankin, J. M., Andres, F. A., & Hinman, C. L. (1999). A preliminary examination of cryotherapy and secondary injury in skeletal muscle. *Medicine & Science in Sports & Exercise, 31*(11), 1516-1521.

Otte, J. W., Merrick, M. A., Ingersoll, C. D., & Cordova, M. L. (2002). Subcutaneous adipose tissue thickness alters cooling time during cryotherapy. *Archives in P hysical Medicine and Rehabilitation, 83*(11), 1501-1505. doi: http://dx.doi.org/10.1053/apmr.2002.34833

Prentice, W. E. (2009a). *Arnheim's Principles of Athletic Training* (13 ed.). Boston, MA: McGraw-Hill.

Prentice, W. E. (2009b). *Arnheim's Principles of Athletic Training: A Competency-Based Approach* (M. Ryan Ed. 13th ed.). New York, NY: McGraw-Hill.

Prentice, W. E. (2009c). *Therapeutic Modalities for Sports Medicine and Athletic Training* (6th ed.). Boston, MA: McGraw-Hill.

Prentice, W. E. (2011). *Rehabilitation Techniques for Sports Medicine and Athletic Training* (5th ed.). New York, NY: McGraw Hill.

Prentice, W. E. (2013). *Essentials of Athletic Injury Management* (10e ed.). New York, NY: McGraw-Hill.

Sims, D. (1986). Effects of positioning on ankle edema. *The Journal of Orthopedic and Sports Physical Therapy, 8*(1), 30-33.

van den Bekerom, M. P., Struijs, P. A., Blankevoort, L., Welling, L., van Dijk, C. N., & Kerkhoffs, G. M. (2012). What is the evidence for rest, ice, compression, and elevation therapy in the treatment of ankle sprains in adults? *Journal of Athletic Training, 47*(4), 435-443. doi:10.4085/1062-6050-47.4.14

Warren, P. J., Hardiman, P. J., & Woolf, V. J. (1992). Limb exsanguination. II. The leg: effect of angle of elevation. *Annals of the Royal College of the Surgeons of England, 74*(5), 323-325.

2

Muscle Activity during Dryland Swimming while Wearing a Triathlon Wetsuit

Ciro Agnelli, John A. Mercer*

Department of Kinesiology & Nutrition Sciences, University of Nevada, Las Vegas, 4505 Maryland Parkway, Box 453034, Las Vegas, NV 89154-3034, USA

Corresponding Author: John A. Mercer, E-mail: john.mercer@unlv.edu

ARTICLE INFO

Conflicts of interest: None
Funding: None

ABSTRACT

Background: Triathletes typically wear a wetsuit during the swim portion of an event, but it is not clear if muscle activity is influenced by wearing a wetsuit. **Purpose:** To investigate if shoulder muscle activity was influenced by wearing a full-sleeve wetsuit vs. no wetsuit during dryland swimming. **Methods:** Participants (n=10 males; 179.1±13.2 cm; 91.2±7.25 kg; 45.6±10.5 years) completed two dry land swimming conditions on a swim ergometer: No Wetsuit (NW) and with Wetsuit (W). Electromyography (EMG) of four upper extremity muscles was recorded (Noraxon telemetry EMG, 500 Hz) during each condition: Trapezius (TRAP), Triceps (TRI), Anterior Deltoid (AD) and Posterior Deltoid (PD). Each condition lasted 90 seconds with data collected during the last 60 seconds. Resistance setting was self-selected and remained constant for both conditions. Stroke rate was controlled at 60 strokes per minute by having participants match a metronome. Average (AVG) and Root Mean Square (RMS) EMG were calculated over 45 seconds and each were compared between conditions using a paired t-test (α=0.05) for each muscle. **Results:** PD and AD AVG and RMS EMG were each greater (on average 40.0% and 66.8% greater, respectively) during W vs. NW ($p<0.05$) while neither TRAP nor TRI AVG or RMS EMG were different between conditions ($p>0.05$). **Conclusion:** The greater PD and AD muscle activity while wearing a wetsuit might affect swimming performance and/or stroke technique during a long distance event.

Key words: Electromyography, Endurance Exercise, Shoulder Muscle Activity, Fatigue, Upper Extremity

INTRODUCTION

Wetsuits have been used among many water sports including SCUBA diving, surfing, open water swimming, and triathlon competitions. Wetsuit design is often unique to the demands of the sport. For example, wetsuits designed for surfing tend to have a thick and rough material to account for how the surfer paddles the surf board. In contrast, a wetsuit designed for swim performance such as a triathlon typically has a smooth surface and thickness needs to be within specific governing body rules. The commonality between wetsuits is that they assist in theromoregulation in part by insulating properties of wetsuit material as well as warming of water between the skin and the material of the wetsuit ultimately providing insulation from cold temperatures (Corona et al., 2017; Naebe, 2013; Wakabayashi, et al., 2006).

During the sport of triathlon, it is very common for athletes to wear a wetsuit to take advantage of both the thermoregulation properties as well as the potential swim performance benefits (Chatard & Millet, 1996; Chatard, Senegas, Selles, Dreanot, & Geyssant, 1995). For example, Chatard et al. (1995) reported that triathlete subjects were on average 19 s faster during a 400 m swim using a wetsuit

vs. no wetsuit. However, it is important to note that not all swim performances will be improved when wearing a wetsuit (Chatard et al., 1995; Cordain & Kopriva, 1991; Ulsemar, Rust, Rosemann, Lepers, & Knechtle, 2014). For example, Chatard et al. (1995) also reported that 400-m swim performance was not influenced by wearing a wetsuit for swimmers. It was concluded that the influence of wetsuit on swim performance was related to swim ability – that is, faster swimmers did not benefit from the wetsuit whereas slower swimmers did. Similarly, Cordain & Kopriva (1991) reported that body composition was related to the influence of wetsuit on swim performance. These observations indicate that a single wetsuit design does not benefit swim performance of all people equally and has led to the development of a wide variety of wetsuit models that incorporate different design features. Two main general categories of wetsuit design are full-sleeve (Figure 1a) and sleeveless (Figure 1b) wetsuits.

Anecdotally, a widely-discussed topic in the triathlon area is whether a triathlete should use a full-sleeve or sleeveless wetsuit. The debate is typically centered on whether or not a full-sleeve wetsuit causes a possible additional resistance to upper extremity movement due to the neoprene sleeve

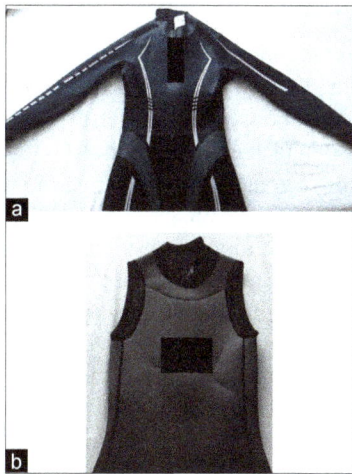

Figure 1. Illustration two main categories of wetsuits used in triathlon: a) Full-sleeve and b) sleeveless.

portion of the wetsuit. An increase in resistance to shoulder movements may influence how active shoulder muscles are. Although it is difficult to relate muscle activity and force during dynamic movements (Deluca, 1997), there is evidence that muscle activity is related to swim performance. For example, Ikuta et al. (2012) demonstrated that swim velocity was related to muscle activity of several muscles combined. Likewise, Figueiredo et al. (2013) reported that upper extremity muscle activity changed during an intense 200 m swim as swimmers experienced fatigue.

Presently, there are no empirical data on the influence of a full-sleeve wetsuit on muscle activity. However, Nessler, Silvas, Carpenter, & Newcomer (2015) investigated the influence of surfing wetsuit design on shoulder movement and muscle activity during simulated surf paddling. In that study, it was reported that shoulder movement pattern and muscle activity were affected by the use of a long sleeve wetsuit when compared to a traditional swimsuit while simulated surfing paddling (Nesser, et al., 2015). However, triathlon wetsuits are designed specifically for swimming (vs. the combination of paddling and surfing) and there are no data on muscle activity during swimming in triathlon wetsuits. Therefore, the purpose of this study was to investigate if shoulder muscle activity was influenced by wearing a full-sleeve wetsuit vs. no wetsuit during simulated dryland swimming. The sleeveless wetsuit was not used in part because funds were not available to purchase additional wetsuits. Nevertheless, it was also considered important to first explore if muscle activity was influenced by the two potentially extreme conditions (i.e., full-sleeve vs. no wetsuit).

METHODS

Participants

Participants (n=10 males; height: 179.1±13.2 cm; mass: 91.2±7.25 kg; age: 45.6±10.5 years) gave written informed consent to participate in the study. In order to be included in the study participants had to fit in at least one of the wetsuit sizes as per manufacturer recommendations. Participants

also had to have swum in a wetsuit and be familiar with the front crawl swimming stroke but not be necessarily swimmers. The level of swimming expertise of participants varied from novice to elite. In addition, participants were free of any acute or chronic shoulder injury.

Experimental Protocol

The experimental approach was a within-subject design where all participants completed two conditions. The two conditions were dryland swimming while wearing a wetsuit and not wearing a wetsuit. Participants were fit to one of four sizes of wetsuit (same model) available for this study (HUUB Design Limited, size: small medium-tall, medium, medium-tall, and medium-large; Aerious model 4 mm:4 mm thickness, Derby, UK) (Table 1). A telemetry EMG system (Noraxon Telemyo, Az) was used to collect muscle activity of four muscles on the right shoulder girdle and arm. An Electrogoniometer was attached to the right elbow joint to track arm flexion and extension with data recorded simultaneously with EMG using the same system.

All dryland swim conditions were completed using a swim ergometer (VASA Inc., Essex Junction, VT) with participants mimicking a crawl stroke technique they would use swimming in water. Participants were given sufficient time to practice using the swim ergometer prior to testing. The swim ergometer was equipped with a digital metronome that was set to 60 strokes per minute (i.e., 1 beat per side per second) with participants asked to maintain that stroke rate for both conditions. Resistance was controlled between conditions with participants self-selecting the resistance needed to maintain a somewhat hard intensity using 60 strokes per minute without wearing the wetsuit.

After practicing and being comfortable using the swim ergometer at the set cadence, the locations for surface EMG were prepared by shaving, abrading, and cleaning the sites where the EMG leads were placed. EMG leads were placed on the right-arm on the surface of the skin of the following muscles: Anterior Deltoid (AD), Posterior Deltoid (PD), Trapezius (TRAP), Triceps Brachii (TRI). Placement of the EMG leads followed the SENIAM guidelines (Hermens, Freriks, Disselhorst-Klyg, 2000). An electrogoniometer was placed on the elbow joint to measure elbow flexion-extension movements. After instrumentation, participants performed a maximal voluntary isometric contraction (MVIC) against maximal scapula elevation load for the trapezius and shoulder press for remaining muscles (anterior, posterior deltoids and triceps Brachii), for 5 second duration. All EMG data were subsequently normalized to the greatest 1-second average from the MVIC per muscle. That is, 100% EMG during a condition means the signal was the same magnitude as during the isometric condition. The normalized EMG data were used for analysis. Following MVIC procedures, Participants completed two dryland swim conditions using a crawl stroke swim technique: 1) with No Wetsuit (NW) and 2) with wetsuit (W). Order of conditions was always NW then W with about 3-5 minutes rest between conditions. The set order was used in order to minimize disrupting EMG lead and electrogoniometer placement when taking the wetsuit off. Each condition lasted 90 seconds with data collected the final 60 seconds of the condition.

Statistical Analysis

EMG data were processed by first removing any zero offset and then full-wave rectifying data. Average (AVG) and Root Mean Square (RMS) EMG was calculated over 45 seconds. Stroke rate was measured by identifying the time to complete 10 right-side strokes by inspecting the elbow flexion-extension data. The dependent variables were AVG and RMS EMG of each muscle (i.e., 8 total dependent variables) as well as stroke rate. Paired t-tests were used to test each dependent variable between conditions using SPSS (IBM SPSS Statistics, version 22.0.0.0; $\alpha = 0.05$).

RESULTS

Stroke rate was not different between conditions (NW: 0.52 ± 0.04 Hz; W: 0.51 ± 0.05 Hz; $t(9)=-1.249$, $p = 0.243$). EMG for PD (AVG: $t(9)=-3.066$, $p = 0.013$; RMS: $t(9)=-2.940$, 0.016) and AD (AVG: $t(9)=-3.491$, $p = 0.007$; RMS: $t(9)=-3.418$, $p = 0.008$) were each different during NW vs. WS (Figure 2, Table 1). Neither TRAP (AVG: $t(9)= -0.079$, $p = 0.939$; RMS: $t(9)=-0.239$, $p = 0.817$) nor TRI (AVG: $t(9)=-0.885$, $p = 0.399$; RMS: $t(9)=-0.587$, $p= 0.572$) EMG were different between conditions (Figure 2, Table 1).

Table 1. Group means and standard deviation of electromyography for each muscle. Data are presented in percentage of the EMG during maximal voluntary isometric contraction (MVIC).

Muscle	No Wetsuit (% MVIC)	Wetsuit (% MVIC)
Trapezius	58.2±45.1	59.5±35.3
Anterior Deltoid	20.9±13.1	34.8±10.7*
Posterior Deltoid	55.6±29.0	77.8±27.4*
Triceps Brachii	46.4±18.3	50.7±21.3

Note: * The Anterior Deltoid and Posterior Deltoid were each different during W and NW (p<0.05)

DISCUSSION

The most important observation of this study was that muscle activity of the PD and AD were each greater while wearing a wetsuit vs. not wearing a wetsuit when simulating swimming on dryland at equivalent stroke rates. On average, PD was about 40% greater while wearing the wetsuit vs. no wetsuit and the AD about 66.8% greater. In contrast, there was no influence of wearing a wetsuit on the muscle activity of the TRAP and TRI muscles. These observations seem to indicate that wearing the wetsuit resulted in increased resistance to shoulder movements.

The observation of greater muscle activity of the PD and AD during simulated swimming while wearing a wetsuit compared to not wearing a wetsuit is similar to what was observed by Nessler, et al. (2015). Although in that study, the muscle investigated was the middle deltoid and the exercise was simulated surf paddling with and without wetsuit. Even though a wetsuit designed for surfing is different than a triathlon wetsuit, Nessler et al. (2015) also reported greater middle deltoid muscle activity while wearing the wetsuit. Although the middle deltoid was not studied in our study, both Nessler et al. (2015) and the results from our study are consistent in that wearing a wetsuit influences shoulder muscle activity. These observations are reasonable given the function of the deltoid muscle as a whole during swimming. Pink, Perry, Browne, Scovazzo, & Kerrigan (1991) studied 12 muscles of the front crawl stroke in order to better understand muscle activity during specific phases of the stroke. Predominately, the AD and PD are recovery phase muscles with its muscle activity peaking during late pulling phase to early recovery for PD, and mid to late recovery for AD. Although we did not analyze the data for different phases of the stroke (i.e. pull and recovery phases), based upon the observations reported by Pink, et al. (1991), it is hypothesized that the difference in the muscle activity of the PD and AD during dryland swimming in wetsuit was mostly during the recovery phase. However, it is important to recognize the individual differences in stroke technique and therefore muscle activity. Martens, Daly, Deschamps, Staes, and Fernandes (2016) analyzed muscle activity during swimming and reported that there is high variability in muscle patterns during swimming. However, in a review of research on muscle activity during swimming, it was noted that the crawl stroke had the least

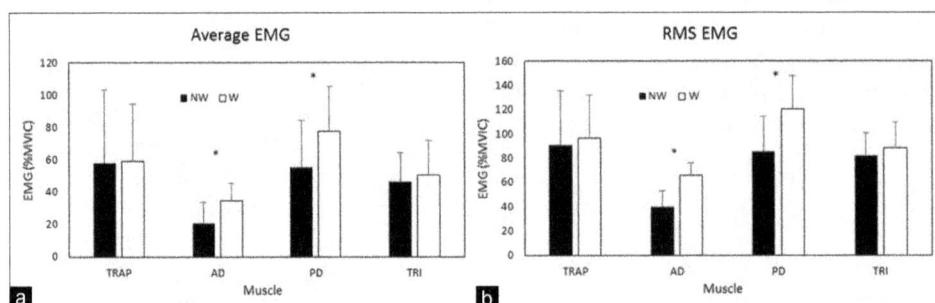

Figure 2. Illustration of Average (a) (AVG) and root mean square (b) (RMS) electromyography (EMG) of the trapezius (TRAP), anterior deltoid (AD), posterior deltoid (PD), and triceps brachii (TRI) during simulated swimming while wearing a wetsuit (W) or no wetsuit (NW). Note: * The AD and PD were each greater during W and NW (p<0.05). Muscle activity of TRAP and TRI were not different between conditions.

variability of muscle activity as compared to other swim strokes (Martens, Figueiredo, & Daly, 2015). Importantly, in the present study, we examined average muscle activity over 45 s vs. comparing patterns. It is important to recognize that it is not clear if the increased muscle activity that we observed while wearing a wetsuit influences swim performance. Hawley et al. (1992) indicated the importance of arm power during swim distances longer than 400 m. Arm power in this work was measured using an arm ergometer (on land). The relationship of predicting front crawl swimming speed based on arm power production was established based on the peak sustained workload during arm ergometer exercise and a 400-m swim comparison. Given the importance of upper body power generation and that triathlon swim segments are typically 750 m and longer, a greater muscle activity of the PD and AD may be an indication that swim performance could be negatively influenced. However, Ikuta et al. (2012) reported that swim velocity was related not specifically to a single muscle but rather velocity was related to the coordination of several muscles. In any case, the added buoyancy of a wetsuit, reduced resistance of water moving along the surface of the wetsuit, and thermoregulation benefits of a wetsuit may negate any potential negative influence of increased shoulder muscle activity. Additional research is needed to determine if an increased muscle activity while wearing a wetsuit would influence swim performance. Although we asked participants to use the same swim technique for each condition, there is the possibility that stroke pattern changed when wearing or not wearing the wetsuit. Qualitatively, it did seem that the stroke pattern changed between conditions. For example, elbow flexion and/or shoulder circumduction may have been different when wearing the wetsuit. Although we measured elbow flexion and extension, we used those data only to check for stroke rate and those data were not sufficient to describe the kinematics of the swim stroke. Future studies should add kinematic analysis to track changes in both sagittal and frontal planes during the recovery phase of the stroke and measure stroke pattern with and without wetsuit. Likewise, we maintained the same swim ergometer resistance setting and controlled stroke rate between conditions. We do not know if participants would have manipulated either of these parameters when using the wetsuit. These controls were put in place to try to isolate a possible influence of wetsuit design on muscle activity. It is also important to recognize that we tested only one model of wetsuit. Furthermore, the wetsuit was dry. It is not known whether or not the wetsuit would influence resistance to shoulder movements the same way if wet or if there was a layer of water between the skin and neoprene (i.e., within the wetsuit). Future studies will need to use water proofed EMG systems to measure muscle activity during swimming in the water. We also recognize that simulated swimming on dry land may not fully replicate swimming movements in the water. For example, Murry, McManus, & Parry (2014) reported that participants achieved similar blood lactate levels during an incremental intensity test on a swim ergometer (VASA) and in the water. However, HR and RPE were different between swimming in the water and on the swim ergometer. Although the present study is the first to measure muscle activity while simulated swimming in a wetsuit – future research is needed to measure muscle activity while swimming in the water using a water proofed EMG system. An advantage of using a swim ergometer, however, is that the resistance and stroke rate could be controlled. With those parameters controlled, we did observe an increase in shoulder muscle activity. It is important to determine if this observation is consistent while swimming in the water.

Finally, we did use a specific order of conditions in that the no wetsuit condition always preceded the wetsuit condition. This was done from a logistic perspective of managing EMG leads – in pilot work, we determined it was easier to put the wetsuit on in a way that minimized any chance to disrupt the EMG set up. We do not know if there was a learning effect; however, the exercise time was short for each condition and participants seemed comfortable using the swim ergometer throughout testing.

Practical Application

When selecting between different brands or models of full-sleeve wetsuits, the athlete should consider shoulder movement allowed by the wetsuit. Some triathlon events favor strong run ability vs. cycling or swimming (Fröhlich et al., 2013). However, considering some swim events involve swimming for over an hour, any added resistance to shoulder movement may cause an athlete to tire sooner. It is important to remember that our study was conducted on land and it may be important for the athlete to try the wetsuit in the water. The athlete should also incorporate regular wetsuit swims in a training program in order to prepare the shoulder muscles for any potential increase in resistance. Furthermore, prior to swimming in a wetsuit, it is important for the athlete to adjust the wetsuit as best as possible to reduce shoulder resistance. This can be partly achieved by pulling the wetsuit up as high as possible as well as adjusting the neoprene around the shoulder/arm region to allow easier shoulder movements. Unfortunately, there are no clear objective criteria for selecting the right sized wetsuit for a triathlete. Although it is common for athletes to be advised to select a wetsuit that is too tight – the athlete must consider selecting a wetsuit to minimize shoulder resistance.

CONCLUSION

It is concluded that muscle activity of the shoulder (i.e., PD, AD) during dryland swimming at a fixed cadence was influenced by wearing a wetsuit. It is important to follow up this study with measuring muscle activity during swimming in the water. As a practical application, it would seem that a wetsuit should be selected that minimizes restrictions to shoulder movements. This could be related to wetsuit size, design, fit, and/or materials used. Manufacturers frequently use a more flexible material on high end wetsuits. However, future research is needed to determine if swim performance is negatively influenced due to increased activity while wearing a full sleeved wetsuit.

REFERENCES

Chatard, J.C., & Millet, G. (1996). Effects of wetsuit use in swimming events: Practical recommendations. *Sports Medicine*, 22(2), 70-75.

Chatard, J.C., Senegas, M., Dreanot, P., & Geyssant (1995). Wet suit effect: A comparison between competitive swimmers and triathletes. *Medicine and Science in Sports and Exercise*, 27(4), 580-586.

Cordain, L., & Kopriva, R. (1991). Wetsuits, body density and swimming performance. *British Journal of Sports Medicine*, 25(1), 31-33.

Corona, L.J., Simmons, G.H., Nessler, J.A., & Newcomer, S.C. (2017). Characterisation of regional skin temperatures in recreational surfers wearing a 2-mm wetsuit. *Ergonomics*, 1-7.

DeLuca, C. (1997). The use of surface electromyography in biomechanics. *Journal of Applied Biomechanics, 13(2), 135-163*.

Figueiredo, P., Sanders, R., Gorski, T., Vilas-Boas, J.P., & Fernandes, R.J. (2013). Kinematic and electromyographic changes during 200 m front crawl at race pace. *International Journal of Sports Medicine*, 34(1), 49-55.

Fröhlich, M., Balter, J., Pieter, A., Schwarz, M., & Emrich, E. (2013). Model-theoretic optimization approach to triathlon performance under comparative static conditions – Results based on the Olympic Games 2012, *International Journal of Kinesiology & Sports Science*, 1(3), 9-14.

Hawley, J. A., Williams, M.M., Vickovic, M.M., Handcock, P.J. (1992). Muscle power predicts freestyle swimming performance. *British Journal of Sports Medicine,* 26(3), 151-5.

Hermens, H.J., Freriks, B., Disselhorst-Klyg, C., Rau, G. (2000). Development of recommendations for SEMG sensors and sensor placement procedures. *Journal of Electromyography and Kinesiology,* 10(5), 361-374.

Ikuta, Y., Matsuda, Y., Yamada, Y., Kida, N., Oda, S., & Moritani, T. (2012). Relationship between decreased swimming velocity and muscle activity during 200-m front crawl. *European Journal of Applied Physiology,* 112(9), 3417-3429.

Martens, J., Daly, D., Deschamps, K., Staes, F., Fernandes, R.J. (2016). Inter-individual variability and pattern recognition of surface electromyography in front crawl swimming. *Journal of Electromyography and Kinesiology*, 31, 14-21.

Martens, J., Figueiredo, P., & Daly, D. (2015). Electromyography in the four competitive swimming strokes: A systematic review. *Journal of Electromyography and Kinesiology*, 25(2), 273-291.

Murry, K., McManus, C., & Parry, D. (2014). The validity of the VAS swim ergometer in the assessment of swimmers in the laboratory. *Journal of Sports Sciences*, 32(s2), 43.

Naebe, M., Robins, N., Wang, X., & Collins, P. (2013). Assessment of performance properties of wetsuits. *Journal of Sports Engineering and Technology*, 227(4), 255-264.

Nessler, J. A., Silvas, M., Carpenter, S., Newcomer, S. C. (2015). Wearing a wetsuit alters upper extremity motion during simulated surfboard paddling. *PLoS ONE*, 10(11), e0142325.

Pink, M., Perry, J., Browne, A., Scovazzo, M. L., Kerrigan, J. (1991). The normal shoulder during freestyle swimming: An electromyographic and cinematographic analysis of twelve muscles. *American Journal of Sports Medicine,* 19(6), 569-576.

Ulsamer, S., Rüst, A.C., Rosemann, T., Lepers, R., Knechtle, B. (2014). Swimming performances in long distance open-water events with and without wetsuit. *BMC Sports Science, Medicine, and Rehabilitation,* 6(20), 1-13.

Wakabayashi, H., Hanai, A., Yokoyama, S., & Normura, T. (2006). Thermal insulation and body temperature wearing a thermal swimsuit during water immersion. *Journal of Physiological Anthropology*, 25(5), 331-338.

3

Race Pattern of Women's 100-m Hurdles: Time Analysis of Olympic Hurdle Performance

Athanasios Tsiokanos[1], Dimitrios Tsaopoulos[2]*, Arsenis Giavroglou[3], Eleftherios Tsarouchas[3]

[1]Department of Physical Education and Sports Science, Laboratory of Biomechanics, University of Thessaly, Trikala 42100, Greece
[2]Institute for Research and Technology Thessaly (IRETETH), Kinesiology Sector, Center for Research and Technology Hellas (CERTH), 51 Papanastasiou St, 41222, Larissa, Greece
[3]Hellenic Sports Research Institute, OAKA, Kifisias 37, Maroussi 15123, Athens, Greece

Corresponding Author: Dimitrios Tsaopoulos, E-mail: dtsaop@gmail.com

ARTICLE INFO

Conflicts of interest: None
Funding: None

ABSTRACT

Background: For control and effective management of training process in women's 100-m hurdles event, the coaches, in addition to detailed biomechanical parameters, need also overall, more comprehensive technical parameters, called direct performance descriptors which are used for planning the distribution of an athlete's efforts over the race. **Purpose:** The aim of this study was the investigation of the race behavior of elite women sprint hurdlers, on the basis of selected time parameters, and the examination of the existence of a common race pattern in high level hurdle performance. **Method:** The time data of the race performance between two consecutive Olympic Games were compared. The analyzing subjects consisted of all women 100-m hurdle finalists in Athens 2004 (n = 6) and all women 100-m hurdle finalists (n = 8) and semi-finalists (n = 14) in Beijing 2008. **Results:** No significant differences were revealed between the two competitions concerning to the means of approach run time, run-in time, intermediate touchdown times, interval times for the hurdle units and the corresponding average velocities. Significant relationship exists between the intermediate times and final performance. The time contribution of the first half of the race to the formation of the final performance is approximately equal to the second one and, generally the standardised time parameters show the existence of a common race pattern in high level hurdle performance. **Conclusion:** The presented biomechanical data provide coaches and athletes with valuable information about hurdle technique for effective interventions in the training process.

Key words: Biomechanics, Track and field, Hurdles, Competition analysis, Women athletes

INTRODUCTION

The women's 100-m hurdles event is a sprint race with ten altered steps needed to clear the barriers (McDonald & Dapena, 1991b). Additionally to sprint velocity, the participant hurdlers is essential to have high level of technical skills, especially concerning the hurdle clearance phase. Therefore, most studies dealing with the technique of the above 100-m hurdles event are focused on the analysis of kinematics (Ryu & Chang, 2011; Iskra & Coh, 2006; Stein, 2000; Wang & Li, 2000; Salo, Grimshaw, & Marar, 1997; Marar & Grimshaw, 1993; McDonald & Dapena, 1991a; Hücklekemkes, 1990) kinetics (McLean, 1994) and energetic characteristics (Ward-Smith, 1997) of the clearance phase. Moreover, There are few studies examining the effects of external conditions on sprint and hurdle performance (Yoshimoto, Takai & Kanehisa, 2016; Hamlin, Hopkins & Hollings, 2015), and a study examining the effects of early sport specialization on the development of a young athlete (Normand, Wolfe & Peak, 2017).

However, for control and effective management of training process in hurdle events, the coaches, in addition to detailed biomechanical parameters describing the clearance phase and inter-hurdle distances (body kinematics, GRF, etc.), need also overall, more comprehensive technical parameters. These parameters (clearance times, horizontal velocity, split times, etc.,) that has been described as direct performance descriptors by Mann & Herman (1985), are used for planning the distribution of an athlete's efforts over the race. For this purpose, the video techniques have established in the major competitions (Graubner & Nixdorf, 2011; Mueller & Hommel, 1997; Brüggemann & Glad, 1990), to provide time parameters during clearance phase and inter-hurdle distances, and indirectly help for the calculation of average running velocities. Hence, with the further statistical analysis of the above parameters, that describe the efforts of world class athletes in the major competitions, theoretical models of effective running performance in hurdle events can be created. These kind of models offer valuable biomechanical informations to athletes and coaches, by enabling the comparison of the statistical models with the data of a hurdler's individual performance in training, control or competition efforts, and by leading to the dynamic adaptation of various intervention method during the training process.

Video techniques analyses of hurdle performances have been carried out either with hurdlers as individuals, Olympic and world champions or world record holders (M Coh & Dolenec, 1996; M Coh, 1987) or with a larger statistical sample of hurdlers (semi-finalists and finalists) included in research projects undertaken at the Olympic Games and IAAF world championships (Graubner & Nixdorf, 2011; Mueller & Hommel, 1997; Brüggemann & Glad, 1990).

According to our knowledge only three biomechanical projects in IAAF world championships (Rome 1987, Athens 1997, Berlin 2009) and only one in Olympic Games (Seoul 1988) have examined the race pattern in high level hurdle performance and the race behavior of elite women sprint hurdlers. After the Olympic Games of Seoul there is no any time analysis study of hurdle performance with Olympic level hurdlers. Hence, the main purpose of this study was to obtain time parameters of 100-m female hurdlers on the basis of video techniques analyses curried out on two Olympic Games (Athens 2004 and Beijing 2008), in an attempt to compare time data of two consecutive Games and reexamine the race pattern of 100-m hurdle performance. Although the official time accuracy for this event is in 1/100 s, all the previous time analyses are based on data collected with cameras recording at 50 Hz. In the present study, the video cameras that selected for race recording, operated at 100 Hz, providing the necessary accuracy in measurements. The fact that the present study concerns in earlier Olympiads does not mean that provide outdated information, because there is no essential performance improvement in the event at the last decade. Actually, conducting a performance comparison among the last four Olympic Games, as shown in table 1, there are neither any differences in the performance of the gold medalists, nor any significant differences among the mean performances of the hurdle finalists in the same Games. Additional aims of the present study were to enrich and update the databases with biomechanical parameters of elite female hurdlers, to provide coaches and athletes with quantitative information on individual techniques, and finally to investigate an existence of a common race pattern in high level hurdle performance.

METHODS

Design and Participation

The data was collected during the Olympic Games of Athens 2004 and Olympic Games of Beijing 2008. The analyzing subjects consisted of all women 100-m hurdle finalists in Athens (n = 6) and all women 100-m hurdle finalists (n = 8) and semi-finalists (n = 14) in Beijing. The efforts of all subjects in their final race were recording by three panned digital video cameras (JVC, GR-DVL 9600 model) with an operating rate of 100 frames per second. The video cameras were set above the spectator stands and were panned to record the sagittal view of the entire race, following the athletes from the start to the finish. The 1st camera was positioned at the line of the 3rd barrier recording mainly the take-off (TO) before and touchdown (TD) after 1st, 2nd and 3rd barriers. The 2nd camera was positioned at the line of the 7th barrier recording mainly TO before and TD after 4th, 5th, 6th and 7th barriers. The 3rd camera was located at the line of the 10th barrier recording mainly TO before and TD after 8th, 9th and 10th barriers. All three camcorders recorded the light signal of the gun, which represented the time of the start of the race, and was the zero point of the time measurements (starting point).

Procedure

In table 2 are presented and defined all variables analysed. All variables were based on video recordings and produced by calculating the passed frames between critical instants, via the Trim Module of the APAS (Ariel Dynamics Inc.). Intermediate times (TH1-10) were calculated from the start to TD of each hurdle. Hurdle unit's times (thu1-9) represent the interval times between two consecutive hurdle TDs. Approach run time is the interval time between the start and first hurdle TD minus the reaction time, while the run-in time is the final time minus the 10th intermediate time. Clearance time represents the time between TO before and TD after each hurdle. Average velocities (Vthu1-9) were calculated by the covered distance (8.50 m) between two consecutive hurdles per corresponding hurdle unit time. For the velocity up to the first hurdle (VTH1) as covered distance was taken the distance from the start to first hurdle (13.00 m) plus 1.05 m to the TD after the hurdle (Mueller & Hommel, 1997) and as time the intermediate time to first hurdle. For the run-in velocity (Vtrin) as covered distance was taken the run-in distance (10.50 m) minus 1.05 m from the 10th hurdle to the TD (Mueller & Hommel, 1997) and as time the run-in time. The relative variables (RTH1, RTH2,…, RTH10, Rtar, Rtrin) were produced from the intermediate times divided by the final time (normalised by the final time). Finally the reaction time and the final time were provided by the official game chronometers.

Statistical Analysis

Statistical analysis, which was performed using SPSS version 18 (SPSS, Chicago, IL), included descriptives (mean, standard deviation), an independent t-test for comparison between Athens and Beijing variable means and a correlation analysis (a Pearson product-moment correlation coefficient) to evaluate relationships between final time and intermediate time variables. The alpha level of significance was set at $p < 0.05$. All procedures performed in the study were in

Table 1. Race performances (in seconds) at the last Olympic Games

	Athens 2004	Beijing 2008	London 2012	Rio 2016
1st finalist	12.37	12.54	12.35	12.48
M±SD	12.61±0.17	12.68±0.12	12.60±0.24	12.68±0.13

M=mean, SD=standard deviation

Table 2. Abbreviation and variable definitions

RT	Reaction time
THi	Time from the start to touchdown after the hurdle i (i=1, 2,..., 10)
FT	Final time at 100-m
thuj	Time for the hurdle unit j (j=1, 2,..., 9)
	(thu1=time interval between 1st and 2nd hurdle touchdown)
	(thu2=time interval between 2nd and 3rd hurdle touchdown)
	(thu9=time interval between 9th and 10th hurdle touchdown)
tar	Approach run time
	(time interval between the start and the 1st hurdle touchdown minus the reaction time)
trin	Run-in time
	(time interval between the 10th hurdle touchdown and the final time)
CTi	Hurdle clearance time of the hurdle i (i=1, 2,..., 10)
	(flight time from take-off before to touchdown after each hurdle)
V-	Estimated average velocity (VTH1, Vthu1, Vthu2, ..., Vthu9, Vtrin)
	(average velocity calculated by the covered distance per corresponding time)
R-	Relative variable (RTH1, RTH2, ... RTH10, Rtar, Rtrin)
	(a variable normalised by the final time)

accordance with the ethical standards of the institutional research committee.

RESULTS

In tables 3a and 3b1 are presented reaction time, final time and intermediate touchdown times of the finalists in Athens 2004 and Beijing 2008 respectively. In both cases the mean data shows that the greater differences between subjects occur in the second half of the race (greater variation of the standard deviation after 5th hurdle). The comparison between Athens and Beijing didn't show any significant differences on the means of the above variables. But it could be seen a better reaction time in Athens 2004 than in Beijing 2008, and the same occurs about final time. In table 3b2 are presented reaction time, final time and intermediate touchdown times of the semifinalists in Beijing. This is an additional sample of top women hurdlers, to enhance the study of the correlation coefficient between the final performance and intermediate times in Beijing Olympic Games.

In tables 4a and 4b are presented approach run time, run-in time and hurdle units' times of the finalists in Athens and Beijing respectively. On average, the hurdlers in Athens and Beijing accelerated from the start to 6th hurdle, indicated by the decreasing hurdle units' times from unit 1 to unit 5. The maximum achieved average velocity in Athens was 8.74 m/s while in Beijing 8.75 m/s (tables 6a and 6b respectively).

In tables 5a and 5b the hurdle clearance times show mean values from 0.28 s to 0.32 s in Athens and 0.29 s to 0.33 s in Beijing. The smallest individual value was 0.24 s and the biggest one 0.36 s. A correlation analysis between the average clearance time of each hurdle and the final time, and also between the mean race clearance time of each athlete and the final time revealed no significant relationship between hurdle clearance time and race performance.

The mean values of relative temporal parameters (tables 7a and 7b) show a similar race pattern of hurdle finalists in both Olympic Games. It is of interest that the time

contribution of the first half of the race is slightly larger than the second one (RTH5 = 0.516 in both Games).

A correlation analysis between the temporal parameters and the final time (table 8) was conducted to identify the decisive points of the race. The analysis revealed no correlation between reaction time and final performance. Regarding to correlation between the final time and intermediate times, the analysis indicated that the size of correlation coefficients increases up to the last intermediate time (TH10), as has been expected. The approach run time showed significant correlation with the final time (r = 0.57) only in analysis with Beijing's data. It is of great interest that after 6th hurdle is determined 67% (r = 0.82) of the variance of the final time. After the 10th hurdle it is determined 94-96% (r = 0.97 and r = 0.98) of the above mentioned variance.

DISCUSSION

The aim of the present study, was 1) to compare the time data of the race performance between the 100-m women hurdle finalists in two consecutive Olympic Games 2) to estimate the average velocities of the hurdlers in an attempt to observe their race behavior and their efforts' contribution during the race and 3) to investigate the existence of a common race pattern in high level hurdle performance.

Reaction Time

In regard to reaction time (RT), although there were no statistical differences between the two events, in Beijing 2008 was appeared greater mean value than in Athens 2004 (0.176 ± 0.031 s vs 0.161 ± 0.019 s), quite greater than the corresponding values in other 100-m hurdle running finals in high level athletic events: In Olympics in Seoul 1988 with RT = 0.164 ± 0.02 s (Brüggemann & Glad, 1990), in IAAF World Championships Athens 1997 with RT = 0.133 ± 0.01 s (Mueller & Hommel, 1997), and in IAAF World Championships Berlin 2009 with RT = 0.143 ± 0.01 s (Graubner & Nixdorf, 2011). Perhaps the finalists in Beijing

Table 3a. Reaction time, final time and intermediate touchdown times (in seconds) in Olympics 2004

	RT	TH1	TH2	TH3	TH4	TH5	TH6	TH7	TH8	TH9	TH10	FT
Hayes J. (USA)	0.169	2.52	3.53	4.50	5.45	6.42	7.36	8.32	9.29	10.27	11.28	12.37
Krasovska O. (UKR)	0.151	2.55	3.55	4.55	5.51	6.48	7.45	8.41	9.39	10.37	11.36	12.45
Morrison M. (USA)	0.145	2.56	3.54	4.50	5.48	6.47	7.48	8.47	9.47	10.47	11.47	12.56
Koroteyeva M. (RUS)	0.195	2.61	3.64	4.63	5.64	6.61	7.57	8.56	9.57	10.58	11.61	12.72
Golding-Clarke (JAM)	0.149	2.54	3.54	4.53	5.49	6.48	7.45	8.45	9.45	10.49	11.54	12.73
Whyte A. (CAN)	0.155	2.56	3.59	4.58	5.57	6.57	7.56	8.53	9.55	10.61	11.64	12.81
M	0.161	2.56	3.56	4.55	5.52	6.50	7.48	8.46	9.45	10.46	11.48	12.61
SD	0.019	0.03	0.04	0.05	0.07	0.07	0.08	0.09	0.10	0.13	0.14	0.17

M=mean, SD=standard deviation

Table 3b1. Reaction time, final time and intermediate touchdown times (in seconds) in final race of Olympics 2008

	RT	TH1	TH2	TH3	TH4	TH5	TH6	TH7	TH8	TH9	TH10	FT
Harper D. (USA)	0.193	2.55	3.59	4.53	5.51	6.50	7.46	8.45	9.44	10.43	11.44	12.54
McLellan S. (AUS)	0.138	2.50	3.51	4.51	5.50	6.50	7.47	8.45	9.45	10.46	11.50	12.64
Lopes-Schliep. (CAN)	0.174	2.57	3.63	4.63	5.60	6.60	7.58	8.54	9.53	10.56	11.58	12.64
Cherry D. (USA)	0.239	2.63	3.66	4.67	5.64	6.61	7.59	8.56	9.55	10.55	11.58	12.65
Ennis-London (JAM)	0.151	2.59	3.59	4.62	5.55	6.52	7.52	8.52	9.47	10.48	11.53	12.65
Foster-Hylton. (JAM)	0.167	2.61	3.63	4.63	5.61	6.59	7.54	8.54	9.52	10.53	11.56	12.66
Jones L. (USA)	0.185	2.57	3.53	4.50	5.44	6.44	7.38	8.34	9.32	10.37	11.46	12.72
Claxton S.(GBR)	0.163	2.59	3.62	4.63	5.63	6.63	7.62	8.62	9.66	10.69	11.77	12.94
M	0.176	2.58	3.59	4.59	5.56	6.55	7.52	8.50	9.49	10.51	11.55	12.68
SD	0.031	0.04	0.05	0.07	0.07	0.07	0.08	0.09	0.10	0.10	0.10	0.12

M=mean, SD=standard deviation

Table 3b2. Reaction time, final time and intermediate touchdown times (in seconds) in semi-final races of Olympics 2008

	RT	TH1	TH2	TH3	TH4	TH5	TH6	TH7	TH8	TH9	TH10	FT
Jones L. (USA)	0.172	2.53	3.52	4.50	5.45	6.40	7.37	8.33	9.33	10.31	11.31	12.43
Ennis-London (JAM)	0.145	2.56	3.58	4.56	5.55	6.54	7.49	8.46	9.47	10.49	11.51	12.67
Lopes-Schliep. (CAN)	0.159	2.51	3.56	4.58	5.57	6.58	7.54	8.50	9.52	10.57	11.59	12.68
McLellan S. (AUS)	0.140	2.54	3.55	4.54	5.53	6.51	7.51	8.52	9.52	10.54	11.57	12.70
Onyia J. (ESP)	0.203	2.60	3.69	4.71	5.72	6.73	7.73	8.72	9.74	10.76	11.79	12.86
Trywianska-Kollasch. (POL)	0.118	2.56	3.69	4.70	5.72	6.73	7.75	8.75	9.76	10.79	11.84	12.96
Nytra C. (GER)	0.144	2.60	3.63	4.66	5.67	6.68	7.70	8.73	9.75	10.79	11.87	12.99
Yanit N. (TUR)	0.201	2.62	3.68	4.70	5.72	6.73	7.76	8.81	9.87	11.10	12.19	13.28
Cherry D. (USA)	0.189	2.59	3.62	4.59	5.55	6.52	7.52	8.52	9.52	10.52	11.54	12.62
Harper D. (USA)	0.191	2.58	3.58	4.55	5.54	6.52	7.48	8.45	9.45	10.49	11.52	12.66
Foster-Hylton. (JAM)	0.162	2.61	3.65	4.66	5.66	6.61	7.59	8.59	9.60	10.62	11.66	12.76
Claxton S. (GBR)	0.145	2.57	3.60	4.59	5.58	6.53	7.53	8.53	9.55	10.61	11.66	12.84
Dixon V. (JAM)	0.237	2.61	3.64	4.64	5.65	6.74	7.77	8.76	9.76	10.75	11.78	12.86
Okori R.F. (FRA)	0.153	2.63	3.70	4.65	5.71	6.73	7.74	8.77	9.80	10.84	11.89	13.05
M	0.168	2.58	3.62	4.62	5.62	6.61	7.61	8.60	9.62	10.66	11.69	12.81
SD	0.032	0.04	0.06	0.07	0.09	0.11	0.13	0.15	0.16	0.20	0.22	0.21

M=mean, SD=standard deviation

have been more cautious in response to the start, and the reason was the track and field's zero-tolerance false start policy. Also, the finding of the present study that there is no any statistically significant correlation between the reaction time and the final performance is consistent with the results of similar studies on elite women hurdlers (Graubner

Table 4a. Approach run time, run-in time, hurdle units' times (in seconds) in Olympics 2004

	tar	thu1	thu2	thu3	thu4	thu5	thu6	thu7	thu8	thu9	trin
Hayes J. (USA)	2.35	1.01	0.97	0.95	0.97	0.94	0.96	0.97	0.98	1.01	1.09
Krasovska O. (UKR)	2.40	1.00	1.00	0.96	0.97	0.97	0.96	0.98	0.98	0.99	1.09
Morrison M. (USA)	2.42	0.98	0.96	0.98	0.99	1.01	0.99	1.00	1.00	1.00	1.09
Koroteyeva M. (RUS)	2.42	1.03	0.99	1.01	0.97	0.96	0.99	1.01	1.01	1.03	1.11
Golding-Clarke (JAM)	2.39	1.00	0.99	0.96	0.99	0.97	1.00	1.00	1.04	1.05	1.19
Whyte A. (CAN)	2.41	1.03	0.99	0.99	1.00	0.99	0.97	1.02	1.06	1.03	1.17
M	2.40	1.01	0.98	0.97	0.98	0.97	0.98	1.00	1.01	1.02	1.12
SD	0.02	0.02	0.01	0.02	0.01	0.02	0.02	0.02	0.03	0.02	0.05

M=mean, SD=standard deviation

Table 4b. Approach run time, run-in time, hurdle units' times (in seconds) in Olympics 2008

	tar	thu1	thu2	thu3	thu4	thu5	thu6	thu7	thu8	thu9	trin
Harper D. (USA)	2.36	1.04	0.94	0.98	0.99	0.96	0.99	0.99	0.99	1.01	1.10
McLellan S. (AUS)	2.36	1.01	1.00	0.99	1.00	0.97	0.98	1.00	1.01	1.04	1.14
Lopes-Schliep. (CAN)	2.40	1.06	1.00	0.97	1.00	0.98	0.96	0.99	1.03	1.02	1.06
Cherry D. (USA)	2.39	1.03	1.01	0.97	0.97	0.98	0.97	0.99	1.00	1.03	1.07
Ennis-London (JAM)	2.44	1.00	1.03	0.93	0.97	1.00	1.00	0.95	1.01	1.05	1.12
Foster-Hylton. (JAM)	2.44	1.02	1.00	0.98	0.98	0.95	1.00	0.98	1.01	1.03	1.10
Jones L. (USA)	2.39	0.96	0.97	0.94	1.00	0.94	0.96	0.98	1.05	1.09	1.26
Claxton S.(GBR)	2.43	1.03	1.01	1.00	1.00	0.99	1.00	1.04	1.03	1.08	1.17
M	2.40	1.02	0.99	0.97	0.99	0.97	0.98	0.99	1.02	1.04	1.13
SD	0.03	0.03	0.03	0.02	0.01	0.02	0.02	0.02	0.02	0.03	0.06

M=mean, SD=standard deviation

Table 5a. Clearance times (in seconds) in Olympics 2004

	CT1	CT2	CT3	CT4	CT5	CT6	CT7	CT8	CT9	CT10
Hayes J. (USA)	0.32	0.32	0.31	0.28	0.30	0.28	0.28	0.29	0.30	0.31
Krasovska O. (UKR)	0.30	0.26	0.27	0.27	0.29	0.29	0.27	0.27	0.30	0.29
Morrison M. (USA)	0.35	0.33	0.33	0.33	0.31	0.33	0.30	0.34	0.36	0.33
Koroteyeva M. (RUS)	0.30	0.33	0.32	0.31	0.32	0.30	0.27	0.28	0.31	0.31
Golding-Clarke (JAM)	0.30	0.31	0.32	0.28	0.31	0.31	0.31	0.32	0.33	0.33
Whyte A. (CAN)	0.26	0.29	0.29	0.28	0.30	0.28	0.28	0.28	0.30	0.30
M	0.30	0.31	0.31	0.29	0.30	0.30	0.28	0.30	0.32	0.31
SD	0.03	0.03	0.02	0.02	0.01	0.02	0.02	0.03	0.02	0.02

M=mean, SD=standard deviation

& Nixdorf, 2011; Mueller & Hommel, 1997; Brüggemann & Glad, 1990). But, generally, in high level sprint running, a short reaction time is considered as a prerequisite for successful performance.

Approach Run Phase

The approach run time was the same in both Games (2.40 ± 0.02 s vs 2.40 ± 0.03 s), nevertheless of the greater final time in Beijing 2008 (FT = 12.68 ± 0.12 s) than in Athens 2004 (FT = 12.61 ± 0.17 s), and also the corresponding relative quantities appeared approximately the same value (Rtar = 0.190 ± 0.002 s in Athens 2004 vs

0.189 ± 0.002 s in Beijing 2008). This fact means that the tar contributes 19% to the formation of final performance. In the present study the time up to the first hurdle was 2.56 ± 0.03 s vs 2.58 ± 0.04 s (respectively for Athens and Beijing) and was at the same level with other studies (Graubner & Nixdorf, 2011; Mueller & Hommel, 1997; Brüggemann & Glad, 1990), representing a mean velocity of 5.44 – 5.49 m/s.

Intermediate Touchdown and Hurdle Units Times

The findings of the present study that hurdle finalists accelerate from the start to 6th hurdle are in agreement with other studies (Graubner & Nixdorf, 2011; Mueller & Hom-

Table 5b. Clearance times (in seconds) in Olympics 2008

	CT1	CT2	CT3	CT4	CT5	CT6	CT7	CT8	CT9	CT10
Harper D. (USA)	0.28	0.30	0.27	0.25	0.30	0.28	0.27	0.30	0.30	0.32
McLellan S. (AUS)	0.39	0.29	0.31	0.31	0.32	0.29	0.29	0.29	0.32	0.32
Lopes-Schliep. (CAN)	0.32	0.37	0.34	0.30	0.34	0.34	0.31	0.33	0.35	0.35
Cherry D. (USA)	0.33	0.31	0.35	0.33	0.32	0.32	0.31	0.29	0.28	0.32
Ennis-London (JAM)	0.33	0.28	0.34	0.28	0.29	0.34	0.33	0.29	0.31	0.34
Foster-Hylton. (JAM)	0.30	0.28	0.34	0.27	0.31	0.34	0.30	0.30	0.31	0.32
Jones L. (USA)	0.30	0.30	0.31	0.28	0.31	0.29	0.28	0.28	0.36	0.35
Claxton S.(GBR)	0.30	0.32	0.34	0.32	0.31	0.24	0.25	0.33	0.33	0.34
M	0.32	0.31	0.32	0.29	0.31	0.30	0.29	0.30	0.32	0.33
SD	0.03	0.03	0.03	0.03	0.01	0.04	0.02	0.02	0.03	0.01

M=mean, SD=standard deviation.

Table 6a. Approach run velocity, run-in velocity, hurdle units' velocities (in m/s) in Olympics 2004

	VTH1	Vthu1	Vthu2	Vthu3	Vthu4	Vthu5	Vthu6	Vthu7	Vthu8	Vthu9	Vtrin
Hayes J. (USA)	6.05	8.42	8.76	8.95	8.76	9.04	8.85	8.76	8.67	8.42	8.50
Krasovska O. (UKR)	5.93	8.50	8.50	8.85	8.76	8.76	8.85	8.67	8.67	8.59	8.50
Morrison M. (USA)	5.89	8.67	8.85	8.67	8.59	8.42	8.59	8.50	8.50	8.50	8.50
Koroteyeva M. (RUS)	5.89	8.25	8.59	8.42	8.76	8.85	8.59	8.42	8.42	8.25	8.35
Golding-Clarke (JAM)	5.95	8.50	8.59	8.85	8.59	8.76	8.50	8.50	8.17	8.10	7.79
Whyte A. (CAN)	5.92	8.25	8.59	8.59	8.50	8.59	8.76	8.33	8.02	8.25	7.92
M	5.86	8.43	8.65	8.72	8.66	8.74	8.69	8.53	8.41	8.35	8.42
SD	0.06	0.16	0.13	0.20	0.12	0.22	0.15	0.16	0.27	0.18	0.33

M=mean, SD=standard deviation.

Table 6b. Approach run velocity, run-in velocity, hurdle units' velocities (in m/s) in Olympics 2008

	VTH1	Vthu1	Vthu2	Vthu3	Vthu4	Vthu5	Vthu6	Vthu7	Vthu8	Vthu9	Vtrin
Harper D. (USA)	5.95	8.17	9.04	8.67	8.59	8.85	8.59	8.59	8.59	8.42	8.43
McLellan S. (AUS)	5.95	8.42	8.50	8.59	8.50	8.76	8.67	8.50	8.42	8.17	8.13
Lopes-Schliep. (CAN)	5.85	8.02	8.50	8.76	8.50	8.67	8.85	8.59	8.25	8.33	8.75
Cherry D. (USA)	5.88	8.25	8.42	8.76	8.76	8.67	8.76	8.59	8.50	8.25	8.66
Ennis-London (JAM)	5.76	8.50	8.25	9.14	8.76	8.50	8.50	8.95	8.42	8.10	8.28
Foster-Hylton. (JAM)	5.76	8.33	8.50	8.67	8.67	8.95	8.50	8.67	8.42	8.25	8.43
Jones L. (USA)	5.88	8.85	8.76	9.04	8.50	9.04	8.85	8.67	8.10	7.80	7.36
Claxton S.(GBR)	5.78	8.25	8.42	8.50	8.50	8.59	8.50	8.17	8.25	7.87	7.92
M	5.85	8.35	8.55	8.77	8.60	8.75	8.65	8.59	8.37	8.15	8.24
SD	0.08	0.25	0.24	0.22	0.12	0.18	0.15	0.21	0.16	0.22	0.45

M=mean, SD=standard deviation.

mel, 1997; Brüggemann & Glad, 1990). The greater average velocity achieved between hurdles in the present study is 8.74 m/s (Athens 2004) or 8.75 m/s (Beijing 2008) and is similar to that from other studies (8.73 m/s in Athens 1997, 8.74 m/s in Berlin 2009) (Graubner & Nixdorf, 2011; Mueller & Hommel, 1997). In Seoul 1988 the biggest average velocity was only 8.67 m/s (corresponding to a mean time of 0.98 s at the 5th hurdle unit). These velocities are much lower than the maximum velocities (10.29 – 10.72 m/s) observed in the 100 m sprint (Mueller & Hommel, 1997). After the achievement of maximum velocity, follows a decline of the running velocity at the next hurdle units up to the last hurdle. It is important for a hurdle runner to minimise the velocity decline. The minimum velocity decline the maximum specific running endurance. In Athens 2004 the average decline of the velocity from the 6th hurdle to the 10th was the 4.46% of the maximum velocity, and the corresponding decline in Beijing 2008 was 6.86% of the maximum.

Regarding to correlation between the final time and intermediate times, the analysis revealed significant relationship between the final performance and touchdown times from the 5th hurdle to 10th hurdle in both Games, with gradually

Table 7a. Relative temporal parameters in Olympics 2004

	RTH1	RTH2	RTH3	RTH4	RTH5	RTH6	RTH7	RTH8	RTH9	RTH10	Rtar
Hayes J. (USA)	0.204	0.285	0.364	0.441	0.519	0.595	0.673	0.751	0.830	0.912	0.190
Krasovska O. (UKR)	0.205	0.285	0.365	0.443	0.520	0.598	0.676	0.754	0.833	0.912	0.193
Morrison M. (USA)	0.204	0.282	0.358	0.436	0.515	0.596	0.674	0.754	0.834	0.913	0.192
Koroteyeva M. (RUS)	0.205	0.286	0.364	0.443	0.520	0.595	0.673	0.752	0.832	0.913	0.190
Golding-Clarke (JAM)	0.200	0.278	0.356	0.431	0.509	0.585	0.664	0.742	0.824	0.907	0.188
Whyte A. (CAN)	0.200	0.280	0.358	0.435	0.513	0.590	0.666	0.746	0.828	0.909	0.188
M	0.203	0.283	0.361	0.438	0.516	0.593	0.671	0.750	0.830	0.911	0.190
SD	0.002	0.003	0.004	0.005	0.004	0.005	0.005	0.005	0.004	0.003	0.002

M=mean, SD=standard deviation.

Table 7b. Relative temporal parameters in Olympics 2008

	RTH1	RTH2	RTH3	RTH4	RTH5	RTH6	RTH7	RTH8	RTH9	RTH10	Rtar
Harper D. (USA)	0.203	0.286	0.361	0.439	0.518	0.595	0.674	0.753	0.832	0.912	0.188
McLellan S. (AUS)	0.198	0.278	0.357	0.435	0.514	0.591	0.669	0.748	0.828	0.910	0.187
Lopes-Schliep. (CAN)	0.203	0.287	0.366	0.443	0.522	0.600	0.676	0.754	0.835	0.916	0.190
Cherry D. (USA)	0.208	0.289	0.369	0.446	0.523	0.600	0.677	0.755	0.834	0.915	0.189
Ennis-London (JAM)	0.205	0.284	0.365	0.439	0.515	0.594	0.674	0.749	0.828	0.911	0.193
Foster-Hylton. (JAM)	0.206	0.287	0.366	0.443	0.521	0.596	0.675	0.752	0.832	0.913	0.193
Jones L. (USA)	0.202	0.278	0.354	0.428	0.506	0.580	0.656	0.733	0.815	0.901	0.188
Claxton S. (GBR)	0.200	0.280	0.358	0.435	0.512	0.589	0.666	0.747	0.826	0.910	0.188
M	0.203	0.283	0.362	0.438	0.516	0.593	0.671	0.749	0.829	0.911	0.189
SD	0.003	0.005	0.005	0.006	0.005	0.006	0.007	0.007	0.006	0.005	0.002

M=mean, SD=standard deviation.

Table 8. Correlation coefficients between final time and temporal parameters

		RT	TH1	TH2	TH3	TH4	TH5	TH6	TH7	TH8	TH9	TH10	tar	trin
Athens 2004	FT	0.10	0.54	0.60	0.61	0.66	0.77*	0.82*	0.86*	0.89*	0.95**	0.98**	0.61	0.79
Beijing 2008	FT	−0.05	0.51*	0.66**	0.68**	0.78**	0.80**	0.82**	0.86**	0.89**	0.95**	0.97**	0.57**	0.07

* $p < 0.05$, ** $p < 0.001$.

rising values of the correlation coefficient ($r = 0.77 - 0.98$). The correlation values were identical in both examined Games and it is remarkable that after the 6th hurdle was determined 67% ($r = 0.82$) of the variance of the final time, while after the 10th hurdle was determined 96% ($r = 0.98$) of the above variance. On the basis of the time data of the Mueller & Hommel (1997) project the corresponding correlation coefficients in Athens 1997 can be calculated, which represent similar values ($r = 0.84$ and $r = 0.97$ for 6th and 10th hurdle, respectively).

Clearance Times

The observed mean values of hurdle clearance times (0.28 ± 0.02 s to 0.33 ± 0.01 s) are in agreement with the findings of Mueller & Hommel (1997) (0.30 ± 0.01 s to 0.31 ± 0.02 s) and of Graubner & Nixdorf (2011) (0.30 ± 0.02 s to 0.33 ± 0.01 s). The absence of a significant relationship between hurdle clearance times and final time, in the present study, does not mean that the hurdle clearance times are not an indicator of the race performance. Contrariwise, a

minimised clearance time is an indicator of high sprinting abilities and top technical level of the hurdle sprinters, and a prerequisite for the elite athletes for successful performance, for the reason that a fast hurdle clearance allows the maintaining of the achieved high horizontal velocity in between the hurdles (Salo et al., 1997).

Run-in Phase

The relative quantity of the run-in time was 0.089 ± 0.003s (1-RTH10 = 1 - 0.911 s) and was the same in both Games, Athens 2004 and Beijing 2008. This fact means that the trin contributed 9.9% to the formation of the final performance. This was in agreement with other studies (Graubner & Nixdorf, 2011; Mueller & Hommel, 1997; Brüggemann & Glad, 1990), and on the basis of these time data the contribution of trin to the formation of the final performance in hurdle races in Seoul 1988 (9.3%), in Athens 1997 (9.0%) and Berlin 2009 (8.8%) can be calculated.

The last part of the race is a net sprint running. Subtracting a distance of 1.05 m (which represents the approximate landing distance after the last hurdle) of the official distance of 10.50 m, the runners are invited to cover an actual distance of 9.45 m, attempting, initially, to carry out the transition from the acyclic movement of the last clearance stride into a cyclic motion (running stride) and then to increase the running velocity up to the finish. The run-in distance, although without hurdles, is not sufficient to develop maximum running velocity, so the achieving run-in average velocity is lower than the velocity in the other hurdle units (except the approach run and 9th hurdle unit). In the present study the run-in average velocities were 8.42 m/s and 8.24 m/s in Athens 2004 and Beijing 2008, respectively. The corresponding velocities were 7.87 m/s in Seoul 1988, 8.30 m/s in Athens 1997 and 8.45 m/s in Berlin 2009 (Graubner & Nixdorf, 2011; Mueller & Hommel, 1997; Brüggemann & Glad, 1990).

Relative Times

Due to the different final performances in the various competitions, as a direct consequence are observed different values in their intermediate times. Thus, to study the temporal distribution of the competitive efforts during the hurdle races and to draw safe conclusions from a comparison among the various competitions, the relative temporal parameters (intermediate times normalised by the final time) were used.

In the present study, the mean values of the relative temporal parameters showed a similar race pattern of the hurdle finalists in both Olympic Games. It is remarkable that the time contribution of the first half of the race was slightly larger than the second one (RTH5 = 0.516 in both Games). On the basis of the time data of top level competitions (Graubner & Nixdorf, 2011; Mueller & Hommel, 1997; Brüggemann & Glad, 1990) could be calculated and produced the corresponding values in Seoul 1988 (RTH5 = 0.512), in Athens 1977 (RTH5 = 0.514) and in Berlin 2009 (RTH5 = 0.516). Additionally, the duration of the hurdle units, as a whole, constituted the 70.8% of the total race time in both Games, Athens 2004 and Beijing 2008. Based again in calculations against the time data of Graubner & Nixdorf (2011), Mueller & Hommel (1997) and Brüggemann & Glad (1990), could be estimated that the corresponding percentages were 72.0% in Seoul 1988, 70.8% in Athens 1977 and 70.7% in Berlin 2009. The remaining percentage, approximately 30%, for formation of the final performance was shared between the first touchdown time (RTH1 = 0.187 to 0.204) and the run-in time (Rtrin = 0.088 to 0.093). The former one contributes 20.3% and the latter one 8.7% for formation of the final race performance, with slight variations on each side in the various races. All the above mentioned, based on the relative temporal parameters, suggest the existence of a common hurdle race pattern, regardless of the final performances in the various competitions. The main limitations of the present study are 1) the absence of physiological characteristics of the subjects (age, body composition, various anatomical characteristics, training experience ets), due to the lack of personal experimental design, 2) the absence of laser instruments for measurement of instantaneous velocities, as well as the no use of high speed cameras to accurate measurement of take-off and landing distances before and after the hur-

dles. Future studies should be focused on linking detailed kinematic and kinetic parameters with the direct performance descriptors of the high level hurdle sprint, and corresponding studies could be conducted in the area of teenagers and young hurdlers.

CONCLUSION

From the direct performance descriptors examined in the present study, it is evident that there aren't any significant differences between the means of time parameters in 100-m women hurdles at two consecutive Olympic Games. In summary, the most important findings are the following:

1. No existence of significant relationship between reaction time and race performance
2. Absence of a significant relationship between hurdle clearance times and race performance
3. Running acceleration from the start to 6th hurdle
4. Identification of the decisive points of the race, especially from the 5th to 10th hurdle (r = 0.77 - 0.98 between the intermediate times and final performance)
5. After the 6th hurdle is determined 67% of the variance of the final time, while after the 10th hurdle 96% of the above variance
6. Finally, the main finding is the existence of a common race pattern in high level hurdle performance, regardless of the final performances in the various competitions. Approximately, to the formation of the race performance the approach run time contributes 19%, the duration of the hurdle units, as a whole, 71% and the run-in time 10%. Additionally, the time contribution of the first half of the race to the formation of the final performance is approximately equal to the second one (51.6% vs 48.4%)

In conclusion the findings of the present study can provide coaches and athletes with valuable quantitative information and offer them the possibility, on the basis of statistical models of technical parameters, to make effective interventions in the training process.

ACKNOWLEDGEMENTS

The authors gratefully acknowledge Prof. Svetoslav Ivanov, Mr. Evaggelos Antzakas and Mr. Nedialko Nedialkov for their assistance during the videotaping session.

REFERENCES

Brüggemann G.-P., Glad B. (1990). Time analysis of the 110 meters and 100 meters hurdles: Scientific Research Project at the Games of the XXIVth Olympiad-Seoul 1988, Final Report. *New Studies in Athletics (supplement)*, 5, 91-131.

Coh, M. (1987). The analysis of the Jordanka Donkova's 100m hurdles world record. *Fizicka Kultura (Belgrade)*, *41 (5)*, 351-353.

Coh M, Dolenec A. (1996). Three-dimensional kinematic analysis of the hurdles technique used by Brigita Bukovec. *New studies in athletics*, 11, 63-70.

Graubner R, Nixdorf E. (2011). Biomechanical analysis of the sprint and hurdles events at the 2009 IAAF World Championships in Athletics. *New studies in athletics, 26 (*1-2), 19-53.

Hamlin, M. J., Hopkins, W. G., & Hollings, S. C. (2015). Effects of altitude on performance of elite track-and-field athletes. *International journal of sports physiology and performance, 10 (*7), 881-887.

Hücklekemkes J. (1990). Model technique analysis sheets for the hurdles. Part VI: The Womens 100 m Hurdles. *New studies in athletics, 5 (*4), 33-58.

Iskra J, Coh M. (2006). A review of biomechanical studies in hurdle races. *Kinesiologia Slovenica*, 1, 84-102.

Mann R, Herman, J. (1985). Kinematic analysis of Olympic hurdle performance: women's 100 meters. *International Journal of Sport Biomechanics, 1 (*2), 163-173.

Marar L, Grimshaw P. (1993). A three-dimensional biomechanical analysis of sprint hurdles. *Journal of Sports Sciences,* 12, 174-175.

McDonald C, Dapena J. (1991a). Angular momentum in the men's 110-m and women's 100-m hurdles races. *Medicine & Science in Sports & Exercise, 23 (*12), 1392-1402.

McDonald C, Dapena J. (1991b). Linear kinematics of the men's 110-m and women's 100-m hurdles races. *Medicine & Science in Sports & Exercise, 23 (*12), 1382-1391.

McLean B. (1994). The biomechanics of hurdling: Force plate analysis to assess hurdling technique. *New studies in athletics*, 4, 55-58.

Mueller H, Hommel H. (1997). Biomechanical research project at VIth World Championships in Athletics, Athens 1997: preliminary report. *New studies in athletics, 12 (*2/3), 43-73.

Ryu J. K., Chang J. K. (2011). Kinematic Analysis of the Hurdle Clearance Technique used by World Top Class Women's Hurdler. *Korean Journal of Sport Biomechanics, 21 (*2), 131-140.

Salo A, Grimshaw P. N., Marar L. (1997). 3-D biomechanical analysis of sprint hurdles at different competitive levels. *Medicine and science in sports and* exercise, *29 (*2), 231-237.

Stein N. (2000). Reflections on a change in the height of the hurdles in the women's sprint hurdles event. *New studies in athletics, 15 (*2), 15-20.

Wang, J. H., & Li., N. (2000). Analysis of the technique of hurdle step and run between hurdles. *Journal of Wuhan institute of physical education, 34 (*1), 92-94.

Ward-Smith, A. (1997). A mathematical analysis of the bioenergetics of hurdling. *Journal of Sports Sciences, 15 (*5), 517-526.

Yoshimoto, T., Takai, Y., & Kanehisa, H. (2016). Acute effects of different conditioning activities on running performance of sprinters. *SpringerPlus*, 5(1), 1203.

Normand, J. M., Wolfe, A., & Peak, K. (2017). A Review of Early Sport Specialization in Relation to the Development of a Young Athlete. *International Journal of Kinesiology and Sports Science*, 5(2), 37-42.

4

Comparison of Body Fat Results from 4 Bioelectrical Impedance Analysis Devices vs. Air Displacement Plethysmography in American Adolescent Wrestlers

Melissa M. Montgomery[1], Risto H. Marttinen[2], Andrew J. Galpin[1]

[1]Center for Sport Performance, Department of Kinesiology, California State University, Fullerton, 800 N. State College Blvd., Fullerton, CA 92831 USA, [2]Department of Kinesiology, California State University, Fullerton, 800 N. State College Blvd., Fullerton, CA 92831 USA

Corresponding Author: Andrew J. Galpin, E-mail: agalpin@fullerton.edu

ARTICLE INFO

Conflicts of interest: None

Funding: The research was funded by the National Wrestling Coaches Association (USA) and the National Federation of State High School Associations (USA).

ABSTRACT

Background: Accurate and accessible methods of body composition are necessary to ensure health and safety of wrestlers during competition. The most valid and reliable instruments are expensive and relatively inaccessible to high school wrestlers; therefore, more practical technology is needed. **Objective:** To compare body fat percentage (BF%) results from 4 bioelectrical impedance analysis (BIA) devices to those from air displacement plethysmography (ADP) in adolescent wrestlers. **Methodology:** 134 adolescent male and female wrestlers (1.72±0.9 m, 66.8±14.3 kg, 15.6±1.1 yrs.) were tested for hydration and then completed 4 body composition tests with different BIA devices and one with Bod Pod. Relative and absolute agreement were assessed between each BIA device and ADP on a single day. **Results:** When compared with ADP, all devices demonstrated excellent reliability (ICC (2,1)) range: 0.88-0.94), but questionable measurement error (SEM range: 2.3-3.6 %BF). Bland-Altman plots revealed that each bioelectrical impedance device we tested over-estimated body fat percent in high school wrestlers (range: 0.8-3.6 %BF) and demonstrated wide 95% limits of agreement (range: 15.0-20.8 %BF) compared to ADP. **Conclusions:** The devices investigated demonstrated reasonable measurement accuracy. However, wide margins of error of each device were noted. Caution should be taken when assessing adolescent wrestlers with lower amounts of body fat, as it may result in failing to identify those who do not meet the minimum body fat percentage for competition. The governing bodies should use the research data in the decision-making process regarding appropriate devices for use in their weight management programs.

Key words: Body Composition, Wrestling, Bioelectrical Impedance, Air Displacement Plethysmography

INTRODUCTION

Because of the danger associated with the unsafe weight loss practices of wrestlers, weight certification programs, such as that developed by the National Wrestling Coaches' Association (NWCA; www.nwca.org) require body composition assessments at the beginning of the season in order to determine the lowest weight class in which each wrestler can safely compete. In the United States, this is determined based on the wrestler's body fat percentage. Currently, the lowest percent body fat at which a wrestler is permitted to compete is 7% for boys and 12% for girls (National Federation of State High School Associations, 2016b). Accordingly, accurate and accessible methods of body composition are necessary to perform these important assessments. Dual energy x-ray absorptiometry (DXA) and air displacement plethysmography (ADP) have been shown to be reliable and valid tools for assessing body composition in adults (Andre-oli, Scalzo, Masala, Tarantino, & Guglielmi, 2009; Fields, Goran, & McCrory, 2002) and adolescents (Fields et al., 2002), but these instruments are expensive and not portable; hence, they are relatively inaccessible to wrestlers. Further, they are impractical for assessing large numbers of wrestlers. Skinfolds are also a considered valid method for predicting body fat; however, the validity of this method relies upon the skill of highly-trained assessors. As such, practical technologies are needed for the purpose of accurately assessing body composition (Utter et al., 2005).

Bioelectrical impedance analysis (BIA) has been adopted by some wrestling governing bodies as a surrogate for the aforementioned methods because of its greater accessibility due to lower price, increased portability, ease of use, and smaller risk of user error compared to other methods. (Utter & Lambeth, 2010) One single frequency leg-to-leg BIA device (Tanita TBF-300WA; Tanita Corporation of America, Inc., Arlington Heights, IL, USA) is currently approved for pre-season assessment of body composition and determination of the minimum wrestling weight by approximately 27 state high school federations in the United States (NFHS. org). This device was approved because it demonstrated acceptable agreement with hydrostatic weighing when measuring fat-free mass in high school wrestlers (Utter et al., 2005). More recently, a multi-frequency BIA device was reported to have a strong correlation and no difference when compared to hydrostatic weighing in high school wrestlers. (Utter et al., 2005) However, the researchers also reported a proportional bias: the BIA device overestimated FFM of wrestlers in the lighter weight classes and underestimated FFM of those in higher weight classes.

With the advances in technology and differences in the design (frequency, electrodes, points of contact, etc.) and proprietary body composition prediction algorithms between manufacturers, one must interpret the findings from individual devices cautiously as the aforementioned factors likely influence our interpretations of accuracy if attempting to extrapolate to new BIA devices. Accordingly, instruments using the most current technology should be investigated in order to determine which instruments are acceptable for assessing body composition, thus ensuring safety for competition. Therefore, the purpose of this study is to compare the body fat percent (BF%) results from 4 BIA devices vs. that from ADP in American high school wrestlers, aged 14-18 years. We chose ADP as the reference because it accepted as a valid method for measuring whole body composition, is not prone to tester error, and is also approved in most states as a final authority for body composition assessment in the case that a wrestler appeals their initial body composition assessment via some other method.

METHODOLOGY

Participants

112 male and 22 female wrestlers from local high schools participated in this study. The proportion of females included in this study (18%) was chosen to ensure that the proportion of secondary school female wrestlers in the United States (~5% nationally (National Federation of State High School Associations, 2016a)) was represented. To be included in the study, they had to be currently competing on their school wrestling team, euhydrated (urine specific gravity <1.025), and had not exercised within 4 hours nor eaten within 3 hours prior to testing. Assent and consent were provided by the participant and parent/guardian, respectively, according to the university Institutional Review Board protocol.

Procedures

Testing took place during the morning hours. Upon arrival, the wrestler was asked to confirm eligibility for participation before being enrolled and provided a subject code. They were then measured for body height with a wall-mounted digital stadiometer (Model DHRWM; *Detecto; Webb City, MO, USA*). Wrestlers were measured in bare feet and were asked to "stand as tall and still as possible with their feet

completely on the floor". This measurement was used for all subsequent body composition tests. Because of the known influence of hydration on body composition assessment devices, all wrestlers were asked to provide a urine sample. Urine specific gravity (USG) was immediately measured with a digital handheld "pen" refractometer (*Atago USA, Inc.; Bellevue, WA, USA*). The wrestler was disqualified from testing if the USG was above 1.025 (Armstrong et al., 1994; California Interscholastic Federation, 2016).

Body composition testing

Properly hydrated wrestlers then completed body composition testing in a randomized order. Because of the known sensitivity of the BIA devices to fluid pooled in the distal extremity (Lozano-Nieto & Turner, 2001), if the ADP measurement was completed before any BIA measurements, investigators ensured the wrestler remained in a standing position for at least 10 minutes before any BIA testing was performed. All participants wore minimal clothing for all testing. For boys, this included: compression shorts, boxer briefs, or a wrestling singlet. For girls, acceptable apparel included: compression shorts and a sports bra, or a singlet. All wrestlers wore the same clothing for each body composition test.

Air displacement plethysmography (ADP) testing

ADP was tested with the Bod Pod (*COSMED USA, Inc., Concord, CA, USA*). (McCrory, Gomez, Bernauer, & Mole, 1995) The manufacturer's complete quality control procedures were performed at the beginning of each testing day. The manufacturer's protocol was followed for each participant, which included approximately 3 minutes of setup and calibration and 2 minutes of actual testing. Briefly, the wrestler's demographic information was input into the software (version 5.4.1), which then prompted the researchers to calibrate the device and scale, weigh the wrestler on the Bod Pod scale, and then perform the ADP measurement. The Brozek equation (Brozek, Grande, Anderson, & Keys, 1963) and predicted thoracic gas volume were used to predict percent body fat from body volume, respectively. The participant was asked to don a swim cap to compress their hair before entering the Bod Pod. They were then instructed to sit still and breathe normally for the duration of the test. The software automatically completed two measurements, with a third in the event that the 1st and 2nd measurements disagreed by more than 3%. Percent body fat was automatically calculated by the software.

Bioelectrical impedance analysis testing

Participants completed body composition assessment with 4 BIA devices: Accuniq BC310 (ACC) (*Accuniq Co., Ltd., Seoul, KOR*), InBody 120 (IB120) (*InBody USA, Cerritos, CA, USA*), InBody 270 (IB270) (*InBody USA, Cerritos, CA, USA*), and the Tanita TBF-300WA plus (TAN) (*Tanita Corporation of America, Inc., Arlington Heights, IL, USA*). Specifications for each device are listed in Table 1.

Before the BIA tests, the participants wiped the palms of their hands and the soles of their feet with wipes soaked with an antibacterial solution (0.9% Sodium Chloride, 15ppm Iso-thiazolinone and 150ppm Didecyldimethylammonium chloride) (InBody Tissue; *InBody US, Cerritos, CA, USA*) in order to ensure clean contacts with the devices and to enhance electrical conductivity. Participants then followed the prompts from each device to complete testing. In brief, these prompts asked the wrestler to step onto the scale and stand still while their body mass was measured. Then the investigators were prompted to enter the wrestler's sex, age/date of birth and height. The wrestler was then asked to align their heels and forefeet with the electrodes on the measurement scale and ensure maximum contact area. For the tetrapolar devices (IB120, IB270, and ACC), the wrestler was also asked to align their thumbs, fingers, and palms to maximize contact area with the electrodes while holding onto the device handles. They were then instructed to extend their elbows and slightly abduct their shoulders to ensure that their arms were not touching their torso. The TAN device was the only bipolar device used and as such, did not have handles. For this test, the wrestler only had to align their feet on the 4 electrodes (heels and forefeet). Once the proper positioning was achieved for each device, the wrestler was then asked to stand still and remain silent while the device completed the body composition measurement, which took 30 seconds on average. The investigators administered and supervised the entire test to ensure that the wrestler maintained the proper position and did not move.

All five body composition assessments were completed within 90 minutes. During that time, the wrestlers were not allowed to eat, drink, or perform physical activity. They were encouraged to empty their bladder if the need arose during the testing appointment. None of the wrestlers needed to urinate during the testing session.

Data Reduction and Statistical Analysis

The percent body fat (%BF) automatically calculated by each device was used for analysis. Intraclass correlation (ICC (2,1))

and standard error of measurement (SEM) were calculated to assess relative agreement. Bland-Altman plots (Bland & Altman, 1986) were created to visually assess the absolute agreement and precision between each device and the Bod Pod. To construct the plots, the difference between each device and Bod Pod was determined by subtracting the BF% value acquired from each device from that acquired from the Bod Pod. Then, the average of the value from the Bod Pod and each BIA device ((BIA+BP)/2) was calculated. Each individual's data were then plotted with the average value measurements (MEAN %BF) on the X-axis and the difference between the two devices (DIFF %BF) on the Y-axis to allow for visualization of the relationship between the difference and the mean. The new MEAN and DIFF variables were inspected and confirmed to conform to a normal distribution. As such, the 95% limits of agreement (±1.96 x SD) were calculated and displayed on each plot as a metric of precision along with the mean difference (bias).

One sample t-tests were first used to determine whether fixed bias (bias is statistically different from zero) existed for the devices. Then, in order to determine whether a proportional bias might be present, the difference in BF% between each device and ADP were regressed on the bias of each device to visually display their relation to one another. In the case that the difference between the BIA and ADP instrument was dependent on the magnitude of BF%, the 95% limits of agreement was recalculated using a regression-based approach. (Bland & Altman, 1999)

All analyses were performed with IBM SPSS version 24 (IBM Corp., Armonk, NY, USA). A significance level of <0.05 was determined a priori.

RESULTS

112 male (1.72±8.4 m; 67.9±15.1 kg; 15.6±1.1 yrs.; 23.0±4.8 BMI; 14.9±7.7% body fat) and 22 female (1.59±6.0 m; 61.1±7.7 kg; 15.5±1.1 yrs.; 24.2±3.3 BMI; 24.2±3.3% body fat) wrestlers participated in this study. For descriptive purposes, wrestlers were classified by the 2017 age division and weight classes (USA Wrestling, 2016) (Figure 1). Descrip-

Table 1. Specifications for Bioelectrical Impedance Analysis (BIA) devices

Device	Accuniq BC310	InBody 120	InBody 270	Tanita TBF-300WA plus
Frequency	Single (50 Hz)	Multiple (20 & 100 kHz)	Multiple (20 & 100 kHz)	Single (50 Hz)
Electrode method	Tetrapolar, 8 electrodes	Tetrapolar, 8 electrodes	Tetrapolar, 8 electrodes	Bipolar, 4 electrodes

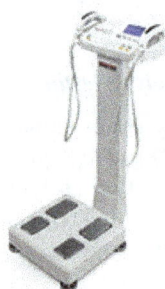

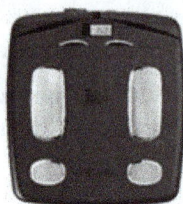

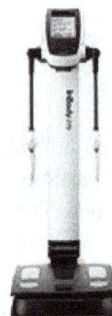

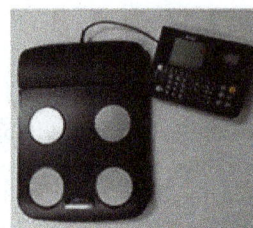

tives for the body fat percentage results from each device are displayed in Table 2.

Intraclass Correlations

The intraclass correlations (Table 3) can be interpreted as the frequency with which the two devices agree within the bounds of the standard error of the measurement (SEM). For example, the results indicate that the %BF results from the IB120 are within 2.3% of the Bod Pod results, 94% of the time. When qualitatively comparing the ICC's, the IB120 and IB270 demonstrated slightly better agreement and precision, compared to the other two devices. However, the ICC for the Tanita device still achieved what is commonly considered as "excellent" agreement, with slightly less precision. While the Accuniq device's ICC was not appreciably worse, the SEM is larger, indicating its precision is about 1% lower than the other devices.

Fixed Bias: One sample T-tests

The t-tests revealed that the bias between each BIA device and ADP was significant (null hypothesis: bias=0) (Table 4). This bias was smallest for the IB120 device, which overestimated body fat by 0.8% and largest for the ACC which overestimated by 3.6% body fat. However, as noted in Table 2,

the effect sizes for the mean difference between each BIA device and the Bod Pod were small (0.08-0.38).

Proportional Bias: Bland-Altman plots and Regression analysis

In order to determine whether the measurement error was uniform across the range of lean body mass values, the Bland-Altman plots were first visually inspected (Figure 3). Then, linear regressions determined whether the mean BF% was a significant predictor of the bias of each instrument. Upon inspection of the plots (Figure 2), outliers were detected for each device, which is typical. In addition to the fixed bias noted, wide limits of agreement, spanning 15.7-20.8% were present for all devices as well (Table 5). In other words, for the IB120, on average we expect about 1% over-estimation of body fat, but we can still reasonably expect anywhere from 8.6% over-estimation to a 7% under-estimation.

The regression analysis revealed no relationship between the difference in BF% and the mean BF% between devices for the IB120 ($F_{1,132}$= 3.80; P=0.05) or the TAN ($F_{1,132}$ = 0.26; P=0.62). However, these relationships were significant for the ACC ($F_{1,133}$= 26.43; P<0.001) and the IB270 ($F_{1,132}$= 8.66; P=0.004). Accordingly, new regression-based 95% LOA's were calculated for these two devices (Figure 2A and 2C).

Table 2. Descriptives for body fat percentage results (mean±SD) for Bod Pod and each bioelectrical impedance analysis device. Mean difference (device-Bod Pod), 95% confidence intervals and effect sizes are provided

Instrument	Mean±SD	Mean difference† and range (Min-Max)	95% CI	Effect size
Bod Pod	16.7±8.4	--	--	--
Accuniq BC310	20.3±10.5	−3.6 (−16.4-14.4)	0.12-1.49	0.38
InBody 120	17.4±9.1	−0.81 (−13.6-11.0)	1.83 − 3.13	0.08
InBody 270	19.2±9.4	−2.5 (−15.6-7.1)	1.38 − 2.98	0.28
Tanita TBF-300WA plus	18.9±8.3	−2.2 (−3.1-13.3)	2.66 − 4.47	0.26

† Negative number indicates overestimation by instrument when compared to air displacement plethysmography

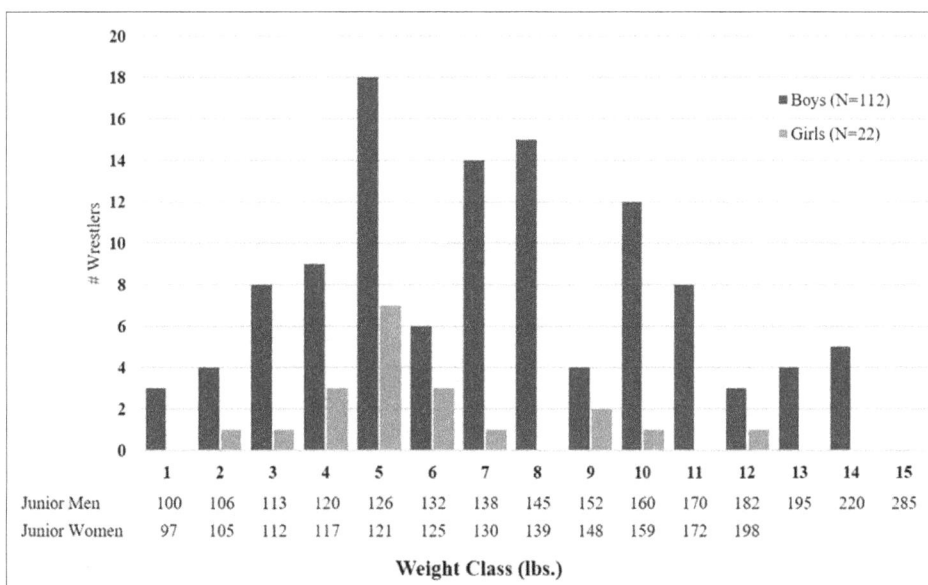

Figure 1: Distribution of wrestlers across weight classes (lbs.)

DISCUSSION

We compared the body fat measurements from 4 bioelectrical impedance devices against results from air displacement plethysmography. Our primary finding was that each of the BIA devices produced significantly higher body fat percentage results than the Bod Pod, which ranged from overestimation of 0.8% to 3.6%. However, despite the statistical significance of the differences, the effect sizes were small. The wide limits of agreement may be somewhat problematic in wrestlers at the lower end of the body fat spectrum, for example when approaching the National Federation of High Schools Association's minimum 7% and 12% cut-offs for boys and girls, respectively.

While several previous studies have evaluated the agreement between BIA devices and a reference standard (e.g. hy-

Table 3. Intraclass correlations (ICC 2,1) and SEM for relative agreement of percent body fat (%BF) results between each device and the Bod Pod

Instrument	ICC (2,1)	SEM (% BF)
Bod Pod	--	--
Accuniq BC310	0.88	3.62
InBody 120	0.94	2.30
InBody 270	0.93	2.43
Tanita TBF-300WA plus	0.90	2.67

drostatic weighing, dual energy x-ray, or air displacement plethysmography), direct comparisons are difficult due to differences in BIA devices and changes in BIA technology (e.g., electrode type, prediction algorithms, etc.), as well as varying methods of assessing agreement (e.g. t-tests, ICC's, correlations, and Bland-Altman plots). Of the previous work in the wrestling population, two studies have reported no difference in the fat-free mass results between single- and multi-frequency BIA devices and hydrostatic weighing in high school (Utter et al., 2005) and college wrestlers (Utter & Lambeth, 2010), respectively. However, a proportional bias was also noted in both datasets, indicating that the BIA devices tended to over-estimate fat-free mass in the lighter individuals, while under-estimating in the heavier wrestlers. Because we compared BF% from the BIA devices in the current study to the ADP reference, our results cannot be directly compared to the previous studies. However, as an illustration of the relative effects of differences in BF% on fat-free mass, Table 6 displays the expected results from each device based on a 150 lb. wrestler with 12% body fat, as assessed by the Bod Pod according to the fat-free mass calculation used in the NCAA Weight Management Program (National Collegiate Athetics Association, 2016) to calculate the lowest allowable weight for competition.

We observed high intraclass correlations for each device, indicating that a measurement from a device would agree with the Bod Pod more than 90% of the time (albeit within an

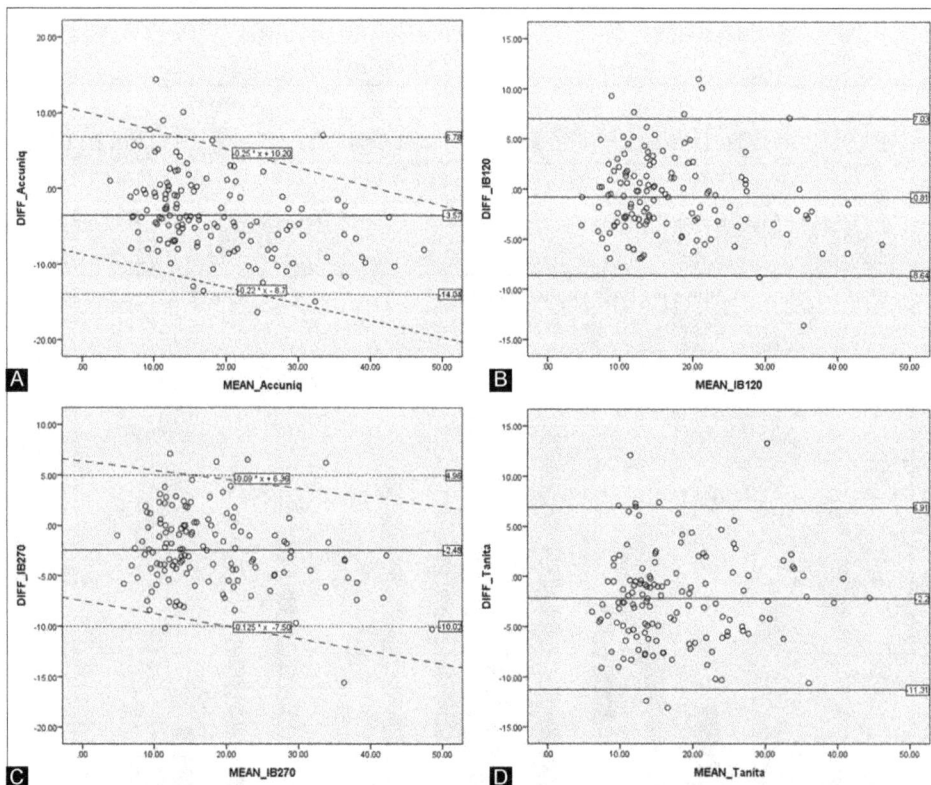

Figure 2: Bland-Altman plots visualize the relationship between the difference in percent body fat result between the Bod Pod and each device (DIFF) and the average percent body fat between the Bod Pod and each device (MEAN): A) Accuniq BC310, B) InBody 120, C) InBody 270, D) Tanita TBF-300WA plus. Solid horizontal line represents the bias (average DIFF). The dotted lines represent the upper and lower boundaries of the 95% limits of agreement (1.96±SD of DIFF). The diagonal dashed lines represent the revised regression-based 95% limits of agreement calculated due to the presence of proportional bias

Table 4. One sample t-test results for bias in percent body fat (%BF; Bod Pod – device) calculated by each device

Instrument	Bias (%BF)	t	P-value	95% CI
Accuniq BC310	−3.63	−7.91	0.00	−4.54 – -2.72
InBody 120	−0.81	−2.33	0.02	−1.49 – -0.12
InBody 270	−2.53	−7.66	0.00	−3.18 – -1.88
Tanita TBF-300WA	−2.20	−5.48	0.00	−2.99 – -1.40

Table 5. Bias and 95% limits of agreement for each device

Instrument	Bias (%)	95% LOA (range %)
Accuniq BC310	−3.63	−14.04 – 6.78 (20.8%)
InBody 120	−0.81	−8.64 – 7.03 (15.7%)
InBody 270	−2.53	−10.02 – 4.96 (15.0%)
Tanita TBF-300WA	−2.20	−11.31 – 6.91 (18.2%)

approximate 2.5% body fat margin of error). Yet, that there were significant differences in the relative agreement (bias) between each device and the Bod Pod provides an illustration of the shortcomings of only analyzing the absolute agreement via ICC's as described by Altman and Bland (Bland & Altman, 1986). The relative agreement (bias) we observed for the devices studied are in accordance with Lee et al (Lee et al., 2017), who reported a 3% and 4.5% bias in school-aged (7-12 years old) boys and girls, respectively, when comparing the InBody 230 multiple frequency BIA device (similar to the IB270 device used in this study) with DXA. An additional study (Utter & Lambeth, 2010) compared fat-free mass measured by a multi-frequency device (InBody 520) to hydrostatic weighing and reported that the device could be expected to measure fat-free mass within 12 lbs. of fat-free mass 95% of the time, which the authors deemed to be within "acceptable range". However, the proportional bias is worth noting, as the device tended to overestimate fat-free mass in the lighter wrestlers and over-estimate fat-free mass in heavier wrestlers.Conversely, our results are contrary to a previous report (Dixon, Deitrick, Pierce, Cutrufello, & Drapeau, 2005) that a leg-to-leg BIA device underestimated the body fat % in college wrestlers by 4.16% when compared to Bod Pod. Another study (Azcona, Koek, & Fruhbeck, 2006) also reported that BIA underestimated BF% by 3.4% and demonstrated limits of agreement spanning 13.7% in obese and non-obese children and adolescents (ages 5-22 years old) when compared to ADP. Another study (von Hurst et al., 2016) reported that the InBody 230 underestimated BF% by an average of 2% in adults in the mid-30 year old range. Interestingly, the previously-mentioned study (Lee et al., 2017) reported a glaring 8.8% overestimation in boys and 9.7% overestimation in girls when measuring with a single-frequency device (Tanita BC-418). We tested two single-frequency devices in this study (Tanita TBF-300WA plus and Accuniq BC310). The Tanita BC-418 is a single-frequency, multi-segment analyzer similar to the specifications of the Accuniq BC310 device used in this study, which was also the least consistent of the four devices we investigated. The Tanita TBF-300WA plus that we tested is a single-frequency, bi-polar (foot to foot) analyzer, which may explain the discrepancy. Perhaps the single frequency is inadequate for tetrapolar, multi-segmental assessments.There is no statistical significance test for the limits of agreement. As such, the acceptable limits of agreement must to be decided by the practitioner in consideration of the particular use. In this dataset, we observed large limits of agreement ranging from 15-20% (Table 6), and crossing zero, which means that while a device on average overestimates %BF, in some cases it will underestimate. These ranges can have a substantial impact on our confidence in the results from any given device. Additionally, we observed a proportional bias in two of the devices (ACC and IB270) whereby the devices showed a tendency to overestimate BF% more so in those with less body fat and to underestimate BF% in those with more body fat. Although these limits of agreement are objectively wider than would be preferable, they are similar to those reported in the only recent study comparing BIA to ADP (von Hurst et al., 2016). In that study of adults, the limits of agreement spanned from -4.3 to 8.4%, which spans 12.7%. It should be considered that there is error inherent to the device comparisons, since the referent measurement by air displacement plethysmography is itself, an estimate based on an indirect measurement of body composition. We chose the Bod Pod as the referent in this study because it is more accessible for the purposes of body composition assessment than DXA or hydrostatic weighing. For example, the California Interscholastic Federation (CIF) wrestling weight management program protocol (California Interscholastic Federation, 2016) allows for a Bod Pod assessment in the event that a wrestler disputes his or her body composition results with the approved BIA device. The most recent study investigating the validity of Bod Pod vs. DXA (Lowry & Tomiyama, 2015) reported 95% limits of agreement in under-, normal, and overweight/obese adults that are similar (under: 0.7-13.2% BF; normal: -5.2-8.9 %BF, overweight/obese: -5.87 – 8.81 %BF) to our BIA 95% limits of agreement which again emphasizes the amount of error that we should consider as inherent in any indirect measurement of body composition.

Implications of Overestimating Body Fat

Despite questions of the overall accuracy of these devices, when applied to the current purpose of evaluating the validity for high school wrestlers, the bias and wide limits of agreement primarily have importance for athletes at the lowest end of the body composition spectrum since the eligibility guidelines only apply to male and female wrestlers with <7% and <12% body fat, respectively. Particular caution should be taken when interpreting BIA (or any body composition test) in this group. For example, if an instrument measures a male at 8% but their true body fat percentage was 6%, they would still be allowed to wrestle and even lose weight (e.g. a 125 lb. wrestler would still be permitted to lose 1.25 pounds of body fat to get down to 7%). The initial inclination is to simply subtract the device's bias to account for the systematic (absolute) overestimation of percent body fat. However, the wide limits of agreement make this strategy problematic. To illustrate the effect of the wide limits of agreement, Table 7 shows the range of results that we could get from the different devices in the case of an individual that has 12% body fat (A), according to the Bod Pod. The "device result" (C) below is the simple result after accounting for the device's bias (B). The (D) device 95% limits of agreement are then applied and the adjusted 95% limits of agreement shows that it is possible that an individual might actually be below the 7% body fat threshold that would exclude him from competition. Re-inspection of the Bland-Altman plots (Figure 3) shows that some individuals in this study would be in that situation. This underscores the need to pay particularly close attention to the wrestlers whose body fat is in the lower ranges, regardless of the type of body composition test that is used.

While this illustration points wide limits of agreement, the lack of precision is similar to the validation study (Utter et al., 2005) of the BIA device that is currently approved for assessing body composition in high school wrestlers in which wide (~15 kg. (33 lb.) of fat-free mass) limits of agreement were reported as well. The researchers illustrated in their dataset, a 20 lb. underestimation of fat-free mass in one wrestler and a 26 lb. overestimation in another. The authors concluded that while the precision of the BIA device was not optimal, it was still a viable option when comparing it to the limitations associated with other body composition analysis techniques. We acknowledge limitations in our study. First, that we used a criterion method that is itself, an indirect method of body composition assessment. We chose the Bod Pod as the criterion method since some high school federation rules (e.g. California Interscholastic Federation) allow for ADP testing when the wrestler disputes their BIA results. However, while hydrostatic weighing or DXA may be considered "gold standards" of body composition assessment, they too are indirect methods of estimating body composition and are too subject to error. The second limitation of our study was that we analyzed males and females together. Due to our attempt to maximize external validity for the high school wrestling community, we only included males and females who were actively competing on their respective school teams. Because of the small proportion of female wrestlers in the community, our sample was not large enough to achieve the statistical power to perform all analyses by sex. Future work should attempt to recruit a larger sample of female wrestlers. Additionally, although recommended by BIA manufacturers, we did not exclude females who were menstruating. This was again, to increase the external validity of our results since oftentimes, wrestlers do not have the ability to choose the date that they are assessed for body composition and as such, cannot avoid testing during menses.

CONCLUSIONS

Each bioelectrical impedance device that we tested over-estimated body fat percent in high school wrestlers.

Table 6. Illustration of relationship between body fat percent on fat-free mass based on an example 150 lb. wrestler. The bias from each device was used to adjust the body fat percentage and accordingly, the fat-free mass

	Example Wrestler	Accuniq BC310	InBody 120	InBody 270	Tanita TBF- 300WA plus
Body mass (lbs.)	150	150	150	150	150
Body fat %	12.0%	15.6%	12.8%	14.5%	14.2%
Fat mass (lbs.) (BF% x Body mass)	18.0	23.4	19.2	21.8	21.3
Fat-free mass (lbs.) (Body mass – Fat mass)	132.0	126.6	130.8	128.2	128.7

Table 7. Illustration of the effect of the limits of agreement on the potential range of "true" body fat percentage of a wrestler with 12% body fat, as measured by Bod Pod

Bod Pod result: 12%BF						
(A) Device	(B) Bias	(C) Device result	(D) 95% LOA		(E) Adjusted 95% LOA	
			Lower	Upper	Lower	Upper
Accuniq BC310	−3.63	15.6%	*		9.3%	27.8%
InBody 120	−0.81	12.8%	−8.64	7.03	5.8%	21.4%
InBody 270†	−2.53	14.5%	†		9.4%	23.8%
Tanita TBF-300WA plus	−2.20	14.2%	−11.31	6.91	7.3%	25.5%

*95% LOA are estimated with the regression: -8.7-0.22*mean (lower) and 10.2-0.25*mean (upper), †95% LOA are estimated with the regression: -7.5-0.12*mean (lower) and 6.4-0.09*mean (upper)

Three of the devices (InBody 120, InBody 270, Tanita TBF-300WA plus) over-estimated to a similar degree (0.8-2.5%), compared to air displacement plethysmography. The 4th device (Accuniq BC310) demonstrated the least agreement of the 4 machines. It appears that the accuracy of bioelectrical impedance analysis technology is not uniform across devices and therefore, each device should be investigated before adopting for body composition assessment. The discrepancies we observed are consistent with previous work in wrestlers and reflect the impractical expectation of finding perfect agreement between two indirect methods of assessing body composition. Our results indicate that three of the devices appear to be similar in accuracy and precision to the currently approved device. Given the success of the weight management programs in preventing weight-cutting-related deaths since adopting the BIA device for body composition assessment, governing bodies for wrestling should use the research data in their decision-making process for approving appropriate devices and thus, the opportunity to implement weight management programs more broadly.

REFERENCES

Andreoli, A., Scalzo, G., Masala, S., Tarantino, U., & Guglielmi, G. (2009). Body composition assessment by dual-energy X-ray absorptiometry (DXA). *La Radiologia Medica*, 114(2), 286-300. doi:10.1007/s11547-009-0369-7

Armstrong, L. E., Maresh, C. M., Castellani, J. W., Bergeron, M. F., Kenefick, R. W., LaGasse, K. E., & Riebe, D. (1994). Urinary indices of hydration status. *International Journal of Sport Nutrition*, 4(3), 265-279.

Azcona, C., Koek, N., & Fruhbeck, G. (2006). Fat mass by air-displacement plethysmography and impedance in obese/non-obese children and adolescents. *International Journal of Pediatric Obesity*, 1(3), 176-182.

Bland, J., & Altman, D. (1986). Statistical methods for assessing agreement between two methods of clinical measurement. *Lancet*, 1(8476), 307-310.

Bland, J., & Altman, D. (1999). Measuring agreement in method comparison studies. *Statistical Methods in Medical Research*, 8(2), 135-160. doi:10.1177/096228029900800204

Brozek, J., Grande, F., Anderson, J., & Keys, A. (1963). Densitometric analysis of body composition: Revision of some quantitative assumptions. *Annals of the New York Academy of Sciences*, 110, 113-140.

California Interscholastic Federation. (2016). 2017-2018 Wrestling weight management program manual. Retrieved from http://cifstate.org/sports/boys_wrestling/assessor/CIF_Wrestling_Weight_Management_Handbook.pdf

Dixon, C. B., Deitrick, R. W., Pierce, J. R., Cutrufello, P. T., & Drapeau, L. L. (2005). Evaluation of the BOD POD and leg-to-leg bioelectrical impedance analysis for estimating percent body fat in National Collegiate Athletic Association Division III collegiate wrestlers. *Journal of Strength and Conditioning Research*, 19(1), 85-91. doi:10.1519/14053.1.

Fields, D. A., Goran, M. I., & McCrory, M. A. (2002). Body-composition assessment via air-displacement plethysmography in adults and children: a review. *American Journal of Clinical Nutrition*, 75(3), 453-467.

Lee, L. W., Liao, Y. S., Lu, H. K., Hsiao, P. L., Chen, Y. Y., Chi, C. C., & Hsieh, K. C. (2017). Validation of two portable bioelectrical impedance analyses for the assessment of body composition in school age children. *PloS One*, 12(2), e0171568. doi:10.1371/journal.pone.0171568.

Lowry, D., & Tomiyama, A. (2015). Air displacement plethysmography versus dual-energy x-ray absorptiometry in underweight, normal-weight, and overweight/obese individuals. *PloS One*, 10(1), e0115086. doi:10.1371/journal.pone.0115086.

Lozano-Nieto, A., & Turner, A. A. (2001). Effects of orthostatic fluid shifts on bioelectrical impedance measurements. *Biomedical Instrumentation and Technology*, 35(4), 249-258.

McCrory, M. A., Gomez, T. D., Bernauer, E. M., & Mole, P. A. (1995). Evaluation of a new air displacement. plethysmograph for measuring human body composition. *Medicine and Science in Sports and Exercise*, 27(12), 1686-1691.

National Collegiate Athletics Association. (2016). 2016-2017 NCAA Wrestling Weight Management Program. Retrieved from https://www.ncaa.org/sites/default/files/2017DIMWR_Wrestling_Weight_Management_Program_Information_20160929.pdf

National Federation of State High School Associations. (2016a). 2015-16 High School Athletics Participation Survey.

Retrieved from http://www.nfhs.org/ParticipationStatistics/ParticipationStatistics.

National Federation of State High School Associations. (2016b). 2016-2017 NFHS Wrestling Rules Book.

USA Wrestling. (2016). Rule Book and Guide to Wrestling: 2017 edition. Retrieved from https://docs.google.com/document/d/1ZXYP9ZG_rFRH6hRglZMrAp8rt-jn1yE1NxaOjl4w0dus/edit?pli=1.

Utter, A. C., & Lambeth, P. G. (2010). Evaluation of multifrequency bioelectrical impedance analysis in assessing body composition of wrestlers. *Medicine and Science in Sports and Exercise*, 42(2), 361-367. doi:10.1249/MSS.0b013e3181b2e8b4.

Utter, A. C., Nieman, D. C., Mulford, G. J., Tobin, R., Schumm, S., McInnis, T., & Monk, J. R. (2005). Evaluation of leg-to-leg BIA in assessing body composition of high-school wrestlers. *Medicine and Science in Sports and Exercise*, 37(8), 1395-1400.

von Hurst, P., Walsh, D., Conlon, C., Ingram, M., Kruger, R., & W, S. (2016). Validity and reliability of bioelectrical impedance analysis to estimate body fat percentage against air displacement plethysmography and dual-energy X-ray absorptiometry. *Nutrition and Dietetics*, 73, 197-204.

5

Differences In Male Collegiate and Recreationally Trained Soccer Players on Balance, Agility, and Vertical Jump Performance

Nicole M. Sauls, Nicole C. Dabbs*

Department of Kinesiology, California State University, San Bernardino, 5500 University Parkway, San Bernardino, CA 92407
Corresponding Author: Nicole C. Dabbs, E-mail: ndabbs@csusb.edu

ARTICLE INFO

Conflicts of interest: None
Funding: None.

ABSTRACT

Objective: The purpose of this investigation was to determine the differences in collegiate and recreationally trained soccer players in sprint, vertical jump, and balance performance. **Methods:** Twenty-one soccer players, twelve Division II collegiate and nine recreationally trained volunteered to participate. Session one acted as a familiarization day, where the participants were familiarized with testing day protocols. During testing day, participants performed a dynamic warm-up, followed by balance measurements, three countermovement vertical jumps, and pro-agility shuttle test. **Results:** There were no significant (p>0.05) differences between groups in the all balance variables. Collegiate soccer players had a significantly (p<0.05) greater peak velocity in vertical jump then recreationally trained soccer players. There were significant differences (p<0.05) between groups for maximum for split velocities, where collegiate soccer players were greater than recreationally trained soccer players. There were no significant (p>0.05) differences in groups in all other variables. **Conclusion:** These results indicate that collegiate, Division II, soccer players had greater vertical jumping and sprinting velocities when compared to recreationally trained soccer players. These results may have been impacted by the lack of resistance training background in either of the two groups. With the addition of more time on a collegiate resistance training program, it is very likely the Division II athletes will see a significant increase in all balance, sprint, and vertical jump performance measures compared to recreationally trained players who receive little to no specialized resistance training.

Key words: Postural Stability, Sprint Performance, Power Output, Jumping

INTRODUCTION

Distinguishing athletic performance between levels of competition in sports is essential in determining athlete success (Cometti, Maffiuletti, Pousson, Chatard, & Maffulli, 2001), establishing normative values (Butler, Southers, Gorman, Kiesel, & Plisky, 2012; Reilly, Williams, Nevill, & Franks, 2010), assessing risk for injury (Agel, Evans, Dick, Putukian, & Marshall, 2007), and designing strength and conditioning programs specific to the needs of its players (Gissis et al., 2006; Kaplan, Erkmen, & Taskin, 2009; Wisløff, Castagna, Helgerud, Jones, & Hoff, 2004). Soccer is imperative to investigate due to its high rate of injury (Agel et al., 2007) and unique performance demands. Regardless of competition level, elements necessary for player success include the ability to sprint short distances at high velocities (Cometti et al., 2001; Davis, Brewer, & Atkin, 1992; Gissis et al., 2006; Kaplan et al., 2009; Reilly et al., 2010; Jason D. Vescovi, 2012)subelite and amateur soccer players to clarify what parameters distinguish the top players from the less successful. We tested 95 soccer players from the French first division (elite, rapidly change direction (Salaj & Markovic,

2011; D. P. Wong, Chan, & Smith, 2012), dynamically maintain a stable position to avoid injury during movement(Butler et al., 2012), and produce large amounts of explosive power (Cometti et al., 2001; Jovanovic, Sporis, Omrcen, & Fiorentini, 2011). These factors should be included in a testing protocol if athletic performance is assessed across levels of play in soccer. Previous research shows sprint performance distinguishes between levels of play in soccer (Cometti et al., 2001; Gissis et al., 2006; Kaplan et al., 2009; Reilly et al., 2010; Jason D. Vescovi, 2012). Although generally recognized as aerobic sport, matches are interspersed with several short (10-30 m) sprints roughly every 90 seconds (Jason D. Vescovi, 2012; Wisløff et al., 2004) which constitutes about 1-11% of the total distance traveled (Wisløff et al., 2004) in a game. Studies using linear sprint testing protocols have discriminated between elite levels of soccer athletes, where the more advanced level produced significantly faster times (Haugen, Tønnessen, & Seiler, 2013; Jason D. Vescovi, 2012) and higher velocities (Kalapotharakos et al., 2006). Researchers using similar testing protocols also distinguished elite level soccer athletes from recreationally trained players (Cometti et al., 2001; Gissis et al., 2006; Reilly et al., 2010). It's important to include recreationally trained players since the sport is not limited to high level athletes. Desires to decrease injury and increase athletic performance should extend to the amateur level. Although existing literature holds significance, testing protocols have only included linear sprints. In a game situation, soccer players are required to sprint while rapidly changing direction (Salaj & Markovic, 2011; D. P. Wong et al., 2012). How quickly a player is able to change directions without slowing down is a vital performance variable (Salaj & Markovic, 2011; D. P. Wong et al., 2012). Designing a protocol to include a pro-agility shuttle test may more accurately simulate game situation sprinting demands. Furthermore, previous research indicates dynamic balance performance to be another classifying variable between levels of competition in soccer (Bressel, Yonker, Kras, & Heath, 2007; Butler et al., 2012; Davlin, 2004)professional, elite, or Olympic levels, or their individual coaches believed the athlete performed comparably to these levels. High level male and female gymnasts (n = 57, M age = 17.3 yr., SD = 4.1. Rapidly changing directions while sprinting requires balance and the capacity to dynamically maintain a stable position over a body's center of mass (Butler et al., 2012). Inadequate dynamic balance capability in soccer players has been correlated with a greater risk for injury (Butler et al., 2012). Having a reliable means to evaluate dynamic balance across all classes of experience in soccer is necessary due to an elevated injury risk to the lower extremities.

Researchers have used a number of methods to measure dynamic balance (Bressel et al., 2007; Butler et al., 2012; Davlin, 2004), so the challenge becomes finding a reliable measurement. One system proven in literature to produce reliable values is the Biodex Balance System SD (Parraca et al., 2011). This method has not yet been used to discriminate between levels of play in soccer; however, it has been used in several studies to assess balance and injury risk. Using the Biodex Balance System SD will increase the reliability and decrease the likelihood of errors in measurement. Moreover, vertical jump measures are able to distinguish levels of competition in soccer (Cometti et al., 2001; Wisløff et al., 2004). Explosive lower body power is required while rapidly changing directions during a sprint (Gissis et al., 2006; Wisløff et al., 2004). Previous research examining lower body power in young soccer players indicate the more elite levels having greater countermovement vertical jump heights (VJH) compared to other sub-elite, and recreationally trained players (Gissis et al., 2006). These analyses used the Vertec® to record vertical jump height and made calculated lower body power estimations (Gissis et al., 2006); however, other exact measures of peak power, peak force, peak velocity, and rate of force development can be recorded with the utilization of a force plate.

Due to existing gaps in literature concerning the means of distinguishing athletic performance between levels of play in soccer, the purpose of our study was to investigate the differences in male collegiate and recreationally trained soccer players on balance, sprint, and vertical jump performance measures. Assessments will be made for dynam-

ic balance using the Biodex Balance System SD (Balance System™ SD, Shirley, NY, USA), vertical jump measures using a Vertec® (floor model) and force plates (AMTI model BP600900, Watertown, MA, USA), and sprint performance using timing gates (Swift Performance Speedlight Timing Systems, Wacol, Australia) during a pro-agility shuttle test. We hypothesize our results will be consistent with existing literature and predict the collegiate level athletes to perform better across all performance variables in comparison to recreationally trained players.

METHODS

Participants

Twenty-one soccer players, twelve Division II collegiate (age 20.33 ± 1.66yrs; height 178.02 ± 6.63cm; weight 74.63 ± 5.73kg) and nine recreationally trained (age 23.22 ± 3.41yrs; height 174.32 ± 5.43cm; weight 72.14 ± 11.79kg) volunteered to participate in one familiarization session and one testing session, separated by at least 24hrs each. Recreationally trained players were required to have at least one year of amateur soccer experience. Division II athletes were recruited from California State University of San Bernardino's collegiate soccer team. An informed consent describing the testing protocol and a Physical Activity Readiness Questionnaire (PARQ) was completed on familiarization day. Participants were healthy and free of any lower body musculoskeletal or orthopedic injuries. The protocol was verbally described and anthropometrics (age, height, and weight) were recorded.

Protocol

Following the completion of an informed consent, PARQ, and collection of anthropometrics on familiarization day, a dynamic warm-up was performed including: two sets of a 15m jog, exaggerated lunges, high knees, walking planks, and leg swings. Next, participants were familiarized with balance, vertical jump, and sprint protocols. Balance tests were completed on the Biodex Balance System SD and consisted of three practice trials each of Static Balance (SB), Limits of Stability (LOS), and Single Leg Balance (SLB) tests. Next, three practice trials of a countermovement vertical jump (CMJ) were performed using a Vertec® and force plate. Lastly, three practice trials of a pro-agility sprint protocol were completed with a 3-minute rest between each trial. Participants returned to the laboratory at least 24 hrs following familiarization for testing session.

Biodex Balance System SD

SB, LOS, and SLB tests were completed on the BioDex Balance System SD. The SB and the SLB test consisted of three successful trials at 20s each with a 10s rest between each trial. The LOS test consisted of three trials until completion of task, with a 10s rest between each trial. A trial was deemed successful if the participant did not touch the side hand rails and kept only one leg on the platform for single leg protocols. The level of each test was determined using a very unstable to static spectrum. Level one is the most difficult and allows for the maximum degrees of variation from horizontal in platform movement and there is no platform movement in the static level. SB was set to static, LOS to level 6, and SLB to level 4. SLB measured Overall, Anterior/Posterior, and Medial/Lateral degrees from horizontal. The LOS test measured Overall, Forward, Backward, Right, Left, Forward/Right, Forward/Left, Backward/Right, Backward/Left degrees from horizontal as well as time to completion. Since there is no movement in the platform, SB outcome variables measure anterior, posterior, right, and left sway from a center point (Oliver & Di Brezzo, 2009).

Vertec and Force Plate

Three successful CMJ trials were performed with 15s rest between each jump (Dabbs, Brown, & Garner, 2014). Participants were instructed to jump as high and as quickly as possible using a countermovement arm swing during each jump. A Vertec® was used to measure VJH and an AMTI force plate was used to measure peak force (PF), peak power output (PPO), peak velocity (PV), and rate of velocity development (RVD). In between each jump, the force plate was zeroed out to ensure accurate measurements.

Timing Gates

Participants performed three successful trials of a pro-agility shuttle test requiring a change in direction twice during the sprint (Vescovi, Brown, & Murray, 2006). The protocol included a 20yd sprint with four, 5yd split times. Swift Performance Speed Light laser timing gates were used to record exact split and total times. Participants were instructed to stand as close to the starting point as possible marked by a taped line and go on the sound of a beep set off by the first set of timing gates. Minimum reaction time (RT), minimum split times (ST), minimum total times (TT), maximum split time velocities (STV), and maximum total velocity (TV) were calculated.

Statistical Analysis

To analyze differences between the recreational and collegiate soccer players, independent t-tests were conducted for each variable in SB, LOS, and SLB balance measures. RT, ST, TT, and STV were calculated from the pro-agility test. The Vertec® was used to measure VJH and the AMTI force plate measured vertical forces and calculated PPO, PV, PF, and RVD.

RESULTS

There was a significant (p= .049) difference between groups with collegiate athletes (3.05 ± .27 m/s) being greater than recreationally trained (2.8 ± .25m/s) soccer players for PV during the vertical jump (Figure 1). There were no significant (p> 0.05) differences between groups in all other vertical jump measures. There were no significant (p> 0.05)

differences in balance measures between groups in all balance measures. There were significant differences (p= 0.02) between groups for sprint TV, where collegiate soccer players (3.85 ± .13m/s) were greater than recreationally trained (3.69 ± .16m/s) soccer players. There were significant differences (p= 0.03) between groups for sprint maximum STV one, STV two, and STV four where collegiate soccer players (3.80 ± .2m/s) were greater than recreationally trained (3.11 ± .1.0m/s) soccer players. There were no significant (p> 0.05) differences between groups for in all other sprint measures (Table 1).

DISCUSSION

The objective of our study was to examine the differences in male collegiate and recreationally trained soccer players on balance, sprint, and vertical jump performance measures. Significant differences were found between levels of play for peak velocity during a vertical jump, maximum total sprint velocity, and maximum sprint velocity during time split one. Significant differences were not found between levels of play for all other balance, sprint, and vertical jump measures.

Previous research examining lower body power in young soccer players indicated more elite levels having greater CMJ height compared to other sub-elite, and recreationally trained players (Gissis 2006); however, studies recording force and velocity vertical jump measures using similar soccer populations could not be found. The current investigation measured peak power, peak velocity, and peak force variables while performing a CMJ and found differences between the two groups was higher in collegiate athletes for peak velocity. Power is the product of force times velocity, where increases in both force and velocity result in an increase in power production capability (Cormie, McBride, & McCaulley, 2009). Although the DII soccer athletes were able to produce higher velocities and move more quickly, the lack of significant difference in peak force and peak power may be explained by their inability to generate enough force to change the power output. Other subsequent research determined dynamic balance performance to be a classifying

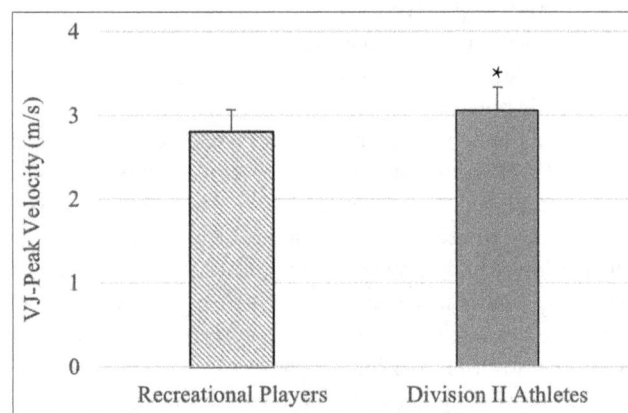

Figure 1: Means ± Standard Deviations for Division II soccer athletes and Recreationally Trained soccer players, indicating a significantly (* p<0.05) greater Peak Velocity during a vertical jump.

Table 1. Differences between recreational players and Division II Athletes in balance, vertical jump, and sprint performance measures

Measure	Recreational players		Division II Athletes	
	Mean	**SD**	**Mean**	**SD**
SB				
Overall	0.69	0.68	0.59	0.56
A/P	0.54	0.7	0.48	0.47
M/L	0.33	0.38	0.24	0.26
SLB right				
Overall	2.06	1.22	1.86	0.7
A/P	1.34	0.66	1.33	0.56
M/L	1.46	1.1	1.13	0.48
SLB left				
Overall	2.04	0.91	1.71	0.52
A/P	1.44	0.63	1.24	0.33
M/L	1.23	0.62	1	0.44
LOS				
Overall	27.56	9.34	25.75	6.81
Forward	36.67	15.43	40	10.94
Backward	43.56	13.24	46.08	15.28
Right	31.56	14.06	27.33	10.19
Left	32.22	13.05	26.5	9.43
F/R	31.89	11.47	29.5	10.06
F/L	28.67	13.24	31.08	8.31
B/R	35.22	12.34	30	9.21
B/L	34.78	8.54	34.58	9.42
VJH (cm)	54.61	7.4	60.21	8.65
PPO (W)	4527.79	516.69	4981.3	670.92
PF (N)	1807.57	304.81	1984.95	376.2
RVD (m/s^2)	7685.73	2712.91	8711	3888.96
Max TV (m/s)	3.69*	0.16	3.85	0.13
Max STV 1 (m/s)	3.12*	1.01	3.81	0.2
Max STV 2 (m/s)	2.97*	1.04	3.65	0.26
Max STV 3 (m/s)	4.06	1.75	4.86	0.38
Max STV 4 (m/s)	2.92*	0.87	3.6	0.29
Min ST 1	1.29*	0.11	1.19	0.07
Min ST 2	1.19	0.11	1.21	0.09
Min ST 3	0.94	0.07	0.92	0.06
Min ST 4	1.33	0.12	1.22	0.16
Min RT	0.49	0.13	0.48	0.11
Min TT	4.76	0.3	4.54	0.22

SB=static balance; SLB=single leg balance; A/P=anterior/posterior; M/L=medial/lateral; LOS=limits of stability; F/R=Forward/Right; F/L=forward/left; B/R=backward/right; B/L=backward/left; VJH=vertical jump height; PV=peak velocity; PPO=peak power output; PF=peak force; RVD=rate of velocity development; STV=split time velocity; ST=split time; RT=reaction time. * Indicates a significant difference, where Division II Soccer Athletes had a greater PV, Max TV, Max STV 1, Max STV 2, and Max STV 4 than Recreationally Trained Soccer Players

variable between levels of competition in soccer (Bressel et al., 2007; Butler et al., 2012; Davlin, 2004) yet the current investigation concluded no significant differences between the two groups in all balance measures. A previous study also indicate balance performance and force production measures to simultaneously increase following resistance training programs (Manolopoulos et al., 2016). Our lack of differences found between levels may be due to a relatively new university strength and conditioning program prior to data collection for the Division II athletes, which may have resulted in a decrease in performance, specifically balance and force production.

Levels of play in soccer have also been distinguished through linear sprint performance (Cometti et al., 2001; Gissis et al., 2006; Kaplan et al., 2009; Reilly et al., 2010; Jason D. Vescovi, 2012); however, similar research utilizing change in direction protocols did not exist which may more closely simulate game situation demands. Our study's methodology included a pro-agility test resulting in collegiate level soccer athletes having significantly higher maximum and split-one velocities in comparison to the recreationally trained players. Although it may have been too early in the newly implemented strength and conditioning program to attribute resistance training to higher velocity measures in the Division II athletes, the measures may be accredited to a more extensive time period of soccer experience and pure exposure to a higher level of competition. Once again, the study's results may have been partially impacted by the lack of resistance training background in either of the two groups. With the addition of a longer time spent resistance training, it is very likely the Division II athletes will see a significant increase in all balance, sprint, and vertical jump performance measures compared to recreationally trained players who receive little to no specialized resistance training. If improvements are shown, this further validates the performance benefits and need of a quality resistance training program for soccer players (Grieco, Cortes, Greska, Lucci, & Onate, 2012; Negra, Chaabene, Hammami, Hachana, & Granacher, 2016; P. Wong, Chaouachi, Chamari, Dellal, & Wisloff, 2010).

Some limitations in the current investigation may be the differences between levels of the soccer players, for instance if the recreationally trained athletes were compared to Division I or professional level team, results may have been different. Additionally, testing the Division II athletes further along in their new strength and conditioning program would have been more representative of their overall performance. Although our study observed differences in velocity measures between Division II collegiate soccer athletes and recreationally trained participants, more research is needed evaluating performance measures in all levels of play. This would contribute to improving resources at hand for professionals working with soccer athletes, so they can properly make assessments of injury risks, normative values, and athlete performance across all divisions of competition. Future research would include investigating Division II soccer players following more routine resistance training and agility training when compare to recreationally trained players. Additionally, investigating a variety of sports comparing highly trained athletes and recreationally trained players.

CONCLUSION

In conclusion, it appears that there is a distinct difference between Division II and recreationally trained soccer athletes in vertical jump and sprint performance. However, training level seems to have no effect on balance performance in the

current investigation. These results may have been impacted by the lack of resistance training background in either of the two groups. With the addition of more time on a collegiate resistance training program, it is very likely the Division II athletes will see a significant increase in all balance, sprint, and vertical jump performance measures compared to recreationally trained players who receive little to no specialized resistance training.

REFERENCES

Agel, J., Evans, T. A., Dick, R., Putukian, M., & Marshall, S. W. (2007). Descriptive Epidemiology of Collegiate Men's Soccer Injuries: National Collegiate Athletic Association Injury Surveillance System, 1988–1989 Through 2002–2003. *Journal of Athletic Training*, 42(2), 270.

Bressel, E., Yonker, J. C., Kras, J., & Heath, E. M. (2007). Comparison of Static and Dynamic balance in female and collegiate soccer, basketball, and gymnastics. *Journal of Athletic Training*, 42, 42–46.

Butler, R. J., Southers, C., Gorman, P. P., Kiesel, K. B., & Plisky, P. J. (2012). Differences in Soccer Players' Dynamic Balance Across Levels of Competition. *Journal of Athletic Training*, 47(6), 616.

Cometti, G., Maffiuletti, N. A., Pousson, M., Chatard, J. C., & Maffulli, N. (2001). Isokinetic strength and anaerobic power of elite, subelite and amateur French soccer players. *International Journal of Sports Medicine*, 22(1), 45–51.

Cormie, P., McBride, J. M., & McCaulley, G. O. (2009). Power-time, force-time, and velocity-time curve analysis of the countermovement jump: impact of training. *Journal of Strength and Conditioning Research*, 23(1), 177–186.

Dabbs, N. C., Brown, L. E., & Garner, J. C. (2014). Effects of Whole Body Vibration on Vertical Jump Performance Following Exercise Induced Muscle Damage. *International Journal of Kinesiology and Sports Science*, 2(1), 24–30.

Davis, J. A., Brewer, J., & Atkin, D. (1992). Pre-season physiological characteristics of English first and second division soccer players. *Journal of Sports Sciences*, 10(6), 541–547.

Davlin, C. D. (2004). Dynamic Balance in High Level Athletes. *Perceptual and Motor Skills*, 98(3_suppl), 1171–1176.

Gissis, I., Papadopoulos, C., Kalapotharakos, V. I., Sotiropoulos, A., Komsis, G., & Manolopoulos, E. (2006). Strength and speed characteristics of elite, subelite, and recreational young soccer players. *Research in Sports Medicine*, 14(3), 205–214.

Grieco, C. R., Cortes, N., Greska, E. K., Lucci, S., & Onate, J. A. (2012). Effects of a Combined Resistance-Plyometric Training Program on Muscular Strength, Running Economy, and VO2 Peak in Division I Female Soccer Players. *Journal of Strength Conditioning Research*, 26(9), 2570–2576.

Haugen, T. A., Tønnessen, E., & Seiler, S. (2013). Anaerobic performance testing of professional soccer players

1995-2010. *International Journal of Sports Physiology and Performance, 8*(2), 148–156.

Jovanovic, M., Sporis, G., Omrcen, D., & Fiorentini, F. (2011). Effects of speed, agility, quickness training method on power performance in elite soccer players. *Journal of Strength and Conditioning Research, 25*(5), 1285–1292.

Kalapotharakos, V. I., Strimpakos, N., Vithoulka, I., Karvounidis, C., Diamantopoulos, K., & Kapreli, E. (2006). Physiological characteristics of elite professional soccer teams of different ranking. *The Journal of Sports Medicine and Physical Fitness, 46*(4), 515–519.

Kaplan, T., Erkmen, N., & Taskin, H. (2009). The evaluation of the running speed and agility performance in professional and amateur soccer players. *Journal of Strength and Conditioning Research, 23*(3), 774–778.

Manolopoulos, K., Gissis, I., Galazoulas, C., Manolopoulos, E., Patikas, D., Gollhofer, A., & Kotzamanidis, C. (2016). Effect of Combined Sensorimotor-Resistance Training on Strength, Balance, and Jumping Performance of Soccer Players. *Journal of Strength and Conditioning Research, 30*(1), 53–59.

Negra, Y., Chaabene, H., Hammami, M., Hachana, Y., & Granacher, U. (2016). Effects of High-Velocity Resistance Training on Athletic Performance in Prepuberal Male Soccer Athletes. *Journal of Strength and Conditioning Research, 30*(12), 3290–3297.

Oliver, G. D., & Di Brezzo, R. (2009). Functional balance training in collegiate women athletes. *Journal of Strength and Conditioning Research, 23*(7), 2124–9.

Parraca, J. A., Sánchez-Toledo, O., Rufino, P., Carbonell Baeza, A., García-Molina, A., A, V., Gusi Fuertes, N. (2011). Test-Retest reliability of Biodex Balance SD on physically active old people. *Journal of Human Sport and Exercise,* 6(2), 444-450.

Reilly, T., Williams, A. M., Nevill, A., & Franks, A. (2010). A multidisciplinary approach to talent identification in soccer. *Journal of Sports Sciences.* 18(9), 695-702.

Salaj, S., & Markovic, G. (2011). Specificity of Jumping, Sprinting, and Quick Change-of-Direction Motor Abilities. *Journal of Strength and Conditioning Research, 25*(5), 1249–1255.

Vescovi, J. D., Brown, T. D., & Murray, T. M. (2006). Positional Characteristics of physical performance in Division I college female soccer players. *Journal of Sports Medicine and Physical Fitness, 46*, 221–226.

Vescovi, J. D. (2012). Sprint speed characteristics of high-level American female soccer players: Female Athletes in Motion (FAiM) Study. *Journal of Science and Medicine in Sport, 15*(5), 474–478.

Wisløff, U., Castagna, C., Helgerud, J., Jones, R., & Hoff, J. (2004). Strong correlation of maximal squat strength with sprint performance and vertical jump height in elite soccer players. *British Journal of Sports Medicine, 38*(3), 285–288.

Wong, D. P., Chan, G. S., & Smith, A. W. (2012). Repeated-Sprint and Change-of-Direction Abilities in Physically Active Individuals and Soccer Players: Training and Testing Implications. *Journal of Strength and Conditioning Research, 26*(9), 2324–2330.

Wong, P., Chaouachi, A., Chamari, K., Dellal, A., & Wisloff, U. (2010). Effect of Preseason Concurrent Muscular Strength and High-Intensity Interval Training in Professional Soccer Players. *Journal of Strength and Conditioning Research, 24*(3), 653–660.

6

Leveling the Playing Field: Assessment of Gross Motor Skills in Low Socioeconomic Children to their Higher Socioeconomic Counterparts

Megan M. Adkins[1]*, Matthew R. Bice[1], Danae Dinkel[2], John P. Rech[1]
[1]Kinesiology and Sport Science, University of Nebraska- Kearney, 2504 9th Ave, Kearney, NE 68849, United States
[2]Health and Physical Education, University of Nebraska- Omaha 6001 Dodge Street, Omaha, NE 68182, United States
Corresponding Author: Megan M. Adkins, E-mail: adkinsmm@unk.edu

ARTICLE INFO

Conflicts of interest: None
Funding: None

ABSTRACT

Background: Fundamental movements (FM) of children influence the willingness to engage in physical activity (PA). Thus, proper FM skills are the foundation for a lifespan of PA. **Objective:** This study examined what factors may affect children's PA in relation to FM pattern capabilities. **Methods:** The study examined the influence of SES when three low-income schools were provided additional PA opportunities on days PE was not taught. FM patterns in relation to object control (OC) and locomotor skill (LC) development were evaluated on K (n = 871), 1st (n = 893), and 2nd graders (n = 829) using the Test of Gross Motor Development-2 (TGMD-2) instrument (Ulrich, 2000). Schools were dichotomized and categorized as being low SES (n = 2008) and high SES (n = 578) status. **Results:** A significant relationship was revealed with LC (r = 0.264; p = 0.001), OC (r = 0.171; p = 0.001), and total TGMD-2 (r = 0.264; p = 0.001). Low and high SES schools significantly improved overall TGMD-2 scores. High SES schools children were significantly higher in LC [F, (2, 1272) = 29.31, p = 0.001], OC [F, (2, 1272) = 23.14, p = 0.001], and total TGMD-2 [F, (1, 1272) = 38.11, p = 0.001]. **Conclusion:** Low SES schools need to concentrate on PA-based activities to engage students in FM patterns, to help narrow the gap in FM capabilities. In addition, the increase in PA opportunities for lower SES schools could positively impact brain function, cardiovascular fitness, and overall well-being.

Key words: Physical Education, TGMD, Fundamental Motor Skills, Low Socioeconomic Students

INTRODUCTION

According to the Centers for Disease Control (2010, 2013), children who meet the recommendation of 60 minutes of physical activity everyday have a lower chance of developing chronic diseases later in life and achieve greater levels of cardiorespiratory fitness and bone strength. Additionally, children who are physically active tend to have increased self-esteem, reduced levels of anxiety and depression, and show improved brain function, academic scores, and have better attendance rates in school (Tremblay, Inman, & Williams, 2000; United States Department of Health and Human Services, 2016; Centers for Disease Control and Prevention, 2010; Strauss, Rodzilsky, Burack, & Colin, 2001). Although the correlation between physical activity, health, and learning performances is widely supported in research, the lack of children meeting the physical activity recommendation of 60 minutes of daily moderate-to-vigorous physical activity is a global concern (Troiano et al., 2008; Guthord, Cowan, Autenrieth, Kann, & Riley, 2010). Specifically within the United States, a report by the National Physical Activity Plan Alliance (NPAPA; 2016) found only one-fourth of children are currently meeting physical activity recommendations.

Due to this lack of physical activity, 75% of children are at an increased risk for future obesity, diabetes, and related chronic illness (NPAPA, 2016).

From birth, children develop movement skills through moving, balancing, stabilizing, and controlling their bodies. These elements of movement are crucial for the developmental progression of a child to successfully perform more complex physical tasks such as combined moves utilized in sports (shooting a lay-up in basketball) later in adolescents (Catenassi et al., 2007). Children with developed motor skills have a greater willingness and desire to engage in physical activity in comparison to children with poorer motor skill development (Wrotniak, Epstein, Dorn, Jones, & Kondilis, 2006). Thus, proper fundamental movement skills are the foundation for a lifespan of physical activity. Having well-developed movement skills may greatly influence a person's level of desire and confidence to partake in physical activity later on in life (Gallahue & Ozmun, 1998).

Decades of research have demonstrated numerous factors that can influence children's physical activity opportunities and relatedly fundamental movement skills. Some of these barriers emerge from issues such as safety of the neighborhood, parental perspective of the need for physical activity, and lack of transportation for children to and from physical activity opportunities (Centers for Disease Control and Prevention, 2003; Kerr et al., 2006; National Safe Routes Task Force, 2008). While disparities have been revealed in physical activity levels of children, little research has examined this potential in motor skills. Schools and Physical education classes are often seen as the time to develop motor skills but it is not known if increased time in school would help improve acquisition of motor skills (Centers for Disease Control and Prevention, 2010; Janz, Dawson, & Mahoney, 2000; National Center for Chronic Disease Prevention and Health Promotion, Division of Adolescent and School Health, 2010). Researchers hypothesize additional time to practice during the school day will improve motor skill development of children.

The number of opportunities for children to participate in physical activity opportunities outside of school is growing daily, with new club and recreational teams being formed all over the United States. Both free play and vigorous physical activity participation rates are lower in children of low SES families (Hansen & Chen, 2007; Inchley, 2005). However, research indicates before and after school time frames are when children are being less physically active (Smith, Hannon, Brusseau, Fu, Burns, 2016). Parents may arguably be the biggest influence on a child's involvement in behaviors due to their control over what activities their children partake in and what resources (i.e., money) are available that allow for participation to occur (Welk, Wood, & Morss, 2003). Children from low-income families have significant key barriers such as the cost of the recreation program, and lack of support from home due to transportation issues, which may hinder them from being a part of recreational activities outside of school (Canadian Fitness and Lifestyle Research Institute, 2015).

Students are in school seven to eight hours a day, thus the school environment can be another influential factor in physical activity levels of children. The majority of this time is in a sedentary environment in the regular classroom. Within schools, there are numerous barriers to physical activity promotion and implementation, but they do differ by school level, experience of the specialist teachers, and can be teacher or student-related (Jenkinson & Benson, 2010). Physical activity can also be influenced by the overall school facility provisions (e.g., amount of facilities available) and equipment (e.g., loose equipment, balls) used during recess (Ridgers, Salmon, Parrish, Stanley, & Okely, 2012).

Physical education is looked upon as a class that can enhance a child's fundamental movement skill development and knowledge of sports and activities as well as be a major contributor to the accumulation of physical activity (Society of Health and Physical Educators of America (SHAPE, 2014). Changes have occurred in the last 25 years making many schools reduce or eliminate recess and Physical education (SHAPE of the Nation, 2016). However, students who attend higher SES schools continue to receive a better quality Physical education experience and spend more time participating in Physical Education (Sallis, Zakarian, Hovell, & Hofstetter, 1996). This is concerning as involvement in complex activities during Physical Education courses aid in the development and improvement of fundamental movement skills (SHAPE of the Nation, 2010). Further, regardless of SES, children who participate in Physical education have better coordination and biomechanics allowing them to perform complex activities required in physical activities (Ketelhut, Bittmann, & Ketelhut, 2003). According to Fairclough and Stratton (2005), children with higher developed movement patterns engaged in more physical activity during Physical education lessons.

One evaluation piece used in Physical education to determine fundamental movement proficiency levels is the Test of Gross Motor Development, second version (TGMD-2). This test scores a child in grades Kindergarten-2nd grade (K-2) on their ability to perform fundamental movement skills, such as running, jumping, throwing, skipping, and catching, that require the use of large muscle groups (Gallahue & Ozmun, 1998; Wrotniak et al., 2006). Since the development of these skills are positively associated with physical activity, and inversely associated with sedentary behaviors and obesity it is critical to evaluate children's movement skills at an early age to ensure lifelong physical activity habits (Khalaj & Amri, 2013; Wrotniak et al., 2006). Unfortunately, low SES children may be at a disadvantage due to decreased opportunities for physical activity outside of school and receiving less Physical education time during school. Given the disparity between what has been established in the literature about the significant role of physical activity for children, the declining number of children meeting the recommended physical activity levels, and the need for developed fundamental movement skills; this study aims to examine what factors may affect children's physical activity in relation to fundamental movement pattern capabilities. Specifically, the current manuscript attempts to answer the following questions.

Does socioeconomic status (SES) level influence fundamental movement patterns of children?

Does additional fundamental movement skill practice time during the school day improve overall fundamental movement abilities for low socio-economic children in grades K-2?

METHOD

Participant

In 2011, public schools within one school district in central Nebraska were notified of the opportunity for their students in grades K-2 to be tested on fundamental movement patterns using the TGMD-2 assessment. Three low socio - economic Title I schools, defined as having a school population with a poverty level (determined by free and reduced meal counts) 40% or above free and reduced lunch, which is an indicator of poverty level, selected to participate (United States Department of Education, 2013). Two high socio - economic schools, defined as having a school population with a poverty level (determined by free and reduced meal counts) between 0% - 14.9% also agreed to participate

(United States Department of Education, 2013). All schools within the district had comparable gymnasium spaces and Physical Education teachers who had been in the field for more than five years. Socio-economic status is the measure of influence that the social environment has on individuals, families, communities, and schools. The definitions of SES emphasize that, as a construct, (a) it is conditional, (b) it is imposed on people, (c) it is used for comparisons, and (d) it is based on economics, opportunity, and means of influence. The SES levels per school were defined by the Nebraska Department of Education in the Handbook for Continuous Improvement in Nebraska Schools (2012). Title I schools are defined as having student enrollment of at least 40 percent of children from low- income families. Title 1 is designed to help students served by the program to achieve proficiency on challenging state academic achievement standards. Schools receive funds from the Federal government to operate "school wide programs" to upgrade the instructional program for the entire school (United States Department of Education, 2017).

Instrument

Trained research assistants conducted the TGMD-2 assessments at all of the participating schools located in central Nebraska during Physical education class in the Fall (2011), and Spring (2012). Training of the assistants included a professional development taught by professors from a local University to learn about the various assessment pieces and then practice assessments on children from the local preschool. During 2012-2014 school years the low SES schools (n = 3) were the only schools that elected to continue with TGMD-2 testing of their students. Prior to beginning testing at the school sites the local University conducting the research received IRB approval. For consistency and accuracy, the TGMD-2 protocol manual, which provides specific instructions to conduct each of the TGMD-2 assessment components, was used by the research assistants to standardize procedures and for quality assurance.

The TGMD-2 has been shown and established as a valid and reliable measure to assess fundamental movement patterns of children (Ulrich, 2000). The TGMD-2 includes six locomotor (run, gallop, hop, leap, horizontal jump, slide) and six object-control (striking a stationary ball, stationary dribble, kick, catch, overhand throw, underhand roll) skills. Participants performed each skill three times. Each skill includes several movement components. If the participant performed all movement components correctly they received a score of 1; if they performed any component incorrectly they received a score of 0. This procedure was completed for each of the trials, and scores were summed to obtain a total raw skill score. Raw skill scores were then added to obtain a raw locomotor subtest score and a raw object-control subtest score. Inter-rater reliability (89% agreement rate) was established by all at the same time by assessors practicing the assessments with children at a local pre-school before movement skills were assessed at the elementary schools.

Intervention

After the fall (2011) TGMD-2 data collection, all three low SES schools, received the traditional Physical education class two times a week, similar to the other schools but on days the children did not have Physical education, each K-2 class received a twenty minute structured physical activity time, taught by a senior level Physical Education major student from the local University. During the physical activity time the K-2 students played low organized games, which require minimal explanation, that emphasized the fundamental movement patterns found in the TGMD-2 test manual. The physical activity instructors were provided access to the research based physical activity curriculum SPARKÒ, for ideas for class physical activities. SPARK® has been identified as a national model for programs designed to increase physical activity and includes a variety of activities designed to improve student physical activity and movement skills (Partnership & Prevention, 2008). For example, the game "junk yard" is a game where students work on overhand or underhand throwing patterns and throw the "junk" to the other side of the gym to "clean" up their half side of the basketball court that is cluttered by bean bags that are thrown by the opposing team on the opposite side of the basketball court. The University Physical education major followed an outline of the class time provided by the lead researcher for the physical activity time at the three schools. The outline included the following for the 20 minute time frame: (a) three minute warm-up incorporating the fundamental movement patterns, (b) two and a half minute introduction to the activity and reminder of proper skill execution, (c) thirteen minutes of playing the physical activity of the day (focusing on at least two fundamental movements), and (d) one and a half minute closure. The three low SES elementary schools continued the physical activity portion for K-2 along with regularly scheduled Physical education in their school day for three years (2011-2014). The TGMD-2 data were assessed every Fall and Spring during those years (2011-2014). The high SES schools, whom did not receive the additional physical activity time elected to only have the TGMD-2 testing completed in the Fall, 2011 and Spring, 2012 school year. This was due to lack of interest from Physical Educators and the concern of the amount of time needed to complete the TGMD-2 test during Physical education class without receiving the benefit of the additional physical activity class like the low SES schools received.

Statistical Analysis

Descriptive statistics were analyzed per student frequencies in each grade (Kindergarten, 1st, and 2nd grade). Pearson product correlations were used to analyze associations between school SES and TGMD-2 (Locomotor, Object Control, and total TGMD). A univariate analyses were used to examine TGMD change and direction between the Fall and Spring among each of the different schools and adjoining years. Low SES schools A, B, and C was analyzed for Year 1, 2, and 3. No data exists for Schools D and E for 2012-2014;

therefore, only Year 1 could be analyzed. Further, multivariate analyses assessed rating of TGMD between low and high SES schools. Data were deemed significance at 0.05.

RESULTS

School Demographics

A total of 2,586 scores of elementary aged students were used in data analysis. Schools were dichotomized and categorized as being low SES (n = 2008) and high SES (n = 578) status. Further the sample includes a range of students that included kindergarten (n = 871), 1st grade (n = 893), and 2nd grade (n = 829) (See Table 1).

Movement Skills and SES Level

Table 2 describes the relationship between TGMD and SES. TGMD data were only available during Year 1 for high SES schools. A significant relationship was revealed with the construct locomotor (r = 0.264; p = 0.001), object control (r = 0.171; p = 0.001), and total TGMD (r = 0.264; p = 0.001). The positive relationship suggests students with high SES yield higher ratings of TGMD.

A multivariate analysis revealed that during Year 1, students that attended high SES schools had significantly higher ratings of locomotor skills [F, (2, 1272) = 29.31, p = 0.001], object control [F, (2, 1272) = 23.14, p = 0.001], thus yielding significantly higher total TGMD [F, (1, 1272) = 38.11, p = 0.001] (See Table 3).

Impact of Additional Movement Skill Practice

ANOVA was performed to analyze change in ratings of locomotor, object control, and overall TGMD. Table 4 provides the mean scores for the TGMD-2 in relation to locomotor, object control, and overall score for each school. The low SES schools completed the TGMD-2 analysis after the first year of data collection to determine if TGMD-2 scores improved with additional physical activity opportunities to practice the fundamental movement skills. Analysis revealed that both low and high SES schools significantly improved overall TGMD (See Table 4).

DISCUSSION

The primary purpose of this study was to assess the motor proficiency (TGMD-2) of children in grades K-2 attending low and high SES schools. The secondary purpose of the study was to subsequently compare changes in motor proficiency of children at low SES schools when 20 minutes of physical activity were added on days Physical Education was not offered at the schools. To our knowledge this is the first study to assess the motor proficiency changes of K-2 grade children when provided a structured physical activity time on days Physical Education was not offered. Overall, findings demonstrated that in year 1, (2011-2012) children at the higher SES schools scored higher than all low SES schools when completing the TGMD-2 both in the Fall and in the Spring. This would be expected due to research indicating higher quality of Physical education and more involvement in external physical activity opportunities outside of the school day (Center for Disease Control and Prevention, 2017). These findings coincide with previous research findings worldwide that typically have found that higher SES children score better on assessments related to fundamental or gross motor skills because of a combination of additional practice time, resources, and outside opportunities that students of high SES school children have compared to low SES schools (Hardy, King, Espinel, Okely, & Bauman, 2010).

Interestingly, low SES schools consistently increased fundamental movement pattern scores between the fall and spring during year 1, 2, and 3 (2011-2014). However, students who attended high SES schools were still at a significant higher proficiency rate in regards to fundamental movement patterns when tested with the TGMD-2. These results provide evidence that physical activity programs emphasizing fundamental movement patterns, along with Physical education, should be implemented, but additional opportunities are still needed outside of school to improve fundamental movement pattern levels for children at low SES schools to meet the level of movement patterns of chil-

Table 1. School demographics

	High SES			Low SES		Total amount
	A	B	C	D	E	A-E
Kindergartens	674	680	661	248	323	2586
1st graders	248	245	220	93	65	871
2nd graders	209	233	214	83	154	893
Total amount=n	217	202	227	72	111	829

Table 2. Correlations between TGMD and SES

TGMD-2 sub categories	SES		
	n	r	p
Locomotor	2586	0.264	0.001
Object control	2586	0.171	0.001
Total TGMD	2586	0.264	0.001

*Denotes significance at P < .01

Table 3. Analysis of variance of TGMD-2: motor skills among low and high SES schools during Year 1

TGMD-2 sub categories	Low SES			High SES			F	p
	n	M	SD	n	M	SD		
Locomotor	703	3.56	1.71	571	4.08	1.73	29.313	0.000
Object control	703	2.39	1.29	571	2.76	1.38	23.14	0.000
Overall	703	5.96	6.84	571	6.35	2.58	38.11	0.000

Table 4. Analysis of change between fall and spring among Year 1, 2 and 3

			Low SES		Year 2		Year 3	
			M	p	M	p	M	p
Low SES								
School A	Locomotor	Fall	2.844	0.001	0.811	0.000	2.000	0.000
		Spring	3.394		2.396		3.916	
	Object control	Fall	2.293	0.419	1.273	0.000	1.546	0.000
		Spring	2.156		2.207		2.444	
	Overall	Fall	5.137	0.11	2.084	0.000	3.546	0.000
		Spring	5.55		4.603		6.361	
School B	Locomotor	Fall	2.720	0.000	1.250	0.000	1.972	0.000
		Spring	5.300		4.310		4.065	
	Object control	Fall	2.090	0.000	1.857	0.009	1.906	0.000
		Spring	3.000		2.367		2.607	
	Overall	Fall	4.820	0.000	3.112	0.000	3.875	0.000
		Spring	8.300		6.680		6.672	
School C	Locomotor	Fall	2.778	0.000	0.960	0.000	1.477	0.000
		Spring	4.053		3.465		3.697	
	Object control	Fall	2.256	0.160	1.376	0.000	1.688	0.000
		Spring	2.490		2.613		2.513	
	Overall	Fall	5.035	0.000	2.336	0.000	3.165	0.000
		Spring	6.548		6.079		6.211	
High SES								
School D	Locomotor	Fall	4.795	0.010				
		Spring	5.278					
	Object control	Fall	2.549	0.000				
		Spring	3.440					
	Overall	Fall	7.344	0.000				
		Spring	8.721					
School E	Locomotor	Fall	2.730	0.000				
		Spring	4.000					
	Object control	Fall	2.323	0.002				
		Spring	2.810					
	Overall	Fall	5.055	0.000				
		Spring	6.816					

dren from higher SES schools. While the direct relationship between the proficiency of fundamental movement patterns and level of participation in physical activity remains inconclusive, the need for future research to determine perceived relationships of physical activity in children's ability to access a range of movement experiences still needs to be explored (Jaakkola & Washington, 2013; Lai et al., 2014). Low SES schools could provide additional opportunities to their students to improve fundamental movement patterns by incorporating classroom activity breaks, before or after school physical activity programs, or creating cross-curricular activities during the school day. For instance, in science class,

students could learn about biomechanics and practice the various fundamental movement patterns. Physical Educators could be utilized to educate classroom teachers in physical activities they could incorporate into their current teaching curriculum.

The current study has a number of strengths including the number of years of testing at the low SES schools, the relatively large sample size, the standard additional amount of time of 20 minutes provided to all low SES schools, and the use of a qualitative, valid assessment of fundamental movements. Limitations of the study should be noted. The assessment of the fundamental movement patterns were only assessed in the high SES status schools during year one 2011. Although the same core curriculum, SPARKÒ was taught by all Physical education and University majors teaching physical activity class physical activity teachers in the district assessed, activities and development of specific components of the curriculum were not regulated. In addition, the University Physical education majors teaching the classes at the low SES schools had free reign over activities the teacher incorporated as long as the activity incorporated at least two fundamental movements. The fundamental movement patterns selected may not have been the areas in which the students needed to focus to improve their TGMD-2 score. Due to the design of this study a cause-and-effect relationship between physical activity and fundamental movement patterns cannot be concluded but only inferred.

CONCLUSION

The current findings suggest that schools, especially lower SES schools, need to concentrate on additional opportunities for physical activity-based activities to engage students in fundamental movement patterns throughout the school day. This could be accomplished through short classroom activity breaks conducted by classroom teachers, by adding a before or after school physical activity program, and/or if available, a program similar to the one outlined in this article where a physical activity class was added in the school day. By adding additional physical activity time, not only could the fundamental movement patterns improve, but brain function and cardiovascular fitness would potentially improve as well. Resources, personnel knowledgeable, and school administration may play into the success of the incorporation of the physical activity time. Overall, by providing physical activity and motor development opportunities for children, whether it is housed during school hours or after school, can be beneficial to helping improve all motor functioning and development of all children, regardless of SES.

REFERENCES

Canadian Fitness and Lifestyle Research Institute, Participation. (2015). *The influence of socio-demographic factors on children's physical activity and sport.* [Online] Available http://www.cflri.ca/sites/default/files/node/1397/files/RF_EN_March_2015_final.pdf.

Catenassi, F. Z., Marques, I., Bastos, C. B., Basso, L., Ronque, E. R. V., & Gerage, A. M. (2007). Relationship between body mass index and gross motor skill in four to six year-old children. *Revista Brasileira de Medicina do Esporte*, 13, 227-230. doi:10.1590/S1517-86922007000400003

Center for Disease Control and Prevention. (2017). *Components of the whole school, whole community, whole child (WSCC).* [Online] Available https://www.cdc.gov/healthyschools/wscc/components.htm.

Centers for Disease Control and Prevention. (2010). Childhood obesity and overweight. [Online] Available http://www.cdc.gov/obesity/childhood/

Centers for Disease Control and Prevention. (2013). Youth Risk Behavior Surveillance—United States, 2013. MMWR 2014;63 (SS-4).

Centers for Disease Control and Prevention. (2010). *The Association Between School-Based Physical Activity, Including Physical Education, and Academic Performance.* Atlanta, GA: U.S. Department of Health and Human Services, 2010.

Centers for Disease Control and Prevention (2008). *Make a difference at your school.* [Online] Available http://www.cdc.gov/HealthyYouth/KeyStrategies/pdf/make-a-difference.pdf.

Centers for Disease Control and Prevention. (2003). Physical activity levels among children aged 9-13 years—United States, 2002. *Morbidity and Mortality Weekly Report*, 52, 785-788.

Fairclough, S., & Stratton, G. (2005). Physical activity levels in middle and high school physical education: A review. *Pediatric Exercise Science*, 17(3), 217-236. doi:10.1123/pes.17.3.217

Gallahue, D. L., & Ozmun, J. C. (1998). *Understanding motor development: Infants, children, adolescents, adults.* New York, NY: McGraw-Hill Humanities, Social Sciences & World Languages.

Guthold, R., Cowan, M. J., Autenrieth, C. S., Kann, L., & Riley, L. M. (2010). Physical activity and sedentary behavior among school children: A 34-country comparison. *The Journal of Pediatrics*, 157, 43-49. doi:10.1016/j.jpeds.2010.01.019

Hanson, M. D., & Chen, E. (2007). Socioeconomic status and health behaviors in adolescence: A review of the literature. *Journal of Behavioral Medicine*, 30, 263-285. doi:10.1007/s10865-007-9098-3

Hardy, L., King, L., Espinel, P., Okely, A., & Bauman, A. (2011). Methods of the NSW schools physical activity and nutrition survey 2010 (SPANS 2010). *Journal of Science and Medicine in Sport*, 14, 390-396. doi:10.1016/j.jsams.2011.03.003

Inchley, J. C. (2005). Persistent socio-demographic differences in physical activity among Scottish schoolchildren 1990-2002. *The European Journal of Public Health*, 15, 386-388. doi:10.1093/eurpub/cki084

Jaakkola, T., & Washington, T. (2013). The relationship between fundamental movement skills and self-reported physical activities during Finnish junior high school. *Physical Education and Sport Pedagogy*, 18(5), 492-505.

Janz, K. F., Dawson, J. D., & Mahoney, L. T. (2000). Tracking physical fitness and physical activity from childhood to adolescence: The muscatine study. *Medicine & Science in Sports & Exercise*, 32, 1250-1257.

Jenkinson, K. A., & Benson A. C. (201). Barriers to providing physical education and physical education and physical activity in victorian state secondary schools. *Australian Journal of Teacher Education*, 35, 1-17.

Katzmarzyk, P. T., Denstel, K. D., Beals, K., Bolling, C., Wright, C., Crouter, S. E., & Sisson, S. B. (2016). Results from the United States of America's 2016 report card on physical activity for children and youth. *Jour-

nal of Physical Activity and Health, 13, S307-S313. doi:10.1123/jpah.2016-0321

Ketelhut, K., Bittmann, F., & Ketelhut, R. G. (2003). Relationship between motor skills and social status in early childhood. *Medicine & Science in Sports & Exercise*, 35, 179. doi:10.1097/00005768-200305001-00993

Kerr, J., Rosenberg, D., Sallis, J. F., Saelens, B. E., Frank, L. D., & Conway, T. L. (2006). Active commuting to school: Associations with environment and parental concerns. *Medicine & Science in Sports & Exercise*, 38, 787-794. doi:10.1249/01.mss.0000210208.63565.73

Khalaj, N., & Amri, S. (2013). Mastery of gross motor skills in preschool and early elementary school obese children. *Early Child Development and Care*, 184, 795-802. doi:10.1080/03004430.2013.820724

Lai, S. K., Costigan, S. A., Morgan, P. J., Lubans, D. R., Stodden, D. F., Salmon, J., & Barnett, L. M. (2013). Do school-based interventions focusing on physical activity, fitness, or fundamental movement skill competency produce a sustained impact in these outcomes in children and adolescents? A systematic review of follow-up studies. *Sports Medicine*, 44, 67-79. doi:10.1007/s40279-013-0099-9

Morley, D., Till, K., Ogilvie, P., & Turner, G. (2015). Influences of gender and socioeconomic status on the motor proficiency of children in the UK. *Human Movement Science*, 44, 150-156. doi:10.1016/j.humov.2015.08.022

National Physical Activity Plan Alliance. (2016). *2016 United States report card on physical activity for children and youth.* [Online] Available http://www.physicalactivityplan.org/projects/reportcard.html.

National Safe Routes Task Force. (2008). *Safe routes to school: A transportation legacy. A national strategy to increase safety and physical activity among American youth.* [Online] Available http://www.saferoutesinfo.org/sites/default/files/task_force_report.web_.pdf

Nebraska Department of Education (2012). *A handbook for continuous improvement in Nebraska schools: Equity and diversity focus.* [Online] Available https://www.education.ne.gov/.

Partnership for Prevention. (2008). *School-based physical education: Working with schools to increase physical activity among children and adolescents in physical education classes—an action guide.* The community health promotion handbook: Action guides to improve community health. Washington, DC: Partnership for Prevention.

Ridgers, N. D., Salmon, J., Parrish, A., Stanley, R. M. & Okely, A. D. (2012). Physical activity during school recess: A systematic review. *American Journal of Preventive Medicine*, 43, 320-328. doi:10.1016/j.amepre.2012.05.019.

Sallis, J. F., Zakarian, J. M., Hovell, M. F., & Hofstetter, C. (1996). Ethnic, socioeconomic, and sex differences in physical activity among adolescents. *Journal of Clinical Epidemiology*, 49, 125-134. doi:10.1016/0895-4356(95)00514-5

Smith, C., Hannon, J., Brusseau, T., Fu, Y., Burns, R. (2016). Physical Activity Behavior Patterns during School Leisure Time in Children. *International Journal of Kinesiology and Sport Science,* 4(1), 17-25.

Society of Health and Physical Educators of America. (2014). National standards & grade- level outcomes for K-12 physical education. *Human Kinetics.* Champaign, IL.

Society of Health and Physical Educators of America. (2010,16). *Shape of the nation report: Status of physical education in the USA.* [Online] Available https://www.shapeamerica.org/shapeofthenation

7

Acute Exercise-Associated Skin Surface Temperature Changes after Resistance Training with Different Exercise Intensities

Martin Weigert*, Nico Nitzsche, Felix Kunert, Christiane Lösch, Lutz Baumgärtel, Henry Schulz
Institute of Human Movement Science and Health, Chemnitz University of Technology, Thüringer Weg 11, 09126 Chemnitz, Germany
Corresponding Author: Martin Weigert, E-mail: martin.weigert@hsw.tu-chemnitz.de

ARTICLE INFO

Conflicts of interest: None
Funding: European Social Fund

ABSTRACT

Background: Studies showed, that changes in muscular metabolic-associated heat production and blood circulation during and after muscular work affect skin temperature (T) but the results are inconsistent and the effect of exercise intensity is unclear. **Objective:** This study investigated the intensity-dependent reaction of T on resistance training. **Methods:** Ten male students participated. After acclimatization (15 min), the participants completed 3x10 repetitions of unilateral biceps curl with 30, 50 or 70% of their one-repetition-maximum (1RM) in a randomized order. Skin temperature of the loaded and unloaded biceps was measured at rest (T_{rest}), immediately following set 1, 2 and 3 (T_{S1}, T_{S2}, T_{S3}) and 30 minutes post exercise ($T_1 - T_{30}$) with an infrared camera. **Results:** Two-way ANOVA detected a significant effect of the measuring time point on T (T_{rest} to T_{30}) of the loaded arm for 30% (Eta²=0.85), 50% (Eta²=0.88) and 70% 1RM (Eta²=0.85) and of the unloaded arm only for 30% 1RM (Eta²=0.41) (p<0.05) but time effects were independent of the exercise intensity (p>0.05). The T values at the different measuring time points ($T_{rest} - T_{30}$) did not differ between the intensities at any time point. The loaded arm showed a mean maximum T rise to T_{rest} of 1.8°C and on average, maximum T was reached approximately 5 minutes after the third set. **Conclusion:** This study indicate a rise of T, which could be independent of the exercise intensity. Infrared thermography seems to be applicable to identify the primary used functional muscles in resistance training but this method seems not suitable to differentiate between exercise intensity from 30 to 70% 1RM.

Key words: Thermography, Skin Temperature, Thermoregulation, Resistance Training, Muscle, Skeletal

INTRODUCTION

Infrared thermography (IRT) is a safe, quick and effective non-contact method to examine the distribution of temperature at the skin surface (T) by measuring the infrared radiation of a person (Costello et al., 2013). Hyperthermic areas may be caused by increased blood flow, inflammation, growing tumor or other tissue lesions.

In medicine, IRT is used as a breast cancer screening method and for the diagnosis of inflammations (e.g. arthritis), vascular diseases (e.g. Raynaud's phenomenon, diabetes, deep vein thrombosis) and dermatological disorders, (Jiang et al., 2005; Lahiri et al., 2012; Ring & Ammer, 2012; Wang et al., 2004). Compared to the aforementioned applications, IRT has been rarely used in sports medicine, but it can be important for an early identification and localization of inflammations, traumatic injuries and overuse injuries (Das, Vardasca, & Mendes, 2017; Hildebrandt, Raschner, & Ammer, 2010; Sillero-Quintana, Gomez-Carmona, & Fernández-Cuevas, 2017).

Apart from the applications in medicine, IRT may play an important role as a noninvasive diagnosis method in sports science. With IRT, it is possible to determine changes in T as a result of heat generation, induced by muscle contraction during physical activity due to temperature changes of body surfaces, concerning to active muscles (Chudecka, 2013). Within this context, IRT can be used to evaluate the symmetry of muscle activity in various types of exercises (Chudecka et al., 2015). For instance, it is important, that the muscles of scullers are equally involved in the performed movement to reach maximum velocity (Chudecka et al., 2015). Furthermore, studies tried to evaluate IRT as a tool for monitoring thermoregulation during and after endurance exercises (Balci, Basaran, & Colakoglu, 2016; Fröhlich et al., 2015; Merla et al., 2010; Priego Quesada et al., 2015; Priego Quesada et al., 2016).

Another possible application area is the use of IRT for analyzing changes in T during and after resistance exercise. Here, IRT could offer indirect hemodynamic recruitment information of muscle masses during exercise-related thermal adjustment. Temperature changes that occurred in working muscle areas are transferred to superficial tissue and can be measured as skin surface temperatures via IRT. Several studies have already dealt with changes in T after resistance exercise but the results have been inconsistent. Fröhlich et al. (2014) studied the T changes of different muscle groups after different resistance exercises. They found a decrease in T after sit ups, back extensions and lat pulls in the corresponding skin areas and almost unchanged T following bench press and squats. Neves et al., (2016) showed a strong acute and 15 minutes lasting decrease of T after biceps curls and half squat exercises whereas Formenti et al. (2016) and Neves et al. (2014) showed an acute T drop after resistance exercise followed by a rise of T over basal values. Further studies showed increased T values after biceps curl (Bartuzi, Roman-Liu, & Wisniewski, 2012; Neves et al., 2015; Neves et al., 2016) and standing calf raise (Formenti et al., 2013).

Most of the studies to date investigating thermographic images during and after resistance training observed, that it is possible to identify the primary used muscles via IRT (Formenti et al., 2013; Formenti et al., 2016; Fröhlich et al., 2014; Neves et al., 2014; Neves et al., 2015; Neves et al., 2016). So far it is not clear how intense a load must be to cause changes in T and if different intensities lead to different T patterns during and after resistance exercise. For instance in reaction to very intense resistance training, a particularly increase or an acute drop in T occurs due to a vasoconstriction of the cutaneous blood vessels (Formenti et al., 2016; Fröhlich et al., 2014; Neves et al., 2014) is possible.

For this reason, the present study investigated the intensity-dependent reaction of T on the resistance exercise unilateral biceps curl in a strongly standardized protocol. We hypothesize a T rise of the loaded arm during and following the resistance exercise, which is augmented with increasing intensity. Furthermore, we expect no changes of T of the unloaded arm.

MATERIALS AND METHODS

Participants

10 healthy male students (age 24.5±2.0 years; height 1.84±0.07 m; body weight 82.8±7.1 kg; BMI 24.3±1.6 kg/m²) participated in the study (Table 1). Participation was voluntary and did not involve any financial compensation. Informed consent was obtained from all students involved in the study. As exclusion criteria, the following aspects were considered for every test day: infections, consumption of alcohol, caffeine or nicotine, exercise, body lotion, therapeutic treatment or massage of the upper limb region, and a meal eaten within the last two hours before the test. The study was

approved by the Ethics Committee of the Chemnitz University of Technology.

Study Procedure

During the first visit, participants were informed about the procedure and the potential risks of the study and provided their written consent. Anthropometric data was collected, body weight, body mass index (BMI), and proportion of body fat calculated with the body composition analyzer InBody 720 (InBody Co., Ltd., Seoul, South Korea). Biceps skinfold thickness (BST) was measured in the middle of the muscle belly of the biceps brachii (area of the largest arm circumference) with a skinfold caliper.

Before the 1RM test, based on the procedure by (Baechle & Earle, 2008), the participants performed a short individual warm up for the upper limbs and were familiarised with the 1RM exercise biceps curl by performing a warm-up set of 10 repetitions at approximately 50% 1RM and 5 repetitions at approximately 75% 1RM. After the warm up, the participants performed a series of single repetitions to determine the dynamic concentric 1RM of the dominant right arm for the resistance exercise biceps curl with the cable pulley with two movable pulleys on a scott bench (1RM defined as the maximum amount of weight lifted with proper form through a 90° range of motion for a single repetition).

During the second, third and fourth visits, the participants came to laboratory and sat for 15 minutes with naked upper body in a relaxed position for acclimatization. The room temperature during testing was 22.1±0.5°C and humidity 35-40%. During acclimatization, the muscle belly of the right and left biceps brachii was marked with cork discs (Figure 1a), which possesses a low thermal conductivity (λ=0.036 W·m^{-1}·K^{-1}) and is visible in thermal imaging.

The training protocol consisted of three sets with 10 repetitions biceps curl to a flexion angle of 90° with the right arm (Figure 1b). Rest between the sets was two minutes. After acclimatization, the participants completed one protocol per visit on nonconsecutive days with 30, 50 or 70% of the 1RM in randomized order. For randomization, the participants drew a number to determine the exercise intensity on each measurement day. The frequency of movement was controlled by a metronome and standardized as 1.5s for concentric and 1.5s for eccentric movement phase. If the participants could not finish a set, they got minimum support by the supervisor, so that all 10 repetitions were performed in the prescribed velocity.

Table 1. Participant characteristics (N=10), data presented as mean, standard deviation, minimum, maximum (BMI=body mass index, BST=biceps skinfold thickness, 1RM=one-repetition-maximum of biceps curl).

	Age [years]	Height [m]	Weight [kg]	BMI [kg/m²]	Body fat [%]	BST [mm]	1RM [kg]
Mean	24.5	1.84	82.8	24.3	14.9	4.9	62.5
SD	2.0	0.07	7.1	1.6	5.3	1.4	10.1
Min	23.0	1.74	70.6	21.7	6.2	3.0	50.0
Max	30.0	1.95	91.3	26.9	22.2	7.0	80.0

Measurement

Thermographic images were taken with the infrared camera FLIR A35 (FLIR Systems, Inc., USA) during the following time points: at rest after 15 minutes of acclimatization (T_{rest}), immediately after the first, second and third set (T_{S1}, T_{S2}, T_{S3}), and at 1,2,3,4,5,6,7,8,9,10,15,20,25,30 minutes post the third set (T_1-T_{30}). Participants stood at a distance of 1.50m from the camera in front of a white uniform background, in order to ensure that the markers of the upper body and arms were visible (Figure 1a). There was constant intensity of light and no direct ventilation in the test room during the measurement procedure because this can influence the skin temperature measurements. In addition, the methodological aspects of infrared thermography in human assessment were considered (Priego Quesada, 2017).

All thermographic images were analyzed by the same examiner with FLIR ResearchIR 4 Software (FLIR Systems, Inc., USA). This software is a tool to calculate mean skin surface temperature in a defined area by averaging the detected temperature values. To determine the mean temperature of the biceps surface at every measuring time point, a line was fitted between the two cork markers at the right arm and at the left arm in the muscle belly region of the biceps brachii. Each of this lines consisted of approximately 50 pixels with 50 temperature values between the markers and the software calculated the mean temperature of this 50 values (Figure 2). When the fitted line ran along the Vena cephalica, the line was positioned medial of the vein, because temperatures at the skin surface of blood vessels are much higher than in other skin areas. Hence a line along a vein does not represent the mean surface temperature.

For an accurate measurement of T of a particular region, a minimum of 25 pixels is recommended (ISO 2009). Therefore, in this study the number of pixels of the region of interest was between 40 and 60.

Table 2 shows the parameters that were calculated for the loaded and unloaded arm.

Statistical Analysis

Data are presented as means ± SD. Normal distribution was checked by Shapiro-Wilk test and homogeneity of variances by Levene test. Two-way ANOVA was used to test the effect of measuring time point and intensity on the surface temperature. One-way ANOVA with repeated measurements tested the time points with a significant temperature difference compared to T_{rest} and the influence of the intensity on

T_{rest}, T_{S3}, T_{max}, time to T_{max}, T_{30}, and T_{max} - T_{30}. P-values were Bonferroni corrected. To determine the relationship of biceps skinfold thickness (BST) and 1RM to T_{S3} and T_{max} the correlation coefficient Spearmans Rho was calculated. The level of significance was 0.05. Statistical analysis was performed using SPSS (Version 23.0 IBM, New York, USA). For graphical representation, Grapher 4.0 (Golden Software Inc., Golden, USA) was used.

RESULTS

The measuring time point had a significant effect on ΔT of the loaded arm for all intensities together and for 30, 50 and

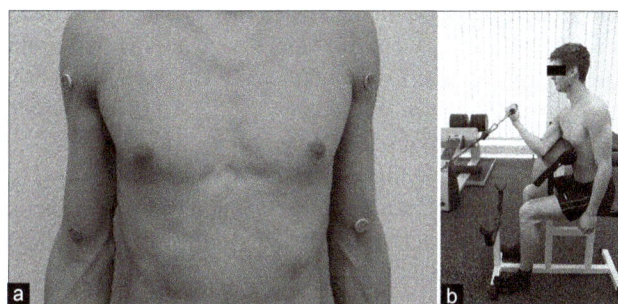

Figure 1. a) Standing position for thermographic images with fixed cork markers at the muscle belly of the right and left biceps brachii, b) Endposition of the resistance exercise biceps curl on a scott bench on the cable pulley

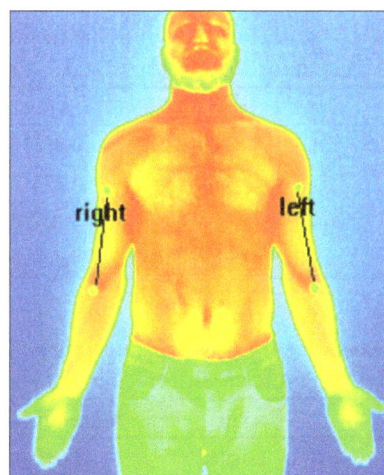

Figure 2. Thermographic image with a fitted line between the cork markers

Table 2. Parameters used to characterize the time profile of biceps surface temperature (T).

Index abbreviation	Definition	Units
Basal temperature (T_{rest})	temperature value prior to the training	°C
Δtemperature to T_{rest} (ΔT)	difference of measured temperature and T_{rest}	°C
T_{S1}, T_{S2}, T_{S3}	Δtemperature to T_{rest} following set 1, 2 and 3	°C
T_1, T_2, T_3, T_4, T_5, T_6, T_7, T_8, T_9, T_{10}, T_{15}, T_{20}, T_{25}, T_{30}	Δtemperature to T_{rest} 1 – 30 min after set 3	°C
T_{max}	maximumΔtemperature	°C
Time to T_{max}	time after T_{S3}, when T_{max} was recorded	min
T_{max} - T_{30}	difference of T_{max} and T30	°C

70% of the 1RM. For the unloaded arm, the measuring time point had a significant effect for all intensities together and for 30% 1RM. The time effects were independent of the intensity (Table 3).

For the loaded arm, the ANOVA of the factor intensity showed no effect for any of the measuring time points or for T_{max}, time to T_{max} and $T_{max} - T_{30}$ (Table 4). Lower intensities showed an earlier significant increase of the biceps surface T of the loaded arm compared to T_{rest}: ANOVA showed a significant higher T of the biceps surface at T_{S2} to T_{15} (30% 1RM), T_{S3} to T_{20} (50% 1RM) and T_1 to T_{15} (70% 1RM) (p<0.05). On average, T_{max} was reached approximately 5 minutes after the third set (T_5) and the time to T_{max} tended (p>0.05) to increase with a higher intensity (Table 4). After reaching T_{max}, a slow temperature decrease on the loaded arm was observed up to the 30th minute (T_{30}), but rest values were not reached again after 30 minutes and T was still increased by 0.4°C (p<0.05).

The unloaded arm showed no significant difference of T to T_{rest} at any time point (p>0.05).

At 30% 1RM positive correlations of the 1RM with T_{S3}, (r=0.842; p=0.002) and T_{max} (r=0.661; p=0.038) were found. BST showed a negative correlation with T_{S3} at 50% 1RM (r=-0.737; p=0.015).

4. DISCUSSION

The present study investigated the influence of a unilateral biceps curl with different exercise intensities on the re-

action of T in the biceps brachii muscle region. In the loaded arm, T increased significantly independent of the exercise intensity. The curves of the different intensities showed qualitatively similar patterns (Figure 3b). Looking at the individual profiles of the surface temperature on the loaded arm, a homogeneous pattern is shown (Figure 3c). All participants showed a rise of T after 30, 50 and 70% 1RM. Therefore, previous studies that observed, that it is possible to identify the primary used muscles via IRT during and after resistance training (Formenti et al., 2013; Formenti et al., 2016; Fröhlich et al., 2014; Neves et al., 2014; Neves et al., 2015; Neves et al., 2016) can be confirmed. Figure 4 shows an example for the visualization of the heated biceps brachii after three sets of biceps curl with the right arm.

Since blood flow was not measured in this study, we assume that the T changes are the result of a higher skin perfusion (Schlager et al., 2010) and/or of muscle contractions due to a change in the muscular blood circulation and muscle heat production during and after exercise (Kenny et al., 2003; Kenny et al., 2008; Krustrup et al., 2003). The resulting muscle heat is transferred to the surrounding tissue and can be measured at the surface.

Interestingly, a slight and non-significant drop in temperature was observed at 70% 1RM after the first set. This has already been described by Formenti et al. (2016) and Neves et al. (2014) and could result from a reactive vasoconstriction of the skin vessels and may indicate a redistribution of the blood immediately after intense exercise into

Table 3. Eta² (p-value) by ANOVA of the factors time (measurement time point) and time x intensity for Δtemperatures of the loaded and unloaded arm (*p<0.05)

	Arm	All intensities	30% 1RM	50% 1RM	70% 1RM
Factor time	loaded	0.863* (p<0.001)	0.853* (p<0.001)	0.879* (p<0.001)	0.863* (p<0.001)
	unloaded	0.273* (p<0.001)	0.411* (p=0.002)	0.254 (p=0.075)	0.239 (p=0.057)
Factor time x intensity	loaded	0.132 (p=0.067)			
	unloaded	0.046 (p=0.686)			

Table 4. Means±SD of selected parameters of the loaded and unloaded arm and differences between loaded and unloaded arm (*significant difference of the loaded arm to the unloaded arm, #significant difference to T_{rest})

	Arm	All intensities	30% 1RM	50% 1RM	70% 1RM	P-value of intensity
T_{rest} [°C]	Loaded	32.6±0.8	32.3±0.7	32.7±0.9	32.9±0.9	0.266
	Unloaded	32.7±0.8	32.3±0.7	32.7±0.9	33.1±0.9	0.137
T_{S3} [°C]	Loaded	0.8±0.5*#	0.9±0.4*#	0.9±0.5*#	0.8±0.6*	0.801
	Unloaded	-0.1±0.4	0.1±0.3	-0.2±0.3	-0.3±0.4	0.064
T_{max} [°C]	Loaded	1.8±0.4*	1.7±0.3*#	1.9±0.5*#	1.8±0.5*#	0.570
	Unloaded	0.4±0.4#	0.5±0.3#	0.3±0.3#	0.2±0.4	0.076
time to T_{max} [min]	Loaded	5.4±2.1*	4.6±1.8*	5.2±2.5	6.4±1.6	0.143
	Unloaded	8.6±6.7	9.7±7.3	8.6±6.9	7.4±6.4	0.785
$T_{max} - T_{30}$ [°C]	Loaded	1.3±0.5*	1.3±0.6*	1.5±0.5*	1.3±0.4*	0.601
	Unloaded	0.5±0.4	0.5±0.3	0.6±0.5	0.5±0.4	0.879
T_{30} [°C]	Loaded	0.4±0.6*#	0.4±0.6	0.4±0.5*	0.6±0.6*	0.650
	Unloaded	-0.2±0.6	0.1±0.6	-0.2±0.5	-0.3±0.6	0.337

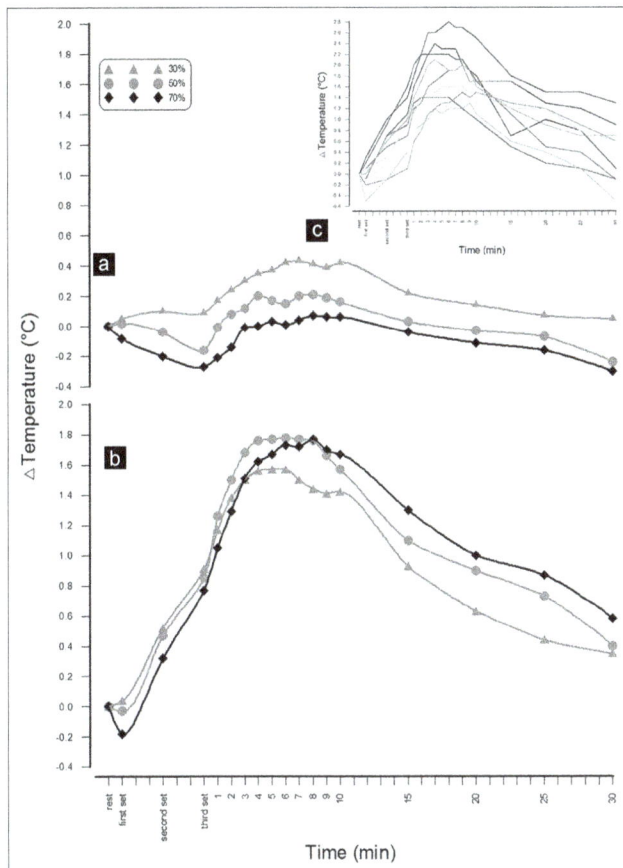

Figure 3. Average biceps surface ΔT at 30, 50 and 70% of 1RM of a) unloaded arm, b) loaded arm. c) Individual biceps surface ΔT at 50% 1RM of the loaded arm for all participants.

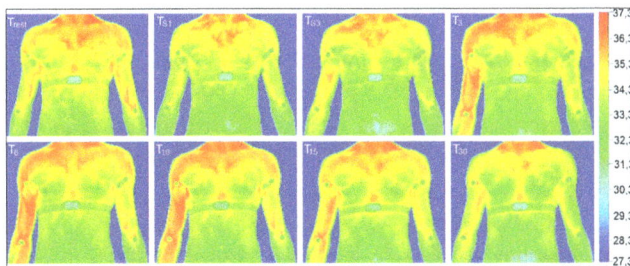

Figure 4. Thermographic images of a representative participant at the time points T_{rest}, T_{S1}, T_{S3}, T_3, T_6, T_{10}, T_{15}, T_{30} (70% 1RM training protocol, right arm = loaded arm)

the stressed muscle. This might be necessary to ensure the energetic and enzymatic processes for muscle contraction because a higher temperature in the muscle results in a higher enzyme activity of the ATPase and creatine kinase in the muscle fiber (Gray et al., 2011; Stienen et al., 1996).

We hypothesized, that the T rise of the loaded arm during and following the resistance exercise is augmented with increasing intensity but temperature changes of the skin surface in the present study were independent of the exercise intensity. In contrast, Bartuzi et al. (2012) found a significant influence of the intensity on T during a biceps exercise. However, it is hard to compare this study with the present one, because the exercise was static and very low intensities were chosen (5, 15, 30% of maximum voluntary contraction), which had to be held for up to 5 minutes. The

temperature differences to T_{rest} was significant higher after the 30% load compared to the 5% load (0.8°C vs 0.2°C). In this context Edwards, Hill, & Jones (1975) showed, that the rate of muscle temperature rise has a positive correlation to the exercise intensity (in % of maximum voluntary contraction). In addition, Krustrup et al. (2003) demonstrate, that muscle heat production is related with the ATP turnover rate and higher intensities showed a higher ATP turnover rate, a higher blood flow and a higher muscle temperature in the stressed muscle. In the present study, higher intensities were also related to higher T_{max} values but due to the small sample size, these findings were not significant but a bigger sample size maybe would show significant differences.

In the unloaded arm, the T patterns were qualitative similar to that in the loaded arm (Figure 3). However, the important quantitative parameters of the study, such as T_{S3}, T_{max}, T_{max} - T_{30} and T_{30} were significantly lower than in the loaded arm (Table 4). Only a significant time effect could be observed at 30% 1RM (Table 3). T rose at 30% 1RM about 0.5°C (T_{max}) whereas at 50% and 70% 1RM, T decreased until T_{S3} and then increased slightly compared to T_{rest}.

For the comparison of the calculated T changes with the values of the existing studies, it must be noted, that the methods in the studies were very different (skin temperature calculation, measurement time points, number of sets, exercise intensity) (Formenti et al., 2013; Formenti et al., 2016; Fröhlich et al., 2014; Neves et al., 2014; Neves et al., 2016). The rise of T to the initial value determined in this study is much higher compared to Formenti et al. (2016), where only one set was performed, whereas in the present study, three sets were completed. This different training load may be the cause of the higher T-values. In other investigations with several sets, an increase of T of 1°C in the biceps area was shown directly after the load (Neves et al., 2015) and in two individual participants, an increase of 2°C and 3.5°C was shown (Neves et al., 2014). In contrast, Neves et al. (2016) found a decrease of T in the biceps region after four sets of biceps curls at 70 and 85% of 10RM. Skin temperature fell by approximately 2°C in the loaded arm and around 2.5°C in the unloaded arm. The author explained this contrasting reaction with the kind of sample, untrained women with larger subcutaneous fat layer and less muscle volume. Therefore, future studies could compare the development of T after resistance exercise in men and women with a large range of subcutaneous fat layer.

This study found also positive correlations of the 1RM and T changes after exercise (T_{S3} and T_{max}). According to Krustrup et al. (2003), individuals with a higher 1RM generate a higher power and have a higher ATP turnover rate and therefore a higher muscle temperature. Despite we did not measured ATP turnover rate, this can possibly explain the higher T-values on the skin surface of the participants with a higher 1RM.

Furthermore, we found correlations of BST and the changes of T after the biceps curls. Lower BST values correlate with higher T_{S3} and T_{max} values but this correlation only reached significance at the 50% 1RM condition. These findings can be confirmed by Priego Quesada et al. (2015), where participants with larger thigh skinfold showed lower

ΔT-values in vastus lateralis and rectus femoris in an incremental cycle exercise (r > -0.7).

The present study was carried out under strict standardized conditions. The frequency of movement was standardized and precisely controlled by a metronome and the room temperature and humidity were maintained at a constant level. A room temperature of 22.1±0.5°C was perceived by the participants as agreeable, to ensure they were not in any discomfort during the 45 minute examination. Furthermore, the 15-minute acclimatization time was exactly maintained so that the unclothed upper body of the participants could adapt to the room temperature. Most studies had acclimatization times of 10 to 20 minutes (Bartuzi et al., 2012; Formenti et al., 2013; Formenti et al., 2016; Fröhlich et al., 2014; Neves et al., 2014; Neves et al., 2016). Marins et al. (2014) recommended an acclimatization time for at least 10 min, but it is uncertain, whether longer periods of acclimatization decisively influence the T patterns. Therefore, following studies should examine the consequences of different acclimatization periods on T during and after exercise.

The study showed that it is possible to visualize the primary used muscles in strength training with a simple and contactless method like IRT and that the stressed muscle groups can be detected through measuring the surface warming of the skin even at low intensities. Due to this measuring method, this visualization can also be used as real-time feedback, because infrared images can be viewed and analyzed in real time.

Future studies should compare the influence on T after resistance exercises with a variation of different load characteristics like number of sets, number of repetitions, movement velocity, rest between the sets and kind of contraction (concentric, eccentric, static). In addition, the influence of the trained muscle group, age, sex, skinfold thickness, acclimatization time, room temperature and humidity on exercise-associated changes of T need further investigation.

CONCLUSION

This study observed an acute increase of T in the stressed muscle region, which could be independent of the exercise intensity. Every participant showed a rise of T at 30, 50 and 70% 1RM and the patterns of the T changes were relatively homogenous and reproducible. Non-contact IRT seems to be applicable to identify the primary used functional muscles in resistance training but this method seems not suitable to differentiate between exercise intensity from 30 to 70% 1RM.

REFERENCES

Baechle, T. R., & Earle, R. W. (Eds.). (2008). *Essentials of strength training and conditioning* (3. ed.). Champaign, IL: Human Kinetics.

Balci, G. A., Basaran, T., & Colakoglu, M. (2016). Analysing visual pattern of skin temperature during submaximal and maximal exercises. *Infrared Physics & Technology, 74*, 57–62. https://doi.org/10.1016/j.infrared.2015.12.002

Bartuzi, P., Roman-Liu, D., & Wisniewski, T. (2012). The influence of fatigue on muscle temperature. *International journal of occupational safety and ergonomics: JOSE,* 18(2), 233–243. https://doi.org/10.1080/10803548.2012.11076931

Chudecka, M. (2013). Use of thermal imaging in the evaluation of body surface temperature in various physiological states in patients with different body compositions and varying levels of physical activity. *Central european journal of sport sciences and medicine, 2*(2), 15–20.

Chudecka, M., Lubkowska, A., Leznicka, K., & Krupecki, K. (2015). The use of thermal imaging in the evaluation of the symmetry of muscle activity in various types of exercises (symmetrical and asymmetrical). *Journal of human kinetics, 49*, 141–147. https://doi.org/10.1515/hukin-2015-0116

Costello, J., Stewart, I. B., Selfe, J., Karki, A. I., & & Donnelly, A. (2013). The use of thermal imaging in sports medicine research: a short report. *International Sportmed Journal, 14*(2), 94–98.

Das, P., Vardasca, R., & Mendes, J. G. (Eds.). (2017). *Innovative research in thermal imaging for biology and medicine. Advances in Medical Technologies and Clinical Practice*: IGI Global.

Edwards, R. H., Hill, D. K., & Jones, D. A. (1975). Heat production and chemical changes during isometric contractions of the human quadriceps muscle. *The Journal of physiology, 251*(2), 303–315.

Formenti, D., Ludwig, N., Gargano, M., Gondola, M., Dellerma, N., Caumo, A., & Alberti, G. (2013). Thermal imaging of exercise-associated skin temperature changes in trained and untrained female subjects. *Annals of biomedical engineering, 41*(4), 863–871. https://doi.org/10.1007/s10439-012-0718-x

Formenti, D., Ludwig, N., Trecroci, A., Gargano, M., Michielon, G., Caumo, A., & Alberti, G. (2016). Dynamics of thermographic skin temperature response during squat exercise at two different speeds. *Journal of thermal biology, 59*, 58–63. https://doi.org/10.1016/j.jtherbio.2016.04.013

Fröhlich, M., Ludwig, O., Kraus, S., & Felder, H. (2014). Changes in skin surface temperature during muscular endurance indicated strain – an explorative study. *International Journal of Kinesiology & Sports Science, 2*(3), 23–27.

Fröhlich, M., Ludwig, O., Zeller, P., & Felder, H. (2015). Changes in skin surface temperature after a 10-minute warm-up on a bike ergometer. *International Journal of Kinesiology & Sports Science, 3*(3), 13–17.

Gray, S. R., Soderlund, K., Watson, M., & Ferguson, R. A. (2011). Skeletal muscle ATP turnover and single fibre ATP and PCr content during intense exercise at different muscle temperatures in humans. *Pflugers Archiv: European journal of physiology, 462*(6), 885–893. https://doi.org/10.1007/s00424-011-1032-4

Hildebrandt, C., Raschner, C., & Ammer, K. (2010). An overview of recent application of medical infrared thermography in sports medicine in Austria. *Sensors (Basel), 10*(5), 4700–4715. https://doi.org/10.3390/s100504700

ISO 2009 Medical electrical equipment-deployment, implementation and operational guidelines for identifying febrile humans using a screening thermograph. TR 13154:2009 ISO/TR 8-600.

Jiang, L. J., Ng, E. Y. K., Yeo, A. C. B., Wu, S., Pan, F., Yau, W. Y., Yang, Y. (2005). A perspective on medical infrared imaging. *Journal of medical engineering & technology, 29*(6), 257–267. https://doi.org/10.1080/03091900 512331333158

Kenny, G. P., Reardon, F. D., Zaleski, W., Reardon, M. L., Haman, F., & Ducharme, M. B. (2003). Muscle temperature transients before, during, and after exercise measured using an intramuscular multisensor probe. *Journal of applied physiology (Bethesda, Md.: 1985), 94*(6), 2350–2357. https://doi.org/10.1152/japplphysiol.01107.2002

Kenny, G. P., Webb, P., Ducharme, M. B., Reardon, F. D., & Jay, O. (2008). Calorimetric measurement of postexercise net heat loss and residual body heat storage. *Medicine and science in sports and exercise, 40*(9), 1629–1636. https://doi.org/10.1249/MSS.0b013e31817751cb

Krustrup, P., Ferguson, R. A., Kjaer, M., & Bangsbo, J. (2003). ATP and heat production in human skeletal muscle during dynamic exercise: Higher efficiency of anaerobic than aerobic ATP resynthesis. *The Journal of physiology, 549*(Pt 1), 255–269. https://doi.org/10.1113/jphysiol.2002.035089

Lahiri, B. B., Bagavathiappan, S., Jayakumar, T., & Philip, J. (2012). Medical applications of infrared thermography: A review. *Infrared Physics & Technology, 55*(4), 221–235. https://doi.org/10.1016/j.infrared.2012.03.007

Ludwig, N., Formenti, D., Trecroci, A., Gargano, M., & Alberti, G. (2014). Comparison of image analysis methods in skin temperature measurements during physical exercise. *Quantitative InfraRed Thermography, Bordeaux 7-11 July*.

Marins, J. C. B., Moreira, D. G., Cano, S. P., Quintana, M. S., Soares, D. D., Fernandes, A. d. A., Amorim, P. R. d. S. (2014). Time required to stabilize thermographic images at rest. *Infrared Physics & Technology, 65*, 30–35. https://doi.org/10.1016/j.infrared.2014.02.008

Merla, A., Mattei, P. A., Di Donato, L., & Romani, G. L. (2010). Thermal imaging of cutaneous temperature modifications in runners during graded exercise. *Annals of biomedical engineering, 38*(1), 158–163. https://doi.org/10.1007/s10439-009-9809-8

Neves, E. B., Cunha, R. M., Rosa, C., Antunes, N. S., Felisberto, I. M. V., Vilaça-Alves, J., & Reis, V. M. (2016). Correlation between skin temperature and heart rate during exercise and recovery, and the influence of body position in these variables in untrained women. *Infrared Physics & Technology, 75*, 70–76. https://doi.org/10.1016/j.infrared.2015.12.018

Neves, E. B., Moreira, T. R., Lemos, R., Vilaça-Alves, J., Rosa, C., & Reis, V. M. (2015). Using skin temperature and muscle thickness to assess muscle response to strength training. *Revista Brasileira de Medicina do Esporte, 21*(5), 350–354. https://doi.org/10.1590/1517-869220152105151293

Neves, E. B., Vilaça-Alves, J., Krueger, E., & Reis, V. M. (2014). Changes in skin temperature during muscular work: a pilot study. *Pan Am J Med Thermol, 1*(1), 11–15.

Neves, E. B., Vilaça-Alves, J., Moreira, T. R., de Lemos, Rui Jorge Canário Alvares, & Reis, V. M. (2016). The thermal response of biceps brachii to strength training. *Gazzetta medica italiana, 175*(10), 391–399.

Priego Quesada, J. I., Carpes, F. P., Bini, R. R., Salvador Palmer, R., Perez-Soriano, P., & Cibrian Ortiz de Anda, R. M. (2015). Relationship between skin temperature and muscle activation during incremental cycle exercise. *Journal of thermal biology, 48*, 28–35. https://doi.org/10.1016/j.jtherbio.2014.12.005

Priego Quesada, J. I. (Ed.). (2017). *Application of infrared thermography in sports science. Biological and Medical Physics, Biomedical Engineering.* Cham: Springer. Retrieved from http://dx.doi.org/10.1007/978-3-319-47410-6

Priego Quesada, J. I., Martínez, N., Salvador Palmer, R., Psikuta, A., Annaheim, S., Rossi, R. M., Pérez-Soriano, P. (2016). Effects of the cycling workload on core and local skin temperatures. *Experimental Thermal and Fluid Science, 77*, 91–99. https://doi.org/10.1016/j.expthermflusci.2016.04.008

Ring, E. F. J., & Ammer, K. (2012). Infrared thermal imaging in medicine. *Physiological measurement, 33*(3), 46. https://doi.org/10.1088/0967-3334/33/3/R33

Sahlin, K., Katz, A., & Henriksson, J. (1987). Redox state and lactate accumulation in human skeletal muscle during dynamic exercise. *Biochemical Journal, 245*(2), 551–556. https://doi.org/10.1042/bj2450551

Schlager, O., Gschwandtner, M. E., Herberg, K., Frohner, T., Schillinger, M., Koppensteiner, R., & Mlekusch, W. (2010). Correlation of infrared thermography and skin perfusion in Raynaud patients and in healthy controls. *Microvascular research, 80*(1), 54–57. https://doi.org/10.1016/j.mvr.2010.01.010

Sillero-Quintana, M., Gomez-Carmona, P. M., & Fernández-Cuevas, I. (2017). Infrared thermography as a means of monitoring and preventing sports injuries. In P. Das, R. Vardasca, & J. G. Mendes (Eds.), *Advances in Medical Technologies and Clinical Practice. Innovative research in thermal imaging for biology and medicine* (pp. 165–198). IGI Global. https://doi.org/10.4018/978-1-5225-2072-6.ch008

Stienen, G. J., Kiers, J. L., Bottinelli, R., & Reggiani, C. (1996). Myofibrillar ATPase activity in skinned human skeletal muscle fibres: Fibre type and temperature dependence. *The Journal of physiology, 493 (Pt 2)*, 299–307.

Wang, H., Wade, Jr., Dwight R., & Kam, J. (2004). IR imaging of blood circulation of patients with vascular disease. In D. D. Burleigh, K. E. Cramer, & G. R. Peacock (Eds.): *SPIE Proceedings, Defense and Security* (p. 115). SPIE. https://doi.org/10.1117/12.545899

8

Effects of Static, Stationary, and Traveling Trunk Exercises on Muscle Activation

Darien T. Pyka, Pablo B. Costa*, Jared W. Coburn, Lee E. Brown

Department of Kinesiology, California State University, Fullerton, 800 N. State College Blvd. USA

Corresponding Author: Pablo B. Costa, E-mail: pcosta@fullerton.edu

ARTICLE INFO	ABSTRACT

Conflicts of interest: None
Funding: None

Background: A new fitness trend incorporates stability exercises that challenges trunk muscles and introduces crawling as an exercise, but has yet to be investigated for muscle activity. **Purpose:** To compare the effects of static (STA), stationary (STN), and traveling (TRV) trunk exercises on muscle activation of the rectus abdominis, rectus femoris, external oblique, and erector spinae using surface electromyography (EMG). **Methods:** Seventeen recreationally active women (mean age ± SD = 22.4 ± 2.4 years, body mass 62.9 ± 6.9 kg, height 165.1 ± 5.8 cm) and twenty-three men (23.6 ±3.9 years, 83.2 ±17.1 kg, 177.1 ± 9.1 cm) volunteered to participate in this study. Subjects performed maximal voluntary contractions for normalization of each muscle's EMG activity. They then performed the three exercises in random order for thirty seconds each with a two-minute rest in between. **Results:** For the rectus abdominis, STA was significantly lower than STN ($P = 0.003$) and TRV ($P = 0.001$). For the external oblique, STA was significantly lower than STN ($P = 0.001$) and TRV ($P = 0.001$) and STN was significantly greater than TRV ($P = 0.009$). For the erector spinae and rectus femoris, STA was significantly lower than STN ($P = 0.001$) and TRV ($P = 0.001$) **Conclusions:** There was greater muscle activation in all muscles tested in the stationary and traveling exercises versus the static. Strength and conditioning coaches and allied health professionals could potentially use stationary and traveling forms of trunk stabilization exercises as a viable strategy to increase muscle activation.

Key words: Electromyography, Exercise Therapy, Torso, Muscle Contraction, Postural Balance, Back Pain

INTRODUCTION

The advancement in research and application of trunk exercises has benefited therapists, trainers, and coaches to improve sports performance, reduce injury risk, and in rehabilitation of their athletes or patients (McGill, 2010; Wheeler, 2015). Research has shown the most effective and safest method to train the trunk is a stabilization exercise, where a neutral spine is maintained against a load (Mendrin, Lynn, Griffith-Merritt, & Noffal, 2016). This is due to increased knowledge that the most common function of the trunk is to prevent motion rather than initiate movement, and the trunk muscles should be trained as stabilizers rather than prime movers (McGill, 2010). McGill (2010) describes a stabilization exercise as any exercise that challenges the spine stability while enforcing trunk co-activation patterns that ensure a stable spine (McGill (2010). These exercises consist of holding the spine in a neutral position while the trunk is loaded through different strategies, such as moving upper and lower limbs in several positions or maintaining the pelvis lifted off the floor against gravity in a hold or stationary position (Vera-Garcia, Barbado, & Moya, 2014). A neutral position is referred to as the natural curvature of

the spine and the pelvis without an anterior or posterior tilt (McGill, 2010).

It is important to have a relatively strong trunk for resistance training and injury prevention (McGill, 2015). In a strongman study, McGill et al. (2009) concluded that strong trunk muscles allow force to dissipate distally to farther areas of the body. A stiff trunk allows power generated from the hips to be transmitted through the torso to the upper body or vice versa. It takes a stiff, stable trunk to allow optimal production, transfer, and control of force during a total body movement (Okada, Huxel, & Nesser, 2011). Hodges and Richardson (1997) found the trunk stabilizers to be activated before any limb movements in a total body exercise, lending the support to the theory that movement control and stability is developed from the trunk to extremity (Okada et al., 2011). Many movements such as pushing, pulling, lifting, carrying, and rotation use power generated from the hips to perform the exercise (McGill, 2010). If a bend in the spine occurs, known as an "energy leak", power is compromised (McGill, 2010).

Chronic disabling low back pain prevalence is 4.2% in individuals between 24 and 39 years of age and 19.6% in those between 20 and 59 years (Meucci, Fassa, & Faria, 2015). There is a direct link between poor movement patterns and low back injuries. Common injuries are a result of excessive spinal flexion and trunk instability. In planning a trunk-strengthening program, stability and endurance exercises have been recommended to be first (McGill, 2010) and the most important (McGill, 2015). Improving the strength of the trunk without these two qualities increases the risk of not performing the exercise correctly with repetition and thereby increases the risk of injury (McGill, 2010). A training program focusing on neuromuscular control for trunk stabilization could be advantageous in a low back injury prevention program (Stevens et al., 2007; Wheeler et al., 2015). Such exercises include the four point kneeling bird dog with extension of the contra-lateral limbs and supine bridging with a single leg extension (Stevens et al., 2007).

Integration core exercises requiring activation of the distal trunk elicit greater activity of the primary abdominal and lumbar muscles compared to isolated exercises (Gottschall, Mills, & Hastings, 2013). In addition, within a trunk stabilization exercise, as instability increases, trunk muscle activity increases proportionally (Anderson & Behm, 2005). Common trunk stabilization exercises that incorporate the above techniques include variations of the prone bridge, side-bridge, quadruped bird-dog, and supine curl-up exercises (McGill, 2010). With the rising popularity of trunk stabilization training and the research on the importance for trunk stability and endurance, there is a new exercise trend known as movement flows that challenge the trunk in a traveling form that has yet to be tested for muscle activity. Part of this trend is the Animal Flow workout, coined by fitness trainer Mike Fitch, which is thought to specifically challenge trunk stability and endurance in a functional manner. In his Animal Flow Coaching Manual (2013) for his level one Animal Flow certification, the author describes the most common position of the Animal Flow workout to be the beast position or more commonly referred to as a bear crawl. This position mimics the bird dog by being a quadruped position but with the knees slightly raised off the ground. The bear position consists of a progression of a static hold, stationary contra-lateral arm and leg lift, and a traveling crawling movement, with the goal of maintaining a neutral spine in each. Accordingly, Mendrin et al. (2016) has already reported the bear crawl as an effective isometric trunk exercise.

In a quadruped position the exercise integrates distal muscle stabilizers and with the knees raised slightly off the ground it serves the same purpose as a plank, to maintain the pelvis position against gravity testing endurance. The exercise loads and challenges trunk coordination, neuromuscular coordination, and balance with the stationary contra-lateral limb lift and traveling crawling movement. This quadruped exercise appears to have the key concepts of a trunk stabilization exercise. However, every trunk exercise studied and listed is either a static hold or in a stationary position. Thus, the question remains of how traveling in a trunk exercise affects muscle activity. Therefore, the purpose of the present investigation was to compare muscle activation of the rectus abdominis, lumbar erector spinae, external oblique, and rectus femoris among static, stationary, and traveling exercises in the quadruped position using surface electromyography.

METHODS

Subjects

Seventeen recreationally active women (mean age ± SD = 22.4 ±2.4 years, body mass 62.9 ± 6.9 kg, height 165.1 ± 5.8 cm) and twenty-three men (23.6 ± 3.9 years, 83.2 ± 17.1 kg, 177.1 ± 9.1 cm) volunteered to participate in this study. An a priori sample size estimate of 28 participants was determined using G*Power software (version 3.1.9.2, Dusseldorf, Germany) with an effect size of 0.25 and a power level set at 0.8. Participants met the inclusion criteria to participate in the study, which included being free of illness, injury, or physical disabilities that may inhibit optimal performance of the tested exercises. They were required to have a minimum of 3 years of recreational activity and have met ACSM's guidelines of 30 minutes of recreational activity at least 3 days a week for at least 3 months.

Research Design

All data were collected over two visits. The first session consisted of reading and signing an informed consent form, filling out a health status questionnaire, and familiarizing the participant with the equipment and exercises. This visit lasted approximately 30 minutes. Participants were instructed to shave areas needed for the surface electrodes before the second session. Areas included the back of their neck, right thigh, area around their navel, and low back. All participants were instructed to wear shorts, to not apply any lotion on their skin prior to the testing session, and women needed to wear a sports bra and remove any umbilicus piercings. The second session consisted of skinfold measurements (Lange Skinfold Caliper, Santa Cruz, CA, USA) on the electrode sites as well as areas for a three-site body composition analysis, electromyography (EMG) electrode attachment, maximal voluntary contractions, and testing of the three exercises for 30 seconds each in random order. Constant speed was set with a metronome at a speed of 55 beats per minute for the stationary and traveling exercise. Data collection for each participant took approximately 45 minutes.

In the first session, anthropometrics of each participant were measured, which consisted of their body mass and height. Body mass was measured and recorded in kilograms with a digital scale (Ohaus ES Series scale, Parsippany, NJ, USA). Height was measured with a stadiometer (Seca stadiometer, Chino, CA, USA) and recorded in centimeters. After, the participant practiced the correct form of the three exercises and became familiar with the cues the researcher would provide during testing. For the static exercise (STA), the participant was instructed to start in a quadruped position (Figure 1), with wrists placed directly under the shoulders, elbows straight, and knees directly under the navel with ankles dorsi-flexed. Once this position was correct, the participant was instructed to raise their knees slightly off the ground such that a neutral spine is maintained. Subjects rested once they performed this position correctly for 30 seconds. Throughout the practice and the start of each testing exercise, participants were given corrective instructions for proper technique. The researcher only provided corrective technique at the start of the testing exercises to assume the quadruped position and did not provide corrective cues during testing. Time was tracked via the EMG software.

After they rested, participants were instructed to get back into the correct static position. When the correct position was assumed, participants began practicing for the stationary (STN) by lifting their right hand off the ground by bending their elbow without losing their trunk position for two seconds. Once this was performed correctly, the participant practiced lifting their left foot off the ground by further flexing their knee without losing their trunk position for two seconds. Once this was performed correctly, they practiced raising their right hand and left foot in the technique they just practiced simultaneously without losing their trunk position for two seconds (Figure 2). The same protocol was followed for the left hand and right foot. When performed correctly, they practiced alternating contra-lateral limbs off the ground to the sound at the metronome. Once they performed this correctly for a total of 30 seconds, they rested for twenty seconds.

After they rested, they practiced the traveling exercise (TRV). Participants were instructed to get back into the correct static position. When the correct position was assumed, participants were instructed to raise their right hand, left foot off the ground simultaneously to the sound of the metronome, in the technique they performed earlier, and place them back down on the ground half a hands length from the stationary hand (Figure 3). They were instructed to raise their left hand, right foot with the same protocol to create a forward crawling movement. They crawled for approximately five to eight yards in the 30 seconds. Form was lost when

trunk position or a neutral spine was not maintained or one wrist was not under the shoulder or one of their knees was not under the navel at all times.

Maximum Voluntary Contraction

In the second session, each participant performed a maximal voluntary isometric contraction of each measured muscle for normalization. Reproducing techniques from McGill and Karpowicz (2009), participants were instructed to push against the manual resistance provided by the research investigator for 10 seconds. For the abdominal muscles, participants assumed a sit-up position and were manually braced at the elbows. Participants then produced a maximal isometric flexor movement. With a 30-second rest period, it was followed by a right twist movement for the external oblique. For the lumbar erector spinae, participants performed a resisted maximum extension in the Biering-Sorensen position. The participant lied prone on a plinth with the upper edge of the iliac crests aligned with the edge of the table (Demoulin, Vanderthommen, Duysens, & Crielaard, 2006). A strap was placed around the knees to anchor the lower body to the table. With arms folded across the chest, participants were instructed to forcefully extend while being manually braced by the research investigator. For the rectus femoris, participants were positioned in a seated position and attempted an isometric knee extension with a simultaneous hip flexion. The same research investigator performed all the tests. The maximal amplitude in any normalizing contraction was used as the maximum for that muscle (McGill & Karpowicz, 2009). After performing maximal voluntary contractions, the participant rested for two minutes. They then performed each exercise in random order for 30 seconds with a rest period of 2 minutes in between exercises to avoid fatigue. Exercises

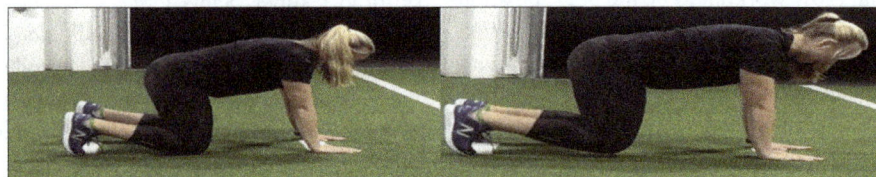

Figure 1. Static exercise (STA)

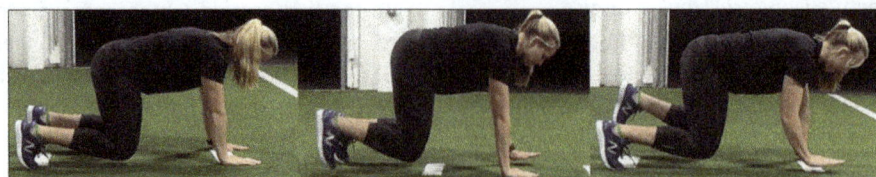

Figure 2. Stationary exercise (STN)

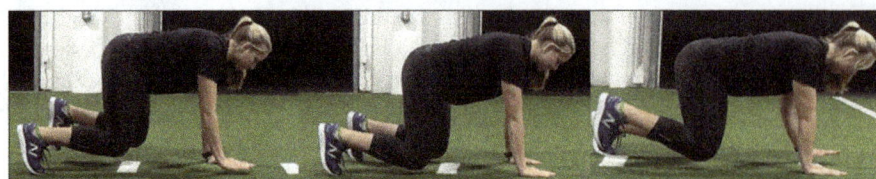

Figure 3. Traveling exercise (TRV)

were performed for 30 seconds based on the recommendation by Mendrin et al. (2016).

All exercises were performed as practiced. If proper form was not maintained, the test was stopped and repeated until a full thirty seconds was performed correctly. Exercises were repeated if the correct form was not performed based on the investigator's (DTP) observations. Examples of incorrect form included not maintaining a neutral spine, raising hips into the air, dropping knees to the ground, or bending the elbows.

Electromyography

The participant's skin was prepared for the use of EMG electrodes prior to their placement, such that the signal was not distorted by exterior variables such as dead skin and excess hair. Excess hair at the site of the electrode placement was shaved and the site cleaned with a swab of isopropyl alcohol. Four preamplified, bipolar surface EMG electrodes (EL254S; Biopac Systems Inc., Santa Barbara, CA; gain = 350) with a fixed center-to-center interelectrode distance of 20 mm were placed in accordance to the SENIAM guidelines (Hermans et al., 2000) and a previous investigation (McGill & Karpowicz, 2009). Electrodes were placed unilaterally on the right side of body for the rectus femoris (RF), rectus abdominis (RA), external oblique (EO), and the lumbar erector spinae longissimus (ES). The RF electrode was placed midway on the line from the anterior superior iliac spine to the superior part of the patella. The RA electrode was placed 1 cm lateral to the navel. The EO electrode was placed 3 cm lateral to the linea semilunaris but on the same level of RA electrode. The ES electrode was placed 3 cm lateral from the spinous process of L1. A single pregelled, disposable electrode (EL501, Biopac Systems Inc., Santa Barbara, CA) was placed on the spinous process of the seventh cervical vertebrae to serve as a reference electrode.

The raw EMG signals were recorded simultaneously with a Biopac data acquisition system (MP150WSW; Biopac Systems Inc., Goleta, CA) interfaced with a laptop computer (Inspiron 8200; Dell Inc., Round Rock, TX) using proprietary software (AcqKnowledge version 5.0; Biopac Systems Inc.). Sampling frequency was set at 1000 Hz and the amplitude of the signals was expressed as root mean square (RMS) values. The EMG signals were bandpass filtered at 10-500 Hz and then normalized to their respective MVC. All analyses were performed with a custom program written with LabVIEW software (version 8.5, National Instruments, Austin, Texas). The middle 10-second epoch of the data collection from each exercise was used for analysis.

Statistical Analysis

Four separate two-way mixed factorial ANOVAs (exercise [static vs. stationary vs. traveling] × sex [men vs. women]) were performed for each muscle. Post-hoc one-way ANOVAs were used when appropriate and necessary. An independent t-test was performed for body fat percentage between men and women. Four separate independent t-tests were performed for skinfold thickness of each site between men and women. An alpha of $P \leq 0.05$ was used to determine sta-

tistical significance for all comparisons. Data were analyzed using SPSS version 23 software (SPSS Inc., Chicago, IL).

RESULTS

Table 1 contains means ± SE for body fat percentage and skinfold thickness of the four electrode sites for men and women. There was a significant difference in body fat percentage between men and women ($P < 0.001$). In addition, there was a significant difference in skinfold thickness for the rectus femoris between men and women ($P = 0.017$). No significant differences in skinfold thickness were found between men and women for external oblique ($P = 0.788$), erector spinae ($P = 0.884$), or rectus abdominis ($P = 0.864$).

Table 2 contains means ± SE for normalized EMG amplitude values for muscle activation under the three exercise conditions collapsed across sex. The results are separated by muscle and their differences in the static (STA), stationary (STN), and traveling (TRV) exercises. There was no significant interactions for sex ($P > .05$); therefore, values are collapsed across sex.

For the rectus abdominis, there was no two-way interaction for exercise × sex ($P = 0.789$). However, there was a main effect for exercise ($P = 0.002$). Normalized EMG amplitude for STA was significantly lower than STN ($P = 0.003$) and TRV ($P = 0.001$) (Figure 4). In addition, there was a main effect for sex ($P = 0.001$), where women had higher activation in all three exercises.

For the external oblique, there was no two-way interaction for exercise × sex ($P = 0.287$). However, there was a main effect for exercise ($P < 0.001$). Normalized EMG amplitude for STA was significantly lower than STN ($P = 0.001$) and TRV ($P = 0.001$) and STN was significantly greater than TRV ($P = 0.009$) (Figure 5). In addition, there was a main effect for sex ($P = 0.012$) where women had higher activation in all three exercises.

For the erector spine, there was no two-way interaction for exercise × sex ($P = 0.713$). However, there was a main effect for exercise ($P < 0.001$). Normalized EMG amplitude for STA was significantly lower than STN ($P = 0.001$) and TRV ($P = 0.001$) (Figure 6). In addition, there was no main effect for sex ($P = 0.513$).

For the rectus femoris, there was no two-way interaction for exercise × sex ($P = 0.169$). However, there was a main effect for exercise ($P < 0.001$). Normalized EMG amplitude

Table 1. Means±SE for body fat percentage and skinfold thickness

Variables	Men	Women
Body fat	12.1±1.1*	21.3±0.8*
RF	15.7±1.5*	20.0±0.8*
AB	16.8±1.4	17.2±1.5
EO	14.7±1.6	14.1±1.6
ES	13.3±1.0	13.1±0.8

RF=Rectus Femoris; AB=Rectus Abdominis; EO=External Oblique; ES=Erector Spinae, *significant difference between sexes

Table 2. Normalized mean±SE for muscle activation under the three exercise conditions collapsed across sex

Muscle	Exercise		
	STA	**STN**	**TRV**
RF	31.46%±2.05%	50.97%±3.45%*	52.07%±3.67%*
AB	18.31%±2.51%	26.52%±3.43%*	24.30%±2.33%*
EO	95.01%±8.11%	171.28%±15.75%*#	139.93%±10.50%*#
ES	6.24%±0.60%	13.18%±1.20%*	12.45%±1.60%*

STA=Static; STN=Stationary; TRV=Traveling, RF=Rectus Femoris; AB=Rectus Abdominis; EO=External Oblique; ES=Erector Spinae, *significant difference from STA exercise, #significant difference among all exercises

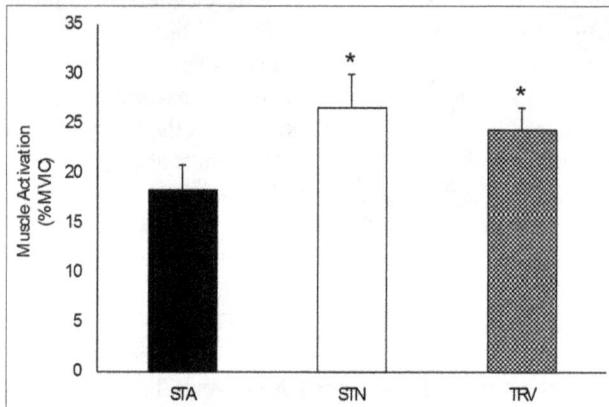

Figure 4. Mean ± SE for normalized EMG amplitude of the rectus abdominis. STA = Static, STN = Stationary, TRV = Traveling, *significant difference from STA

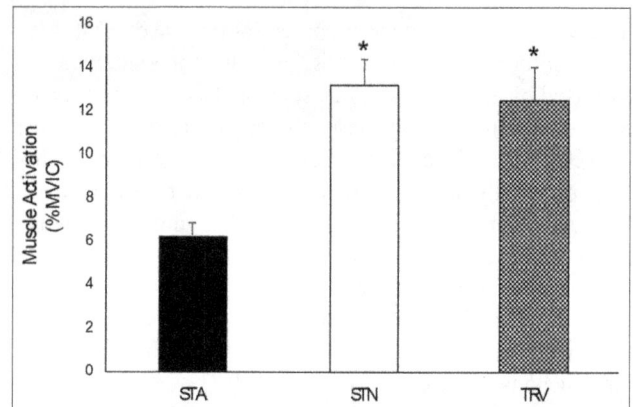

Figure 6. Mean ± SE for normalized EMG amplitude of the erector spinae. STA = Static, STN = Stationary, TRV = Traveling, *significant difference from STA

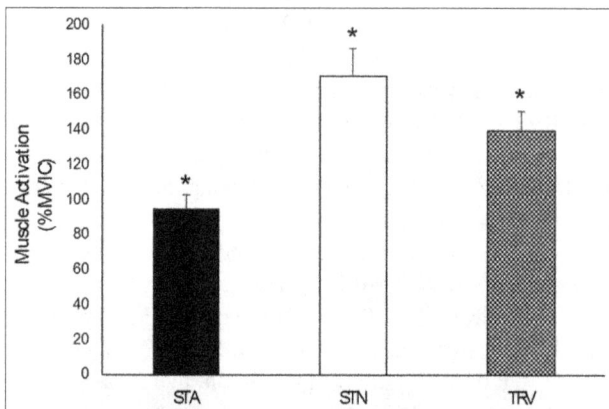

Figure 5. Mean ± SE for normalized EMG amplitude of the external oblique. STA = Static, STN = Stationary, TRV = Traveling, *significant difference from STA

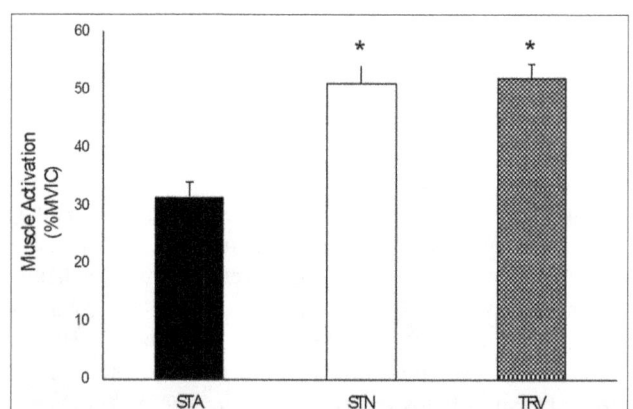

Figure 7. Mean ± SE for normalized EMG amplitude of the rectus femoris. STA = Static, STN = Stationary, TRV = Traveling, *significant difference from STA

for STA was significantly lower than STN ($P = 0.001$) and TRV ($P = 0.001$) (Figure 7). In addition, there was no main effect for sex ($P = 0.886$).

DISCUSSION

The results indicated there were differences in muscle activation among the static, stationary, and traveling trunk exercises. Based upon muscle activity, the exercises requiring movement of the upper and lower limbs elicited greater muscle activity while challenging coordination and balance. These findings are in congruence with Gottschall et

al. (2013) who reported integration core exercises requiring movement of the distal trunk, elicited higher activity of the primary abdominal and lumbar muscles compared to isolation exercises. The movement of the limbs with stabilization of the spine challenged postural stability and balance and resulted in greater muscle activation (Hanney, Pabian, Smith, & Patel, 2013). The current results are also in agreement with Anderson and Behm (2005) who reported as instability increases within a trunk stabilization exercise, trunk muscle activity increases. In addition, women had greater activation than men in all the exercises for the RA and EO. It is evident low back pain and injuries are common and on the rise

(Hanney et al., 2013). A major contributing factor to this is trunk instability and lack of trunk muscle endurance (Mc-Gill, 2010). Exercises focusing on neuromuscular control for trunk stabilization could be advantageous in a low back injury prevention program (Stevens et al., 2007; Wheeler et al., 2015). Such exercises include the four-point kneeling bird dog with extension of the contra-lateral limbs, which contain similar elements as the stationary and traveling exercises tested in the present study.

The progression in muscle activation of static, stationary, and traveling exercises was shown to be correct for the rectus femoris. As for the rectus abdominis and erector spinae, the stationary exercise elicited greater muscle activation than the traveling exercise, albeit not significantly. Only the external oblique; however, showed a significant difference between the stationary and traveling exercise. Overall, the progression in movement from a static to stationary to traveling position did not show the same progression in level of muscle activity for the majority of the muscles tested. There was a main effect for sex for the rectus abdominis and the external oblique muscles. In all three exercises, women had greater relative muscle activation than men. This may be in part due to the exercise being relatively more difficult to perform for the women compared to the men and because of more strength-trained men participants than women. Therefore, the men may have had a stronger trunk and could utilize their strength more effectively in the exercises. Although in this case, greater muscle activation could not be explained by body composition, since women typically have higher levels of subcutaneous fat that could act as a filter. In the present study, women had significantly higher body fat percentage than men. Consequently, they had less fat-free mass and possibly needed greater activation to perform the exercises. Another possibility of women having greater muscle activation may be due to women adopting different motor recruitment strategies than men as reported in a study investigating unanticipated cutting maneuvers where women used different co-contraction strategies to achieve stabilization at the knee (Beaulieu, Lamontagne, & Xu, 2008). However, in regards to muscle activity, no sex differences were found in a study comparing muscle activity in unilateral weight bearing tasks (Bouillon et al., 2012), trunk muscle activation during a squat and a deadlift compared to isometric instability exercises (Hamlyn, Behm, & Young, 2007), and in various popular trunk exercises (Youdas et al., 2008).

McGill (2010) described that a strong and conditioned trunk musculature is needed to produce, control, and transfer force in various if not all movements. If the musculature cannot maintain strength to combat "energy leaks" or sustain a load over a long duration, the tissue will fatigue with each repetition and might eventually result in injury (McGill, 2010). Therefore, a compelling reason to strengthen the trunk musculature for adults or athletes is to decrease the chance of injury, especially low back and hip injuries as well as pain. Injury occurs when the applied load exceeds the strength of the tissue (McGill, 2015). More commonly, the injury results from the accumulation of repetitive micro-traumas when the tissue is fatigued (McGill, 2015). Strengthening the core through stabilization exercises improves postural

control and the ability to land and decelerate the body, which increases the athlete's resistance to injury (Sadeghi, Shariat, Asadmanesh, & Mosavat, 2013). Thus, it is important to incorporate exercises that challenge the strength and endurance of the trunk musculature in maintaining a neutral spine to prevent sub-traumas that will result in injuries. However, for improving sports performance, exercises targeting the trunk musculature might not be as beneficial and incorporating compound movements such as the front and back squats might be enough stress the trunk to improve strength and endurance (Tyler, Adams, & DeBeliso, 2017). Nevertheless, for younger and less fit athletes, developing a proper foundation of trunk strength and endurance is essential to prevent future injury.

It has been researched and reported that the safest manner to train the trunk musculature is to maintain the spine in a neutral position when any load is placed on the body (Mendrin et al., 2016). Different strategies are used to place load on the body, including holding the pelvis off the floor and then moving the limbs in various positions (Vera-Garcia et al., 2014). The static, stationary, and traveling exercises used in this study fulfilled these loading properties. In addition, static exercises may be easier to learn and require less muscle activity. Therefore, static exercises are a good precursor for younger athletes and patients undergoing rehabilitation to acquire a foundation for trunk strength and endurance. Participants were limited to a population of convenience, which consisted of college-age participants from the local university and a strength and conditioning facility. In addition, no comparisons were made between individuals who were experienced in different modes of training (e.g., resistance, aerobic, etc.). Future studies include examining chronic effects of training with the exercises used in the present study and investigating participants already familiar with these exercises. Furthermore, future investigations may compare potential differences in balance and stability between static and stationary exercises training programs.

CONCLUSION

In conclusion, there was greater muscle activation in the stationary and traveling exercises compared to the static exercise. The next progression from a static exercise may be a stationary or traveling exercise. Other than the external oblique, there was no significance difference in muscle activity between stationary and traveling modes of trunk exercises. Due to the significant differences in muscle activity from the static mode, personal trainers, sports coaches, and allied health professionals who are seeking to increase instability during a trunk exercise, may wish to incorporate stationary and traveling variations into their training prescription. Stationary and traveling exercises with the movement of the limbs might potentially offer an alternative when training for trunk stabilization.

REFERENCES

Anderson, K., & Behm, D. G. (2005). The impact of instability resistance training on balance and stability. *Sports*

Medicine, 35(1), 43-53.

Beaulieu, M., Lamontagne, M., & Xu, L. (2008). Gender differences in time-frequency EMG analysis of unanticipated cutting maneuvers. *Medicine Science in Sports Exercise, 40*(10), 1795- 1804.

Bouillon, L. E., Wilhelm, J., Eisel, P., Wiesner, J., Rachow, M., & Hatteberg, L. (2012). Electromyographic assessment of muscle activity between genders during unilateral weight-bearing tasks using adjusted distances. *International Journal of Sports Physical Therapy, 7*(6), 595-605.

Demoulin, C., Vanderthommen, M., Duysens, C., & Crielaard, J.-M. (2006). Spinal muscle evaluation using the Sorensen test: a critical appraisal of the literature. *Joint Bone Spine, 73*(1), 43-50.

Gottschall, J. S., Mills, J., & Hastings, B. (2013). Integration core exercises elicit greater muscle activation than isolation exercises. *The Journal of Strength & Conditioning Research, 27*(3), 590-596.

Hamlyn, N., Behm, D. G., & Young, W. B. (2007). Trunk muscle activation during dynamic weight-training exercises and isometric instability activities. *The Journal of Strength & Conditioning Research, 21*(4), 1108-1112.

Hanney, W. J., Pabian, P. S., Smith, M. T., & Patel, C. K. (2013). Low back pain: movement considerations for exercise and training. *Strength & Conditioning Journal, 35*(4), 99-106.

Hermens, H.J., Freriks, B., Disselhorst-Klug, C., Rau, G. Development of recommendations for SEMG sensors and sensor placement procedures. *J Electromyogr Kinesiol* 2000: 10: 361-374.

Hodges, P. W., & Richardson, C. A. (1997). Contraction of the abdominal muscles associated with movement of the lower limb. *Physical therapy, 77*(2), 132-142.

McGill, S. M. (2010). Core training: evidence translating to better performance and injury prevention. *Strength & Conditioning Journal, 32*(3), 33-46.

McGill, S. M. (2015). *Low Back Disorders, 3E*: Human Kinetics.

McGill, S. M., Grenier, S., Kavcic, N., & Cholewicki, J. (2003). Coordination of muscle activity to assure stability of the lumbar spine. *Journal of Electromyography and Kinesiology, 13*(4), 353-359.

McGill, S. M., McDermott, A., Fenwick, C. M. (2009). Comparison of different strongman events: Trunk muscle activation and lumbar spine motion, load and stiffness. *Journal of Strength & Conditioning Research, 23*(4), 1148-1161.

McGill, S. M., & Karpowicz, A. (2009). Exercises for spine stabilization: motion/motor patterns, stability progressions, and clinical technique. *Archives of Physical Medicine and Rehabilitation, 90*(1), 118-126.

Mendrin, N., Lynn, S. K., Griffith-Merritt, H. K., & Noffal, G. J. (2016). Progressions of isometric core training. *Strength & Conditioning Journal, 38*(4), 50-65.

Meucci, R. D., Fassa, A. G., & Faria, N. M. X. (2015). Prevalence of chronic low back pain: systematic review. *Revista De Saude Publica, 49,* 1-10.

Okada, T., Huxel, K. C., & Nesser, T. W. (2011). Relationship between core stability, functional movement, and performance. *The Journal of Strength & Conditioning Research, 25*(1), 252-261.

Sadeghi, H., Shariat, A., Asadmanesh, E., & Mosavat, M. (2013). The effects of core stability exercise on the dynamic balance of volleyball players. *International Journal of Applied Exercise Physiology, 2(2),* 1-10.

Stevens, V. K., Coorevits, P. L., Bouche, K. G., Mahieu, N. N., Vanderstraeten, G. G., & Danneels, L. A. (2007). The influence of specific training on trunk muscle recruitment patterns in healthy subjects during stabilization exercises. *Manual Therapy, 12*(3), 271-279.

Tyler, R., Adams, K. J., & DeBeliso, M. (2017). The relationship between core stability & squat ratio in resistance-trained males. *International Journal of Kinesiology & Sports Science, 5*(2), 7-15.

Vera-Garcia, F. J., Barbado, D., & Moya, M. (2014). Trunk stabilization exercises for healthy individuals. *Revista Brasileira de Cineantropometria & Desempenho Humano, 16*(2), 200-211.

Wheeler, R. (2015). Limiting lower back injuries with proper technique and strengthening. *Strength & Conditioning Journal, 37*(1), 18-23.

Youdas, J. W., Guck, B. R., Hebrink, R. C., Rugotzke, J. D., Madson, T. J., & Hollman, J. H. (2008). An electromyographic analysis of the Ab-Slide exercise, abdominal crunch, supine double leg thrust, and side bridge in healthy young adults: implications for rehabilitation professionals. *The Journal of Strength & Conditioning Research, 22*(6), 1939-1946.

9

The Effects of High Intensity Neuromuscular Electrical Stimulation on Abdominal Strength and Endurance, Core Strength, Abdominal Girth, and Perceived Body Shape and Satisfaction

John Porcari*, Abigail Ryskey, Carl Foster

Department of Exercise and Sport Science, University of Wisconsin- La Crosse, La Crosse, WI USA
Corresponding Author: John Porcari, E-mail: jporcari@uwlax.edu

ARTICLE INFO	ABSTRACT
Conflicts of interest: None Funding: This study was funded by a grant from Bio-Medical Research, Ltd, Galway, Ireland	**Background:** Neuromuscular electrical stimulation (NMES) has been used clinically for many years as a modality to improve muscular strength and endurance. Recently, equipment manufacturers have developed over-the-counter NMES units to target specific muscle groups, particularly the abdominal region. **Objective:** To study the effects of self-administered neuromuscular electrical stimulation (NMES) on changes in abdominal muscle strength and endurance, core strength, abdominal girth, and subjective measures of body satisfaction and shape. **Methods:** Fifty-three adults were randomly assigned into high intensity (HI: n=27) or low intensity (LI: n=26) groups. The NMES device for the LI group had been altered so that subjects felt some tactile sensation, but the intensity was not sufficient to elicit a muscular contraction. All subjects stimulated their abdominal muscles 5 days per week (30 minutes per session) for 6 weeks. Subjects were tested at Baseline, 2, 4, and 6 weeks. **Results:** The HI group had a significantly greater increase in strength at 4 weeks (19%) and 6 weeks (29%) compared to the LI group and performed significantly more curl-ups than the LI group at 2 weeks (62%). Both groups had a significant increase in core strength over the course of the study, with no difference between groups. There was no change in abdominal girth between groups. Both groups had significant improvements in body satisfaction from Baseline to 4 weeks and Baseline to 6 weeks, with no significant interaction. **Conclusions:** Results of the current study indicate that high intensity NMES can significantly increase abdominal strength and endurance compared to LI intensity (control) stimulation. Results for subjective measures tended to favor the HI group, but were less conclusive, since the LI group also had some positive changes.

Key words: Prone Plank Test, Curl-ups, Slendertone, Placebo |

INTRODUCTION

Neuromuscular electrical stimulation (NMES) is a well-established therapeutic modality that has been used for many years in the practice of physical therapy. When traditional exercise is not possible due to injury or surgery, NMES may be used as a means of maintaining muscular strength and minimizing atrophy due to immobilization (Hainaut & Duchateau, 1992). In the 1960's, Kots (1977) reported using NMES as a training adjunct with elite athletes in the former Soviet Union and reported strength improvement of 30- 40%. He suggested that NMES might be more effective than volitional exercise for strength improvement. In recent years, fitness equipment companies have marketed NMES devices for healthy individuals as an alternative way to improve muscle strength and endurance and improve body composition. These devices are designed for many different muscle groups, but are of particular interest for the abdominal region. The desire of Americans to have a trim waist and

flat stomach without having to exercise is an attractive option for many people. There are conflicting results regarding the effects of NMES on the abdominal musculature. Many studies have demonstrated significant improvements in abdominal strength and endurance, perceived muscle tone, and body satisfaction following NMES training (Alon et al., 1987; Alon et al., 1992, Abendroth-Smith & Sword, 1977; Anderson et al., 2006, Ballantyne & Donne, 1999; Porcari et al., 2005), while others have shown no improvement in these parameters (Aikman, et al., 1985; Porcari et al., 2002).

Whether or not improvements in muscular strength and endurance are seen with NMES is reasonably dependent upon the strength of the resulting contraction. Those studies that have utilized contractions in excess of 60% of maximum voluntary contraction (MVC) have shown positive benefits (Currier & Mann, 1983; Muffiuletti, 2002; Selkowitz, 1989; and Soo et al., 1988). Many over-the-counter NMES devices do not deliver a strong enough stimulus to reach this threshold. A previous study in our laboratory (Porcari et al., 2002) investigated the effects of training with one of these devices (Body Shapers, International, Model BM1012BI) on the strength of various muscle groups, body composition, and physical appearance. No statistically significant improvements in any of the outcome measurements were found. The conclusion of the study was that the stimulator and electrodes used to deliver the stimulation were poorly constructed and did not deliver a strong enough current to elicit a contraction of sufficient strength to induce gains in strength. Additionally, the stimulation was very uncomfortable for subjects. Measures taken during stimulated contractions suggested that the percentage of maximal strength that the muscles were contracting was less than 20% of MVC.

In an attempt to overcome this deficiently and elicit stronger muscular contractions, Bio-Medical Research, Ltd. (Galway, Ireland) developed an NMES belt that targets the abdominal muscles. The device delivers an electrical current to the abdominal region using medical-grade adhesive pads placed over motor units of the abdominal musculature. The belt is cleared by the Food and Drug Administration (FDA) in the United Sates to increase the strength and tone of the abdominal muscles. A subsequent study from our laboratory (Porcari et al., 2005) supported these claims, as abdominal strength improved 49% and abdominal endurance increased 72% compared to a non-stimulation control group. There was also an increase in perceived muscle tone in all subjects in the stimulation group, as well as reduction in abdominal girth. A criticism of the above study was that the control group did not receive any intervention. Thus, it was felt that some of the improvement in the stimulation group, particularly regarding subjective outcome measures, was attributable to the placebo effect. Bio-Medical Research, Ltd. has developed a newer NMES device called the Slendertone® System Abs belt, which has the same indications for use as the Slendertone® FLEX, but with higher intensity levels. The higher intensity levels are purported to elicit stronger, more effective muscle contractions. The purpose of this study was to determine the efficacy of the Slendertone® System Abs belt for increasing abdominal muscular strength and endurance, improving core muscle strength, decreasing abdominal girth, and improving self-perceived body satisfaction and abdominal muscle tone in healthy, middle-aged adults.

METHODS

Subjects

Fifty-six adult volunteers from the La Crosse, Wisconsin area were recruited through an advertisement in the local newspaper. Inclusion criteria required the subjects to be between 25 and 55 years old, to be healthy by their own report, to have a body mass index (BMI) between 18 and 30, and not to have been involved in any type of formal abdominal training program within the previous 6 months. In addition, subjects with any implanted medical devices (pacemaker, pump, catheter, etc.), insertion or removal of an IUD contraceptive

device (i.e. coil) within the previous month, or who were currently pregnant or had given birth in the previous three months were excluded. Subjects were randomly assigned into one of two groups: a high intensity treatment group (HI) or a low intensity treatment group (LI). Group assignment was randomized and training was double-blinded. Both groups were instructed not to alter their diet or engage in any additional exercise over the course of the 6-week study period. All subjects gave written informed consent prior to participating in the study and the protocol was approved by the Institutional Review Board for the Protection of Human Subjects at the University of Wisconsin-La Crosse. Subjects in both groups received a $200 honorarium and a stimulation belt at the conclusion of the study.

Testing

All subjects completed an identical battery of tests at Baseline and at 2, 4, and 6 weeks of the study protocol. Testing included a series of questionnaires, anthropometric measurements, and determination of abdominal muscle strength, abdominal endurance, and core muscle strength. All tests were given in the same order for all subjects. Testers were blinded to group assignment of the subjects.

Questionnaires

Subjects completed two questionnaires: The Body Satisfaction Scale and an Overall Results Questionnaire. The Body Satisfaction Scale has been used in a previous study (Porcari et al., 2005) and assessed responses to 10 opposite descrip-tors of body satisfaction. Each set of descriptors was given a score between one (most negative) and five (most positive). At the final visit, participants in both groups also complet-ed an Overall Results Questionnaire. The questionnaire was a simple 13-item questionnaire that asked for a subject's agreement or disagreement with a set of statements regard-ing their perceived benefits from participating in the study.

Anthropometric Measures

Body weight was measured to the nearest 0.1 kilogram using a standard laboratory beam scale and height was measured to the nearest 0.1 centimeter using a stadiometer. Body mass index (BMI) was calculated from height and weight. Two circumference measurements were taken. One measurement (abdominal measurement) was taken horizontally at the level of the natural waist (the smallest circumference between the ribs and the iliac crest). The second measurement (waist measurement) was taken at the level of the umbilicus. Two measurements were taken at each site. A third measurement was taken if there was greater than one centimeter difference between the first two measurements. The average of the two closest measurements was used in the analysis. All abdominal and waist circumference measurements were made by the same examiner throughout the study using a spring-loaded tape measure.

Abdominal Strength

Abdominal strength was measured by having the subject perform five isometric contractions using an isokinetic dynamometer (Biodex, USA). The subject rested supine on a movable bench in a bent-knee position. The lever arm of the isokinetic dynamometer was set horizontal with the ground (180 degrees) and the padded extension arm was placed just below the nipple line on the lower third of the sternum. The height of the bench was adjusted for each subject so that the extension arm remained at 180 degrees. Each subject was given several practice trials to make sure the position of the lever arm was comfortable on their chest. Subjects then performed five maximal isometric contractions, with 30 seconds rest between repetitions. The average torque measurement of the highest two repetitions was used in the analysis. Reliability of the abdominal strength test in our laboratory is ICC=.96.

Abdominal Endurance

Abdominal endurance was assessed using the American College of Sports Medicine (ACSM) paced curl-up test (ACSM, 2000). The subjects were in a supine position on a mat with the knees bent to 90 degrees (measured with a goniometer). The subject's arms were at the side, palms facing down, with the middle fingers touching a piece of tape. A second piece of tape was placed 8 cm (for those who were ≥ 45 years) or 12 cm (for those who were <45 years) from the first piece of tape. The subject's shoes remained on during the test. The individual completed slow, controlled curl-ups to lift the shoulder blades off the mat (trunk makes a 30-degree angle with the mat) in time with a pre-recorded tape at a pace of 40 curl-ups per minute. The subject performed as many curl-ups as possible without pausing. The test was terminated when the subject could no longer keep up with the pace of the tape or their fingers could not reach the second piece of tape. The reliability of the abdominal endurance test in our laboratory is ICC=.83.

Core Strength

Core strength was measured using the Prone Plank test (Quinn, 2008). Subjects assumed the prone "plank" position, with their full body weight supported only by the forearms and toes. Their body was straight with the elbows parallel to each other and directly under the shoulders. They held this "plank" position for a period of 60 seconds. At the end of the 60 second period, the subjects successively raised each limb individually for a period of 15 seconds each. They then were to raise their right arm and left leg for 15 seconds then their left arm and right leg for 15 seconds. Upon completion of the limb movements, the subjects returned to the plank position for 30 seconds. These series of movements were continued until the subject could no longer continue or was no longer able to maintain a straight body position. The total hold time was measured for each subject. The reliability of the prone plank test in our laboratory is ICC=.90.

Training

All subjects underwent stimulation five times per week for six weeks. Each session was 30 minutes in duration. The NMES device used in the current study was the Slendertone® System Abs belt (Bio-Medical Research, Ltd. (Galway, Ireland). The belt uses three pre-gelled electrodes to deliver an electrical current to the abdominal region. The HI group used the stimulation belt that is currently on the market. The LI group used the same belt, but the stimulator had been altered so that the electrical current was strong enough to cause some tactile sensation, but was not strong enough to elicit a visible muscular contraction. Both groups used program number 3 on the stimulation controller. Each subject was given an individual orientation session, during which they were supervised for their first stimulation session. All other stimulation sessions were completed on their own. Subjects in both groups were encouraged to use the highest tolerable level on their stimulator to achieve the strongest possible contractions. Subjects recorded the maximum intensity reached during each stimulation session in a training log.

Statistics

Standard descriptive statistics were used to characterize the subject population. Changes in anthropometric data, the Body Satisfaction Scale, abdominal strength, abdominal endurance, and core strength were analyzed using a 3-way ANOVA with repeated measures (Group X Gender X Time). Since there were no differences in the responses of male and females, data were collapsed across gender. Data were then analyzed with a 2-way ANOVA with repeated measures (Group X Time). When there was a significant F ratio, Tukey's post-hoc tests were used to isolate pairwise differences. A Mann Whitney-U test was used to compare differences in the frequency of responses between groups for the Shape Evaluation Scale over the four testing periods. Alpha was set at 0.05 to achieve statistical significance for all analyses. Data were analyzed using SPSS version 25.0.

RESULTS

Fifty-three of the original 56 subjects successfully completed the study. One member of the LI group withdrew from the study due to dissatisfaction with the training intensity delivered by the attenuated device and another subject in the LI group was disqualified for doing additional sit-ups during the study period. One subject in the HI group was withdrawn from the study after experiencing heavier than usual blood flow during menses. For the final analysis there were 27 subjects in the HI group (14 male and 13 female) and 26 subjects in the LI group (12 male and 14 female). Descriptive characteristics of the subjects who completed the study are presented in Table 1. There were no significant differences between groups at the start of the study for any of the outcome measures.

Anthropometric Measurements

Results for the anthropometric data collected during the study are presented in Table 2. There were no significant

Table 1. Descriptive characteristics of the subjects who completed the study.

Group	Age (yr)	Height (cm)	Weight (kg)	BMI
High Intensity				
Males	39.7±8.0	178.3±6.4	79.8±7.7	25.2±2.4
Females	39.5±9.8	161.9±5.6	62.1±5.5	23.7±1.9
Overall	39.6±8.7	170.4±10.2	71.4±11.4	24.4±2.2
Low Intensity				
Males	37.3±9.0	178.0±8.1	82.7±8.6	26.2±2.6
Females	40.7±8.2	168.7±6.6	72.3±7.3	25.4±2.3
Overall	38.8±8.5	173.0±8.6	77.2±9.4	25.7±2.5

Values represent mean and standard deviation

Table 2. Changes in body weight, BMI, waist circumference, and abdominal circumference over the course of the study.

Variable	Group	Baseline	Week 2	Week 4	Week 6
Body Weight (kg)	High Intensity	71.4±11.4	71.5±11.4	71.5±11.4	71.7±11.4
	Low Intensity	77.2±9.4	77.3±9.5	77.0±9.7	77.2±9.7
Body Mass Index	High Intensity	24.4±2.2	24.4±2.3	24.4±2.3	25.4±2.4
	Low Intensity	25.7±2.5	25.8±2.4	25.7±2.5	25.7±2.5
Waist Circumference (cm)	High Intensity	82.3±9.2	81.9±9.6	80.4±13.7	82.0±9.5
	Low Intensity	85.0±8.6	84.6±8.7	83.0±8.8	84.3±8.9
Abdominal Circumference (cm)	High Intensity	90.0±7.9	88.4±8.3	88.0±8.6	87.6±8.3
	Low Intensity	94.0±7.5	92.4±7.3	90.5±7.4	90.5±7.4

Values represent mean and standard deviation

changes in body weight, BMI, abdominal circumference, or waist circumference in either group over the course of the study.

Abdominal Strength

Abdominal strength for each group at each time point are presented in Figure 1. There was a significant main effect across testing time ($p<.001$) and a significant interaction between groups across time ($p<.001$). There were no significant changes for the LI group across the 6-week study. The HI group had significant increases in strength at weeks 4 and 6 compared to Baseline. Changes between groups were statistically significant at weeks 4 and 6.

Abdominal Endurance

Curl-up performance of the two groups is presented in Figure 2. There was a significant main effect across testing time ($p<.001$) and a significant interaction between groups across time ($p=.034$). There were no significant increases for the LI group at any time point compared to Baseline. The HI group had significant improvements in curl-up performance after 2, 4, and 6 weeks compared to Baseline. Changes between groups were statistically significant only at week 2.

Prone Plank Test

Changes in prone plank test performance are presented in Figure 3. There was a significant main effect across time ($p=.001$), but there was no significant interaction between groups across time ($p=.27$). There were no significant in-

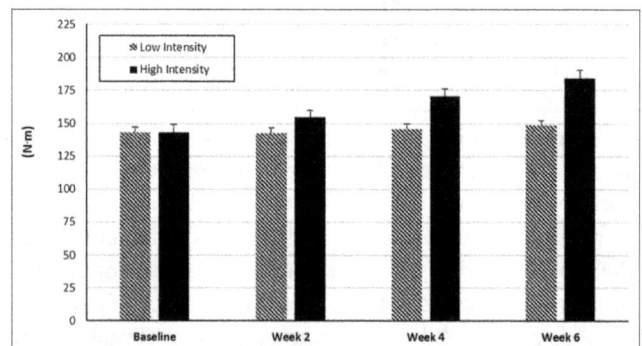

Figure 1. Changes in abdominal strength over the course of the 6-week study. Values represent mean and standard deviation

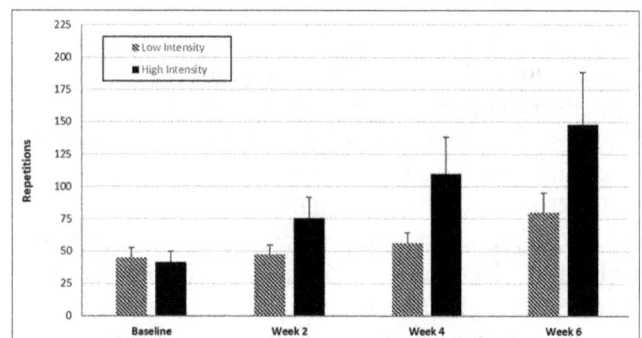

Figure 2. Changes in curl-ups completed over the course of the 6-week study. Values represent mean and standard deviation

creases for the LI group at any time point compared to Baseline. The HI group had significant improvements in prone plank performance at 4 and 6 weeks compared to Baseline, but these differences were not significantly different than the LI group at the same time points.

Questionnaire Data

Summary data for the Body Satisfaction Scale are presented in Table 3. There was a significant main effect across time (p<.001), but there was no significant interaction between groups and time (p=.43). Both groups had significant improvements in the total score at 4 weeks and 6 weeks compared to Baseline.

For the Overall Results Questionnaire, significantly more subjects in the HI group reported that they noticed positive results after using the belt compared to the LI group (96% vs. 56%). Significantly more subjects in the HI group also reported an improvement in the perceived firmness (92% vs. 63%) and tone (81% vs. 56%) of their stomach muscles compared to the LI group. An improvement in perceived strength of the abdominal muscles was reported by 92% of the HI group compared to 70% of the LI group. However, this difference was not statistically significant. Significantly more subjects in the HI group felt that using the belt was as effective as sit-ups compared to the LI group (81% vs. 44%).

DISCUSSION

The present study found 19% and 29% gains in abdominal strength after 4 and 6 weeks of high intensity stimulation, respectively. These results are in line with results from other studies that have used EMS to stimulate the abdominal musculature (Alon et al., 1987; Alon et al., 1992; Ballantyne & Donne, 1999). The results of Alon et al. (1987) and Alon et al. (1992) are virtually identical to those of the current study, as they found increase of 20.8% and 19.6%, respectively, after 4 weeks of EMS training. Since Alon's studies were both 4 weeks in duration, comparisons beyond that point are not

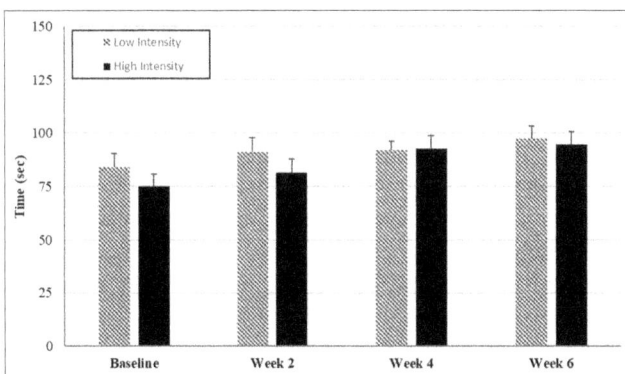

Figure 3. Changes in prone plank time over the course of the 6-week study. Values represent mean and standard deviation

possible. The magnitude of the strength improvements seen in the current study are less than those reported previously in our laboratory using a previous version of the belt (Porcari et al., 2005). In the current study a 19% improvement was apparent after 4 weeks, compared to a 34% strength increase in the earlier study after the same amount of time. In the previous study strength improvement was not measured at 6 weeks; however, using linear extrapolation, improvement would have been approximately 46%, compared to 29% in the current study. It has been suggested that in the earlier study a greater number of training sessions were supervised, which may have led to increased compliance with the treatment protocol; hence greater strength improvement. However, the device used in the current study recorded the frequency of stimulation sessions as well as the peak stimulation level used during each session. Attendance to the number of training sessions for every individual in the study was exactly as prescribed (5 sessions per week for 6 weeks). Peak intensity was slightly lower in the current study versus the earlier study. However, since the available intensity of the stimulator used in the current study (Slendertone® System Abs) was stronger than that used in the previous study (Slendertone® FLEX), the intensity of the achieved contractions were assumed to be similar.

The HI group had significantly greater improvements in abdominal endurance at 2 weeks compared to the LI group. The data at weeks 4 and 6 also indicated a strong trend in favor of the HI group. However, due to the large standard deviation of scores, the difference was not statistically significant at either time point. The percentage increases in the HI group at 2, 4, and 6 weeks were 64%, 133%, and 243%, respectively, compared to 2%, 15%, and 73% for the LI group at the same time points. The difference in improvement between the HI and LI groups were 62%, 118%, and 170% at weeks 2, 4, and 6. The magnitude of the net improvement for the HI group in the current study was larger than previously found in our laboratory (Porcari et al., 2005). When looking at the raw data, it was observed that two male subjects in the HI group did 575 and 600 curl-ups at the 4-week time period. These same individuals did 800 and 797 curl-ups, respectively, at the 6-week testing mark. As the curl-ups for these individuals were conducted according to protocol, their data was included in the final analysis. Had the data for these two individuals been removed from the data set, the net improvement between the HI and LI groups at weeks 4 (the only comparable testing time between the two studies), would have been 40% in favor of the HI group. This is comparable to the 49% improvement seen in the previous study at the same time point.

Another fact to point out was that the LI group had a 15% improvement in curl-up performance at the 4 – Week

Table 3. Total score on the Body Satisfaction Scale for both groups over the course of the study

Group	Baseline	Week 2	Week 4	Week 6
High Intensity	25.1±6.44	27.8±5.36	29.4±5.09*	31.4±5.11*
Low Intensity	24.3±5.86	26.5±5.05	28.9±5.46*	30.4±4.44*

Values represent mean and standard deviation.* Significantly different than Baseline (p<.05).

testing time and a 73% improvement at the 6 – Week testing point. In the previous study by Porcari et al. (2005), a passive control group (no stimulation) had a 28% improvement in curl-up performance after 8 weeks. This would indicate that there is learning effect associated with performance of the curl-up test. However, the magnitude of the improvement over time, coupled with the fact that the subjects in the current study were receiving some simulation, even though it was at a very low level, suggests that the LI group may have had some improvement in muscular performance. Consistent with this finding is the report of Alon et al. (1997) of a 14% increase in strength when subjects received very low levels of abdominal electrical stimulation (just enough to elicit a visible tetanic contraction) for 3 hours per day. Another possibility is that because tests like the curl-up test are effort dependent; improvements may have reflected an increased effort on the part of subjects. If they felt that the belt was providing a benefit, they may have tried harder during the later testing sessions.

Results for core strength testing showed significant improvements for both groups. The HI group improved 18% after 6 weeks and the LI group improved 12% over the same time frame. Since the prone plank test is a novel test for most people, performance on the test depends a great deal on technique and balance. It is plausible that the overall improvement reflected an improvement in technique, which may have masked any therapeutic difference that may have existed between the groups.

There were no significant changes in any of the anthropometric measures over the course of the study. There was a non-significant decrease in abdominal circumference (the smallest circumference between the ribs and the iliac crest) in both groups. This finding is in conflict with the results of a previous study completed in our laboratory (Porcari et al., 2005). That study found a decrease of 2.6 centimeters in abdominal circumferences after 8 weeks of stimulation. The magnitude of the decrease in abdominal circumference in the above study is similar to that found in the current study (2.4 cm for the HI group and 3.5 cm for the LI group). However, because there were changes in both groups and because there were no changes in body weight in either group, the decreases were attributed to a consistent evaluator error. Abendroth-Smith and Sword (1977) also failed to find reductions in abdominal girth following 8 weeks of NMES, despite significant improvements in strength.

Several studies have found abdominal NMES training to have a positive effect on self-perception and body image measures (Anderson et al., 2006; Porcari et al., 2005). This study also found significant improvements in the subjective data. However, positive improvements were seen in both groups. Results of the Body Satisfaction Scale were virtually identical between groups, with both the HI and LI groups improving their scores after 4 and 6 weeks of the study. Additionally, even though the HI group had subjectively greater improvements in perceived abdominal firmness and tone than the LI group, the LI group also perceived some benefit. There are a number of possible explanations as to why the LI group had improvements in

the subjective tests. In the studies by Porcari et al. (2005) and Anderson et al. (2006), subjects in the control group did not receive any intervention. In the current study, the LI group (designed to be the control group) used belts that elicited some tactile sensation, but no visible muscular contraction. It is likely that because the LI group did feel something, they felt like they were getting a benefit. Anderson et al. (2006) attributed improvements in subjective measures to improvements in abdominal and waist circumference. This could have also played a role in the current study. Even though subjects were not told their previous scores at follow-up testing sessions, many of them could remember their previous values. Thus, since some of knew that they had completed more sit-ups or knew that their abdominal circumference was less during the earlier testing sessions; they assumed that the belt was working. Thus, it would be logical for them to feel better about their midsection.

It was also likely that many of the subjects had seen advertising about the positive results from the previous study (Porcari et al., 2005). That study found significant improvements in muscle strength and endurance and 100% of the subjects felt that the NMES device improved their abdominal firmness and tone. Thus, subjects probably entered the current study expecting positive benefits. Because none of the subjects had used electrical stimulation previously, they did not know what NMES was supposed to feel like. Even though subjects in the LI group were receiving a low threshold stimulus, they were fooled into thinking that it was working. It was interesting to note that 81% of the HI group and 44 % of the LI group felt that using the belt was as effective as sit-ups. This further illustrates the magnitude of the placebo effect, since the LI device did not elicit any visible muscle contraction.

The strength of the current study was that the control group actually underwent some sort of intervention, as opposed to just going through all of the testing at the various time points. Additional strengths of the study were that the examiners were blinded to group assignment and the study was overseen by an external study monitor. All facets of data collection and data input were independently verified prior to analysis. The major limitation of the study was that training sessions were carried out independently by subjects and were not monitored. We did not feel monitoring was necessary, since the simulator recorded the number of sessions completed, average intensity of stimulation, and peak intensity. Despite this, future studies may want to include training supervision. Also, since the simulation belt provides an improvement in muscular strength and endurance without having to do traditional abdominal exercises, a similar study could be conducted in individuals in which abdominal exercises may be contraindicated (e.g. people with low back pain).

CONCLUSIONS

High intensity electrical muscle stimulation to the abdominal musculature resulted in greater improvements in abdominal muscular strength and endurance compared to low intensity (control) stimulation. The non-significant improvements in abdominal endurance and core strength in the LI group were thought to be due to a learning effect associated with the tests performed, the placebo effect, or a combination of both factors. It is also possible that these results could have been due to the fact that the LI group was receiving a very low level of electrical stimulation, which could have caused some positive neuromuscular changes. Since the results of the current study and data available in the literature present conflicting results regarding the effect of NMES on body composition and perceived body image, additional well-designed studies are needed to clarify this issue. Additionally, future studies may want to compare the potential benefits of traditional abdominal exercises vs. NMES applied to the abdominal musculature.

REFERENCES

Abendroth-Smith, J., & Sword, K. (1977). Toning and strengthening predominant muscle groups through electrical muscle stimulation. *Medicine and Science in Sports and Exercise, 29(5)*, 165.

Aikman, H.D., Majerus, J.J., Van Wart, K.W., Barr, J.O., & Cook, T.M. (1985). Effects of electrical stimulation vs. sit-ups on abdominal strength and endurance. *Physical Therapy, 65*, 596.

Alon, G., Frederickson, R., Gallagher, L., Rehwoldt, C.T., Guillen, M., Putnam-Pement, M.L., & Barhart, J.B. (1992). Electrical stimulation of the abdominals: The effects of three versus five weekly treatments. *Journal of Clinical Electrophysiology, 4*, 5-11.

Alon, G., McCombe, S.A., Koutsantinis, S., Stumphauzer, L.J., Burgwin., K.C., Parent, M.M., & Bosworth, A. (1987). Comparison of the effects of electrical stimulation and exercise on abdominal musculature. *The Journal of Orthopaedic and Sports Physical Therapy, 8*, 567-573.

Alon, G., & Taylor, D.J. (1997). Electrically elicited minimal visible tetanic contraction and its effect on abdominal muscles strength and endurance. *European Journal of Physical Medicine and Rehabilitation, 7*, 2-6.

American College of Sports Medicine. (2000). ACSM's Guidelines for Exercise Testing and Prescription. 6th Edition. Lippincott Williams & Wilkins, Philadelphia.

Anderson, A.G., Murphy, M.H., Murtagh, E., & Nevill, A. (2006). An 8-week randomized controlled trial on the effects of brisk walking, and brisk walking with abdominal electrical stimulation on anthropometric, body composition, and self-perception measures in sedentary adult women. *Psychology of Sport and Exercise, 7*, 437-451.

Ballantyne, E., & Donne, B. (1999). Effects of neuromuscular electrical stimulation on static and dynamic abdominal strength and endurance in healthy males. *Sports Science*, 431.issue and page number

Currier, D.P., & Mann, R. (1983). Muscular strength development by electrical stimulation in healthy individuals. *Physical Therapy, 63*, 915-921.

Hainaut, K., & Duchateau, J. (1992). Neuromuscular electrical stimulation and voluntary exercise. *Sports Medicine, 14(2)*, 100-113.

Kots, Y. (1977). Electrostimulation of skeletal muscles. *Canadian-Soviet Exchange Symposium*, Concordia University.

Maffiuletti, N.A., Dugnani, S., Folz, M., Di Pierno, E., & Mauro, F. (2002). Effect of combined electrostimlation and plyometric training on vertical jump height. *Medicine and Science in Sports and Exercise, 34*, 1638-1644.

Mueller, E.A. (1959) Training muscle strength. *Ergonomics, 2*, 216-222.

Porcari, J.P., Palmer McLean, K., Foster, C., Kernozek, T., Crenshaw, B., & Swenson, C. (2002). Effects of electrical muscle stimulation on body composition, muscle strength, and physical appearance. *Journal of Strength and Conditioning Association Research, 16*, 165-172.

Porcari, J.P., Miller, J., K. Cornwell., Foster, C., Gibson, M., McLean, K., & Kernozek, T. (2005). The effects of neuromuscular electrical stimulation training on abdominal strength, endurance, and selected anthropometric measures. *Journal of Sports Medicine and Science, 4*, 66-75.

Quinn, E. (2008) Core muscle strength and stability test. [Online] Available: http://sportsmedicine.about.com/od/bestabexercises/a/core_test.htm(October 23, 2007)

Selkowitz, D.M. (1989). High frequency electrical stimulation in muscle strengthening. *American Journal of Sports Medicine, 17*, 103-111.

Soo, C.L., Currier, D.P., & Threlkeld, A.J. (1988). Augmenting voluntary torque of healthy muscle by optimization of electrical stimulation. *Physical Therapy, 68*, 333-337.

10

The Effect of an Isometric Hip Muscle Strength Training Protocol on Valgus Angle During a Drop Vertical Jump in Competitive Female Volleyball Players

Kaitlin M. Jackson[1], Tyson A. C. Beach[2]*, David M. Andrews[1]

[1]*Department of Kinesiology, University of Windsor, 401 Sunset Avenue, Windsor, ON, Canada N9B 3P4, [2]Faculty of Kinesiology & Physical Education, University of Toronto, 55 Harbord St, Toronto, ON, Canada M5S 2W6*

Corresponding Author: Tyson A. C. Beach, E-mail: tyson.beach@utoronto.ca

ARTICLE INFO

Conflicts of interest: None
Funding: None

ABSTRACT

Background: Hip muscle weakness is associated with higher peak knee valgus angles (VA) during drop vertical jumps (DVJ) and linked to ACL injury risk. **Objective:** To determine if isometric strengthening (IST) of the hip extensor, abductor, and external rotator muscle groups would reduce VA exhibited during a DVJ. **Methodology:** Fourteen female volleyball players (7 training (TG), 7 control (CG), VA≥9° during DVJ) participated. Pre- and post-test gluteal, quadriceps and hamstring strength were measured with a digital force gauge. Three-dimensional kinematics were collected during 15 DVJ trials. TG participated in a 6-week IST program that targeted the hip extensor, abductor, and external rotator muscle groups. Two-way mixed ANOVAs compared mean differences of VA and strength. Single-participant analyses examined if athlete-specific adaptations went undetected in the analyses of aggregated data. **Results:** TG hip extension, abduction, and knee flexion strength increased, respectively, by 20.5%, 27.5% and 23.5% (P<0.05). No group-level changes in VA were detected. Unilateral VA decreased for 5 TG participants, and bilateral VA decreased in 2 TG participants. **Conclusions:** IST increased isometric hip muscle strength, but its effect on VA is inconclusive based on group-level analyses. Using single-participant designs, future studies should assess IST and/or dynamic resistance/neuromuscular training in a larger sample to determine its effect on ACL injury risk factors.

Key words: Anterior Cruciate Ligament, Knee Injuries, Sports, Training, Kinematics

INTRODUCTION

Preventing anterior cruciate ligament (ACL) injuries in female athletes has been heavily researched in recent decades due to high injury rates. Female athletes have twice as many ACL injuries (de Loes, Dahlstedt, & Thomee, 2000) and require surgery for ligamentous knee injuries almost twice as often as their male counterparts (Fernandez, Yard, & Comstock, 2007). Female athlete knee injuries predominantly occur during non-contact maneuvers such as deceleration, pivoting, or landing tasks that are associated with high external loads at the knee joint (Bessier, Lloyd, Cochrane, & Ackland, 2001; Boden, Dean, Feagin, & Garrett, 2000; Hewett et al., 2005). There has been an emphasis in the literature placed on sports-related non-contact injuries sustained during landing activities due to the high forces and high risk biomechanical strategies used (Chappell & Limpisvasti, 2008; Ford, Myer, & Hewett, 2003; Hewett et al., 2005; Jacobs, Uhl, Mattacola, Shapiro, & Rayens, 2007; Joseph et al., 2008; Myer, Ford, McLean, & Hewett, 2006). These high-risk landing strategies have prompted a focus on exercise interventions in an attempt to alter landing mechanics and subsequently reduce injury risk (Cammarata & Dhaher, 2010; Ford et al., 2003;

Howard, 2011; Jacobs et al., 2007; Joseph et al., 2011; Myer, Ford, Palumbo, & Hewett, 2005).

The ACL's primary role in knee stabilization is to resist both anterior translation and internal rotation of the tibia relative to the femur (Butler, Noyes, & Grood, 1980; Ellison & Berg, 1985). It is the positive association of knee valgus motion with the occurrence of anterior tibial translation and internal rotation that relates valgus motion to increased knee ligament strain and injury potential (Cooke, Sled, & Scudamore, 2007; Myer et al., 2005). In a non-contact landing, high knee valgus deviation (frontal plane projection angle of 9° or greater) has been found to be one of the strongest links to ACL injury (Hewett et al., 2005; Levine et al., 2013).

Recent research in this area has focused on the effectiveness of various exercise interventions to improve the biomechanics of the knee by strengthening hip muscles (Anwer & Alghadir, 2014; Earl-Boehm & Hoch, 2011; Herman et al., 2008). With the hip being the most proximal joint of the lower extremity closed-kinetic-chain, attaining adequate control of this joint is hypothesized to improve control at the knee (Powers, 2010). Evidence of this is seen with a reported link between hip muscle strength and non-contact ACL injury

(Khayambashi, Ghoddosi, Straub, & Powers, 2015). Specifically, muscle weakness in hip abduction (Jacobs et al., 2007; Nadler et al., 2002), external rotation (Howard, 2011; Khayambashi, Mohammadkhani, Ghaznavi, Lyle, & Powers, 2012), and extension (Nadler et al., 2002) are all associated with higher knee valgus angles during landing. Therefore, strengthening hip muscles to improve control of the femur proximally could help to maintain a more neutral alignment of the distal femur with the tibia at the knee, thereby preventing excessive valgus deviation.

Some studies on the effectiveness of dynamic resistance and/or neuromuscular (plyometrics, agility, balance) exercise protocols have shown that such interventions can improve drop vertical jump (DVJ) mechanics in controlled settings (Hewett et al., 2005; Myer et al., 2005), while other studies show strength improvements but no changes in lower extremity movement mechanics (Chappell et al., 2008; Ferber, Kendall, & Farr, 2011). The inconsistencies in the results between studies could be due, in part, to the variation of exercises and exercise durations utilized.

Isometric resistance training of hip musculature has not been reported in the literature to improve DVJ mechanics. This type of training typically involves constant-length muscle contractions of targeted muscles surrounding one joint at a time, with the focus being on strengthening the muscles primarily responsible for resisting joint rotation when an external force is applied. Studies show that isometric resistance training produces larger strength gains (Duchateau & Hainaut, 1984; Folland, Hawker, Leach, Little, & Jones, 2005) and faster muscle activation timing (Tsao, Galea, & Hodges, 2010) than dynamic resistance training. However, these results were joint position-specific and have yet to be shown to transfer to changes in DVJ mechanics. The majority of resistance training protocols investigated in the literature to date have used dynamic exercises to modify lower extremity biomechanics, in an attempt to improve injury outcomes. Although there is increasing evidence that some of these approaches are efficacious (Chappell et al., 2008; Ferber et al. 2011; Myer et al., 2005), the components of the interventions are inconsistent, leaving questions regarding their independent contributions and/or relative (in) effectiveness. A recent meta-analysis (Donnell-Fink et al., 2015) dubbed the general quality of these studies to be somewhat low, leaving room for future studies to assess the efficacy of the specific components of various interventions. The effect that isometric hip muscle strengthening alone has on ACL injury risk factors has yet to be studied.

Considering all the research completed to date, no study has assessed the effectiveness of an isometric tri-planar hip-strengthening program to control frontal plane knee motion during a DVJ task. Therefore, the purpose of this study was to determine if an isometric strengthening program targeting the hip extensor, abductor, and external rotator muscles would improve the VA during a DVJ. It was hypothesized that there would be an increase in hip joint moment-generating capacity (i.e. hip muscle strength) following isometric hip muscle training, which would result in a decrease in knee valgus motion during a DVJ.

METHODOLOGY

Participants and Study Design

Fourteen female volleyball players (age 22.4 ± 1.6 years, height 1.77 ± 0.09 m, and body mass of 69.5 ± 10.2 kg) (7 training group [TG], 7 control group [CG]), with at least two years of experience on university, college and/or club level volleyball teams, were recruited from the Greater Toronto Area (Ontario, Canada). All participants had no history of lower extremity surgery, no lower extremity injury within 3 months of starting the study, and demonstrated a peak knee valgus angle of 9° or greater (2D projected angle) during drop landings, as determined during a pre-screening protocol (detailed below). This study was approved by the Research Ethics Boards of both the University of Toronto and University of Windsor. Written informed consent was obtained from each participant prior to data collection.

The procedures of this study were executed in four stages described below: pre-screen; pre-test; training; and post-test. During the pre- and post-test data collection sessions, all participants performed 15 trials of a DVJ task approximately 7 weeks apart. The TG participated in 6 weeks (5x/week) of isometric strength training between the pre- and post-test data collection sessions, while the CG continued normal activity during this period.

Test Procedures

The peak knee valgus angles of a total of 109 volleyball players were quantified from frontal plane video records obtained during a pre-screen session in order to determine eligibility for the full study. Players were eligible to participate in the study if the peak knee valgus angle (2D frontal projection angle) during at least two of three DVJ trials was 9° or greater. During the screening session, participants wore spandex shorts, a t-shirt, and the shoes that they typically wear during volleyball participation. An Apple iPad tablet (3rd Gen., Taiwan) was set up on a tripod at knee height, approximately two meters in front of each participant while they performed a DVJ (described below). The frame that corresponded with the highest knee valgus angle observed during the landing of the DVJ task (peak medial deviation) was used to determine eligibility in the study. Each potential participant performed a minimum of three practice trials to familiarize herself with the task. Three trials were recorded for each player with a minimum of 30 seconds rest provided between trials.

For the pre- and post-test data collection sessions, participants were asked to wear athletic shoes in which they would normally play volleyball, and a sports bra and spandex shorts, in order to minimize clothing interference during motion capture. Upon arrival to the laboratory, the participant's body mass (kg) and height (m) were measured when standing on a force platform with a reflective marker (for motion capture) placed at the apex of their head.

To measure the strength of the gluteal, hamstring and quadriceps muscle groups bilaterally, each participant performed three maximum voluntary isometric contraction (MVIC) trials against a digital force gauge (Manual Muscle Testing System, Layfayette Instrument Company, Lafayette, IN) anchored to a custom-made table (MotionBlock™, Toronto, Canada) which had built-in adjustable lever arms to provide the resistance against which the participants contracted (Figure 1).

Each MVIC trial involved a brief ramp up to a maximal effort contraction (held for 5 seconds), followed by a return to rest. A minimum of 60 seconds rest was provided between trials. The researcher provided verbal motivation to encourage maximal effort. Standardized positions of each force measurement for each muscle are outlined in Table 1.

Following the MVIC trials, a total of 45 spherical (14 mm) reflective markers were placed with double-sided tape on: top of the head; C7; sternal notch; xiphoid process; four skin markers placed asymmetrically approximately 5-10 cm from the spine at the T5 and T9 spinal processes; acromion processes; iliac crests; three on the lateral posterior pelvis bilaterally; greater trochanters; frontal thighs at the approximate midpoint of the thigh; lateral thighs halfway between the frontal thigh marker and the knee; medial and lateral femoral epicondyles; tibial tuberosities; anterior midpoints of the shanks; lateral shanks halfway between the anterior shank and ankle joint; medial malleolus; lateral malleolus; posterior calcaneus; intermediate cuneiforms; and the 1st and 5th metatarsals (Figure 2).

After the collection of a static calibration trial during

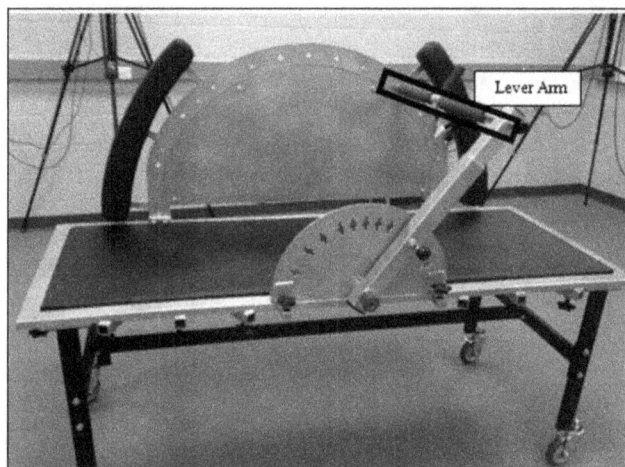

Figure 1. MotionBlock™ table used for MVIC and isometric strength training

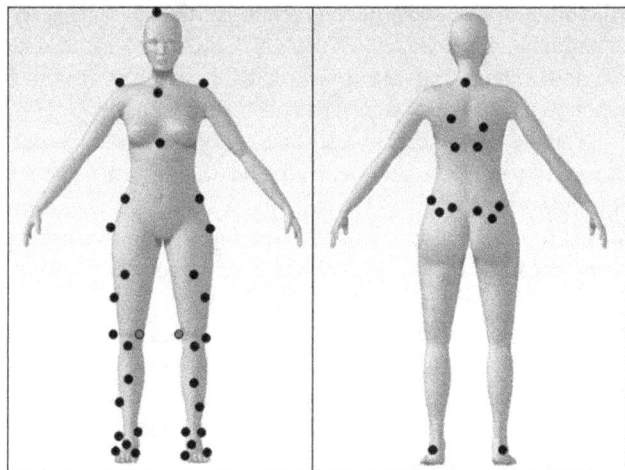

Figure 2. Reflective marker placement for 3D tracking (black dots) and calibration only (red dots)

which participants stood "quietly" in the anatomical position, the medial knee markers were removed to prevent interference during the DVJ trials. Each DVJ trial began with participants standing atop a box 30 cm high, with their feet approximately shoulder-width apart. Participants were instructed to drop down (the stepping foot was not specified) with each foot landing on one of the two force platforms placed directly in front of the box. Immediately following the landing, participants executed a vertical jump with their shoulders fully extended, as if they were performing a maximal block jump. Given that DVJ mechanics are influenced by verbal cueing (Khuu, Musalem, & Beach, 2015), participants were specifically instructed prior to stepping down to "drop down on the force platforms, then immediately jump up as if you are performing a maximal block jump. Focus on pressing your hands over a net, and land with one foot on each platform". The focus for the participant was directed to upper body block jump technique in order to simulate a practice/game situation, as well as to direct their attention away from their lower body mechanics. Several practice trials were permitted to ensure participants were comfortable with the DVJ task. A total of 15 trials were recorded for each participant, with a minimum of 60 seconds rest provided between trials.

An optoelectronic motion capture system (Qualisys AB, Gothenburg, Sweden) with eight Oqus 1 (0.3 MP) cameras collected 3D marker position data at 200 Hz during the DJV trials. A ±10V, 16-bit analog-to-digital conversion system (Analog Acquisition Interface Unit, Qualisys AB, Gothenburg, Sweden) was used to synchronously collect force platform data at 1000 Hz. Qualisys Track Manager (QTM) software was used to acquire marker position and force platform data. An MTD-2 CalTester Rod (Motion Lab Systems, Inc., Baton Rouge, LA) with CalTesterPlus software (C-Motion, Inc., Germantown, MD) was used to spatially locate two force platforms (AMTI-OR6-6-1000, AMTI, Waterdown, MA). Visual3D (C-Motion, Inc., Germantown, MD) was used to smooth marker position and force platform data using a zero-lag Butterworth low-pass filter with an effective cut-off frequency of 10 Hz (Kristianslund, Krosshaug, & van den Bogert, 2012), and to generate a 3D dynamic linked-segment model of the body (as described in Khuu et al., 2015). From the linked-segment model, bilateral peak knee valgus angles were extracted for statistical analyses.

Exercise Protocol

The TG performed a 6-week isometric strength training protocol, consisting of five sessions per week (three supervised and two unsupervised), each lasting approximately 45-60 minutes. During the unsupervised sessions, the TG group was encouraged to train in groups to maximize compliance. There were two missed supervised sessions for four of the participants that occurred in different weeks, resulting in each of those participants having only two supervised and three unsupervised sessions for two of their training weeks.

Each exercise session included five isometric exercises (Table 2), which were completed as three sets of ten maximal effort isometric contractions lasting ten seconds (10

Table 1. Standardized positions for the maximum isometric strength tests during pre- and post-training data collection sessions. The force gauge was attached to a lever at a fixed position tailored to each of the four positions

Target muscle/ Muscle group	Position
Gluteus Maximus	The participant lay prone on the Motionblock™ table with knee flexed to 90° and the ankle in a neutral position. The researcher applied pressure on the participant's lower back to prevent excessive motion. The participant was instructed to extend her thigh off the table while keeping her ASIS in contact with the table. The force gauge was positioned at the midpoint between the popliteal fossa and the gluteal fold and resisted extension
Hip Abductors	The participant lay on the Motionblock™ table on the contralateral side of the gluteus medius being measured. Her hip was in a neutral position. The researcher applied pressure and visually monitored the participant's lower back to prevent excessive motion. The participant was instructed to maximally abduct the leg as the force gauge provided resistance. The force gauge was positioned 4 cm above the knee joint on the lateral aspect of the distal thigh
Hamstrings	The participant lay prone on the Motionblock™ table with the knee flexed to 90°. The researcher applied pressure to the participant's lower back to prevent hip extension and other excessive motion. The participant was instructed to maximally flex the knee as the force gauge provided resistance. The force gauge was adjusted to contact the skin at the posterior aspect of the distal shank at a knee flexion angle of 90°
Quadriceps	The participant was seated at the side of the MotionBlock™ table with knees flexed at 90°. The participant was instructed to maximally extend the knee as the force gauge provided resistance. The force gauge was adjusted to contact the skin at the frontal aspect of the distal shank at a knee flexion angle of 90°

Table 2. Position, action and target muscles associated with the exercises completed during each training session. All positions were completed while lying supine, unless otherwise stated

Exercise	Position	Action	Target muscles
1	Prone 90° knee flexion Ankle in neutral position No lateral movement of limb	Hip extension	Gluteus maximus Biceps femoris
2	Prone Full hip external rotation 90° knee flexion 30° hip abduction Ankle in neutral position	Hip extension	Gluteus maximus Gluteus medius Biceps femoris
3	0° hip abduction 0° hip flexion 0° hip rotation	Hip abduction	Gluteus maximus Gluteus medius
4	30° hip abduction 0° hip flexion Full hip external rotation	Hip abduction and external rotation	Gluteus maximus Gluteus medius
5	0° hip flexion 90° knee flexion	Knee flexion	Biceps femoris

s rest between reps, 60 s rest between sets). Each exercise was performed bilaterally, one side at a time. Stationary resistance was met via the MotionBlock™ while maintaining prescribed position. Participants were coached on where they should expect to feel the contraction, based on the muscle group targeted in each exercise. If the participant felt a non-targeted muscle group becoming active during the contraction, they were instructed to stop and rest for one or two minutes and re-attempt the exercise. All participants verbally indicated that they were able to perform the exercises and feel the target muscle(s) activating.

For exercises 1 and 2, while lying in a prone position on the MotionBlock™ table, participants attempted to raise the thigh being measured off the MotionBlock™ table while keeping both anterior superior iliac spines firmly against the mat. If additional biofeedback was necessary to help the participant, light pressure was applied by the researcher's hand to the low back, and fingers were placed between the mat and the participants' anterior superior iliac spine (on the side of the thigh being raised). Exercises 3 and 4 involved various hip abduction and hip external rotation positions; hip external rotation range varied, therefore each participant's maximum range of motion was used. While lying on the contralateral side to the exercising leg, participants abducted the hip against a rigid adjustable bar frame (MotionBlock™) that was placed at the appropriate distance above the participant to ensure a 30° abduction angle position. For exercise 5, lying prone on the MotionBlock™, the participant attempted knee flexion at a fixed angle of 90° against the adjustable bar frame (MotionBlock™). Lateral thigh movement during the contraction was limited by positioning the body beside the back wall of the MotionBlock™ table. The participant was instructed to keep the exercising leg "lightly touching the wall".

Statistical Analyses

An *a priori* power analysis calculation showed that a participant pool of 22 was required in order to achieve a power level of 0.8. The effect size of 0.6 was based on data and power analyses done in similar studies on lower extremity kinematic changes seen with training (Earl-Boehm et al., 2011; Hewett et al., 2005; Joseph et al., 2008; Snyder, Earl, O'Connor, & Ebersole, 2009). Given that the convenience sample of 14 participants was anticipated to not likely result in statistical significance (i.e., because the study was underpowered for group-level analyses), the results were assessed on both a group and individual basis. Two-way mixed ANOVAs with one between-participant factor (Group = TG vs. CG) and one within-participant factor (Time = pre- vs. post-training) were performed to test for mean differences in the dependent variables (i.e., peak knee valgus angles and muscle strength measures). ANOVAs were performed using SAS system software for Windows (Version 9.3.1, SAS Institute Inc., Cary, NC), with the alpha level set at 0.05.

Single-participant analyses were conducted using a model statistic procedure (Bates, Dufek, & Davis, 1992). The basic approach was to compare differences between dependent variables in the pre- and post-testing conditions to that of a probabilistic critical difference (test statistic) on a participant-by-participant basis (Bates, James, & Dufek, 2004). If the empirically observed mean difference ($|mean_{pre} - mean_{post}|$) was greater than the test statistic (critical value $\times [sd_{pre}^2 + sd_{post}^2/2]^{1/2}$, where sd = standard deviation) for a given participant, then the difference was deemed statistically significant for that participant. Critical values based on the number of trials collected and desired alpha levels (0.01, 0.05, or 0.10) were garnered from a table generated by Bates et al. (1992). Single-participant analyses were performed using Microsoft Excel software.

RESULTS

There were significant group × time interaction effects for hip extension (left P=0.0483, right P=0.0085), hip abduc-

tion (left P=0.0036, right P=0.0255), and knee flexion (left P=0.0026, right P=0.0010) strength from pre- to post-test in the TG. On average (bilaterally), hip extension, hip abduction, and knee flexion force increased by 20.5%, 27.5% and 23.5%, respectively (Figure 3). No significant changes in strength were seen in the CG. Knee extension strength did not significantly change in either group from pre- to post-test (left P=0.3018, right P=0.6871).

At the group-level, there were no significant changes in the mean peak knee valgus angle (left P=0.1038, right P=0.375) from pre- to post-test. In the individual-level analyses, five out of seven TG participants exhibited a significant decrease in peak knee valgus angle on one or both sides from pre- to post-test. Four TG participants significantly decreased their left peak knee valgus deviation (decrease of 8.3^0, 7.2^0, 2.3^0, and 1.3^0), and three TG participants significantly decreased their right knee valgus deviation (decrease of 11^0, 6.8^0, and 1.9^0) (Table 3). Of the five participants who exhibited decreases, two demonstrated a bilateral decrease in knee valgus angle (left knee and right knee valgus angles decreased by 8.3^0 and 7.2^0, and 11^0 and 6.8^0, respectively) (Figure 4). Among the CG, five, two and no participants exhibited unilateral increases (of 2.2^0, 1.3^0, 2^0, 1^0 and 2.2^0 on average), decreases (of 2.3^0 and 2.5^0), and bilateral decreases in knee valgus angle.

DISCUSSION

It was hypothesized that isometric strength training of the hip extensor, abductor, and external rotator muscles would decrease the knee valgus angle during a drop vertical jump task. After a 6-week isometric strength training protocol targeting the hip extensor, abductor, and external rotator muscles, a significant improvement in strength in these muscles was seen in the training group (TG). The mean peak knee valgus angle did not change significantly in either group after training. However, significant individual improvements were seen in 5 out of 7 TG participants (two of which showed a bilateral improvement), and significant negative effects were seen in 5 out of 7 CG participants (note that two CG participants displayed a unilateral improvement in valgus movement).

The strength produced by the hip musculature (extension, hip abduction, and lying prone knee flexion – targeting the

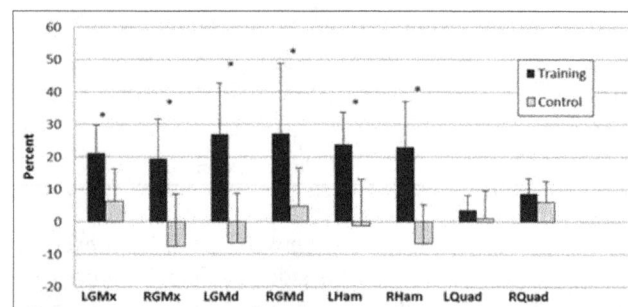

Figure 3. Percent change (error bars = standard deviation) in muscle strength measured against a digital force gauge for the training group and control group between the pre- and post-test. A positive value indicates an increase in strength from the pre- to post-test

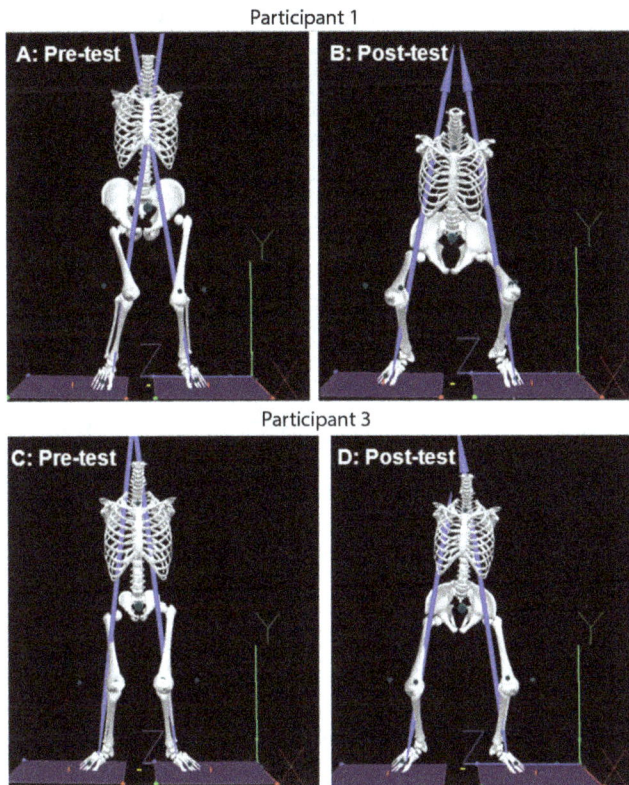

Figure 4. Frontal view at the time of peak knee valgus angle during the initial landing in pre- and post-testing for Participant 1 (pre-test = A and post-test = B) and Participant 3 (pre-test = C and post-test = D)

gluteus maximus, gluteus medius, and hamstrings, respectively) improved significantly by approximately 20.5%, 27.5%, and 23.5%. The percent strength increases seen in this and other isometric training studies were notably higher than increases reported in longer duration dynamic strength training protocols: mean increases of 7% for 12 weeks of training (Delecluse, Roelants, & Verschueren, 2003) and 15.1% for 10 weeks of training (Painter et al., 2012). The results of the current study support the use of isometric training over a 6-week duration as a means by which significant strength gains can be achieved at the trained joint angle. A shorter time to achieve larger strength gains would be beneficial among those seeking to improve strength as fast as possible, such as athletes, and patients undergoing rehabilitation. The isolation of the target muscle groups seems to be an ideal solution to increase the strength without strengthening surrounding non-target muscle groups (i.e., strengthening the gluteal muscles without strengthening the quadriceps), if desired to remedy muscle strength imbalances.

Group-wide, there was no significant change in peak knee valgus angle after training. The training protocol in this study proved to be adequate to generate significant strength gains of the target musculature, thereby allowing for possible connections to be made between changes in strength and changes in kinematics. However, the overall lack of significant group changes in knee valgus angle suggests that isometrically stronger muscles around the hip joint do not necessarily translate into significant changes in dynamic knee kinematics of a DVJ task for the population studied. These

findings could also suggest that the changes observed after isometric training may vary greatly based on each individual, and may require that movement (re)training using combined approaches is needed to more consistently facilitate positive transfer of strength gains (Donnell-Link et al., 2015).

When considered on an individual level, five training group participants exhibited significantly lower peak knee valgus angles for one or both knees following the intervention. Lower knee valgus angles are associated with a decrease in the strain on the ACL and a lower injury risk (Hewett et al., 2005). No control group participants exhibited a bilateral decrease in knee valgus angle, although two demonstrated a unilateral decrease in the right knee. This suggests that isometric strengthening of the hip extensors, external rotators, and abductors could potentially improve the frontal plane kinematics during a drop vertical jump task in certain individuals. However, due to the low number of participants, the effectiveness of the isometric training protocol on frontal plane lower extremity kinematics is inconclusive in this study. The lack of a significant group-wide change in knee valgus angles, or even a consistent trend amongst all training group participants, suggests that strengthening the hip musculature may affect each athlete differently. An exercise program's effectiveness could vary from person to person as each individual may differ in unique physiological and psychological factors that affect performance and response to exercise (Cowley, Ford, Myer, Kernozek, & Hewett, 2006; Eynon et al., 2011; Miller, MacDougall, & Sale, 1993). In addition, gains in isometric strength of specific muscle groups (through position isolation) associated with poor landing kinematics may not generally transfer to dynamic movement patterns. Increasing the isometric strength of the hip muscles could perhaps serve as an initial step in a program which utilizes the benefits of dynamic or neuromuscular training in conjunction with isometric training, since a combined approach has been previously shown to be effective (Donnell-Link et al., 2015; Fontenay et al., 2013). Future studies should assess the efficacy of utilizing a combined intervention with isometric and dynamic resistance training.

One limitation was the low number of participants (14 total), with only seven participants who completed the training program. Based on *a priori* statistical power calculations, it was acknowledged that the study would be under-powered at the outset. As a consequence, it was decided to collect 15 DVJ trials during pre- and post-testing to combine individual- and group-level statistical analyses, which can be considered a strength of the study. It is possible that the lack of significant findings was due to small numbers, and/or attributable to the variability with which the participants executed the DVJ task. There were some trends seen for a number of individual participants in both the TG and CG regarding VA, but no significant group effects were seen. Similar studies assessing the mechanics of a DVJ task after a training protocol had participant pools of 30 (Chappell et al., 2008), 19 (Earl-Boehm et al., 2011), 50 (Cochrane et al., 2010) and 74 (Herman et al., 2008) individuals. Despite our best efforts to recruit, 68 out of 109 athletes did not meet the inclusion criteria. Of the 41 athletes remaining, only 7 were able to commit to the time-intensive nature of the intervention (i.e., 5

Table 3. Mean (standard deviation) 3D peak knee valgus angles for the training (TG) and control (CG) group participants in pre- to post-testing

Group	ID	Mean (SD) Knee Valgus Angle (deg)							
		Left side				Right side			
		Pre		Post		P-value	Pre		Post		P-value
TG	1	4.3	(2.9)	−4.0	(2.3)*	<0.001	−13.2	(1.9)	−2.2	(4.9)*	<0.001
	3	2.7	(1.7)	−4.5	(6.1)*	<0.001	−3.8	(2.1)	3.0	(6.7)*	<0.001
	4	7.2	(1.7)	7.2	(1.4)	0.9893	−7.6	(2.0)	−5.7	(1.8)*	0.0114
	5	−1.9	(2.6)	−4.2	(2.2)*	0.0125	−4.9	(1.6)	−4.3	(2.6)	0.4241
	6	0.6	(2.1)	0.7	(1.6)	0.8902	−0.6	(3.3)	−1.4	(2.6)	0.5018
	8	2.1	(2.1)	7.1	(1.7)*	<0.001	0.2	(2.5)	−2.8	(1.9)*	<0.001
	14	1.8	(1.6)	0.5	(1.7)*	0.0514	−2.3	(1.8)	−3.8	(1.5)*	0.0173
CG	2	0.1	(1.7)	2.3	(2.6)*	0.0320	−2.6	(2.0)	−3.6	(1.5)	0.1120
	7	0.4	(1.4)	1.7	(2.0)*	0.0364	2.2	(1.9)	1.6	(2.5)	0.4492
	9	0.1	(2.0)	0.9	(2.3)	0.3407	−0.4	(1.1)	0.2	(1.3)	0.1562
	10	2.0	(1.6)	4.0	(2.1)*	0.0061	−3.8	(1.1)	−3.6	(2.2)	0.8243
	11	−0.4	(1.4)	−1.2	(1.4)	0.1579	−0.2	(1.3)	2.5	(1.4)*	<0.001
	12	5.1	(2.6)	6.1	(2.2)	0.2795	−2.4	(2.2)	−4.6	(2.3)*	0.0122
	13	4.6	(1.7)	5.6	(1.2)*	0.0585	−2.4	(1.0)	0.1	(1.6)*	<0.001

Positive left side and negative right side value = valgus; negative left side and positive right side value = varus

sessions/week for 6 weeks) due to their volleyball training and competition schedule. It was due to the smaller-than-desired sample size that despite collecting force plate data, we *a posteriori* elected against conducting inverse dynamics analyses; analyzing joint kinetics would have necessitated the application of additional correction factors, which would have further limited our ability to detect changes. Future studies should be designed with sufficient sample sizes to test the effect of isometric strength training on lower extremity joint kinetic and/or muscle activation patterns (using electromyography) during the DVJ.

Another limitation was the inability to strictly control the athletes' activities outside of the isometric training protocol, again due to their competition and training schedule. However, athletes were asked to continue their regular level of volleyball play, and were discouraged from making any changes in their current fitness training. There was a high level of adherence to these requests, established by verbal confirmation.

The reliability of the anatomical landmarking needed for the motion capture markers utilized during the pre- and post-test data collections was controlled by having the same researcher perform the task in all cases. However, the variability in marker placement was not evaluated independently in this study. The overall impact that differences in marker placement has on knee valgus angle calculations pre- and post-test should be considered in future studies, especially given that a number of differences were noted in the pre- and post-test knee valgus angles in the CG.

The participants played volleyball at a highly competitive level. Consequently, their movement patterns (drop-jump skill) may have been more engrained than a younger, less trained cohort, and could therefore be more resistant to change after a 6-week isometric strength training program.

This was not seen as a major limitation to the current study in that the focus was on changing knee valgus angle in competitive players. The changes that were noted for a few individuals are encouraging, and will hopefully translate into reduced injury risk for them. This is viewed as a positive outcome of this work, and a starting point for future studies in this area.

CONCLUSIONS

Although hip extensor, abductor, and external rotator muscle weaknesses are associated with high-risk DVJ mechanics (i.e., uncontrolled frontal plane knee motion), isometric strengthening of these muscle groups did not directly transfer to improved DVJ mechanics based on the group-level analyses conducted in this study. However, improvements in DVJ mechanics were detected in individual participants, which warrant further investigation of the effectiveness of isometric training at the individual level. Moreover, using single-participant experimental designs, future studies should assess combinations of isometric and neuromuscular training to potentially enhance the effectiveness of training to alter DVJ mechanics, and therefore reduce ACL injury risk.

REFERENCES

Anwer, S., & Alghadir, A. (2014). Effect of isometric quadriceps exercise on muscle strength, pain, and function in patients with knee osteoarthritis: a randomized controlled study. *Journal of Physical Therapy Science,* 26(5), 745-748.doi:10.1589/ipts.26.745

Bates, B.T., Dufek, J.S., & Davis, H.P. (1992). The effect of trial size on statistical power. *Medicine and Science in Sports and Exercise,* 24(9), 1059-1068. doi: 10.1249/00005768-199209000-00017

Bates, B.T., James, C.R., & Dufek, J.S. (2004). Single-subject analysis. In N. Stergiou (Ed.), *Innovative Analyses of Human Movement* (pp. 3-28). Champaign, IL: Human Kinetics. 3-28.

Bessier, T.F., Lloyd, D.G., Cochrane, J.L., Ackland, T.R. (2001). External loading of the knee joint during running and cutting maneuvers. *Medicine and Science in Sport and Exercise,* 33, 1168-1175. doi:10.1097/00005768-200107000-00014

Boden, B.P., Dean, G.S., Feagin, J.A. Jr., Garrett, W.E. Jr. (2000). Mechanisms of anterior cruciate ligament injury. *Orthopedics,* 23, 573-578. doi: 10.3928/0147-7447-20000601-15

Butler, D. L., Noyes, F. R., & Grood, E. S. (1980). Ligamentous restraints to anterior-posterior drawer in the human knee. *The Journal of Bone and Joint Surgery,* 62(2), 259-270. Retrieved from http://jbjs.org.myaccess.library.utoronto.ca/content/jbjsam/62/2/259.full.pdf

Cammarata, M. L. & Dhaher, Y. Y. (2010). Evidence of gender-specific motor templates to resist valgus loading at the knee. *Muscle & Nerve,* 41(5), 614-623. doi:10.1002/mus.21509

Chappell, J.D. & Limpisvasti, O. (2008). Effect of a neuromuscular training program on the kinetics and kinematics of jumping tasks. *The American Journal of Sports Medicine,* 36(6), 1081-1086. doi:10.1177/0363546508314425

Cochrane, J. L., Lloyd, D. G., Besier, T. F., Elliott, B. C.m Doyle, T. L. A., & Ackland, T. R. (2010). Training affects knee kinematics and kinetics in cutting maneuvers in sport. *Medicine and Science in Sport and Exercise,* 42(8), 1435-1544. doi:10.1249/MSS.0b013e3181d-03ba0

Cooke, T. D. V., Sled, E. A., & Scudamore, R. A. (2007). Frontal plane knee alignment: A call for standardized measurement. *Journal of Rheumatology,* 34(9), 1796-1801. Retrieved from https://jrheum.com/subscribers/07/09/1796.html

Cowley, H. R., Ford, K. R., Myer, G. D., Kernozek, T. W., & Hewett, T. E. (2006). Difference in neuromuscular strategies between landing and cutting tasks in female basketball and soccer athletes. *Journal of Athletic Training,* 41(1), 67-73. Retrieved from https://www.ncbi.nlm.nih.gov/pmc/articles/PMC1421490

de Loes, M., Dahlstedt, L.J., & Thomee, R. (2000). A 7-year study on risks and costs of knee injuries in male and female youth participants in 12 sports. *Scandinavian Journal of Medical Science and Sports,* 10(2), 90-97. doi: 10.1034/j.1600-0838.2000.010002090.x

Delecluse, C., Roelants, M., & Verschueren, S. (2003). Strength increase after whole-body vibration compared with resistance training. *Medicine and Science in Sports and Exercise,* 6, 1033-1041. doi:10.1249/01.MSS.0000069752.96438.B0

Donnell-Link, L. A., Klara, K., Collins, J. E., Yang, H. Y., Goczalk, M. G., Katz, J. N., & Losina, E. (2015). Effectiveness of knee injury and anterior cruciate ligament tear prevention programs: A meta-analysis. *PLoS One,* 10(12), e0144063. doi:10.1371/journal.pone.0144063

Duchateau, J. & Hainaut, K. (1984). Isometric or dynamic training: differential effects on mechanical properties of a human muscle. *Journal of Applied Physiology,* 56(2), 296-301. Retrieved from http://jap.physiology.org/content/56/2/296

Earl-Boehm, J. E. & Hoch, A. Z. (2011). A proximal strengthening program improves pain, function, and biomechanics in women with patellofemoral pain syndrome. *The American Journal of Sports Medicine,* 39(1), 154-163. doi:10.1177/0363546510379967

Ellison, A. E. & Berg, E. E. (1985). Embryology, anatomy, and function of the anterior cruciate ligament. *Orthopedic Clinics of North America,* 16, 3-14. Retrieved from http://search.proquest.com.myaccess.library.utoronto.ca/docview/75955310?accountid=14771

Eynon, N., Ruiz, J. R., Oliveira, J., Duarte, J. A., Birk, R., & Lucia, A. (2011). Genes and elite athletes: a roadmap for future research. *The Journal of Physiology,* **589,** 3063-3070. doi:10.1113/jphysiol.2011.207035

Ferber, R., Kendall, K. D., & Farr, L. (2011). Changes in knee biomechanics after a hip-abductor strengthening protocol for runners with patellofemoral pain syndrome. *Journal of Athletic Training,* 46(2), 142-149. doi:10.4085/1062-6050-46.2.142

Fernandez, W. G., Yard, E. E., & Comstock, R. D. (2007). Epidemiology of lower extremity injuries among U.S. high school athletes. *Academic Emergency Medicine: Official Journal of the Society for Academic Emergency Medicine,* 14(7), 641-645. doi:10.1197/j.aem.2007.03.1354

Folland, J. P., Hawker, K., Leach, B., Little, T., & Jones, D. A. (2005). Strength training: Isometric training at a range of joint angles versus dynamic training. *Journal of Sports Sciences,* 23(8), 817-824. doi:10.1080/02640410400021783

Fontenay, B.P.D., Lebon, F., Champely, S., Argaud, S., Blache, Y., Collet, C., Monteil, K. (2013). ACL injury risk factors decrease & jumping performance improvement in female basketball players: a prospective study. *International Journal of Kinesiology & Sports Science,* 1(2), 10-18. doi:10.7575/aiac.ijkss.v.1n.2p.10

Ford, K. R., Myer, G. D., & Hewett, T. E. (2003). Valgus knee motion during landing in high school female and male basketball players. *Medicine & Science in Sport & Exercise,* 35(10), 1745-1750. doi:10.1249/01.MSS.0000089346.85744.D9

Herman, D. C., Weinhold, P. S., Guskiewicz, K. M., Garrett, W. E., Yu, B., & Padua, D. A. (2008). The effects of strength training on the lower extremity biomechanics of female recreational athletes during a stop-jump task. *The American Journal of Sports Medicine,* 36(4), 733-740. doi:10.1177/0363546507311602

Hewett, T.E., Myer, G.D., Ford, K.R., Heidt, R.S., Colosimo, A.L., McLean, S.G., van den Bogert, A.J., Paterno, M.V., & Succop, P. (2005). Biomechanical measures of neuromuscular control and valgus loading of the knee predict anterior cruciate ligament injury risk in female athletes. *The American Journal of Sports Medicine,* 33(4), 492-501. doi:10.1177/0363546504269591

Howard, J. (2011). Structure, sex, and strength and knee and kinematics during landing. *Journal of Athletic Training,* 46(4), 376-385. Retrieved from http://www.natajournals.org/doi/full/10.4085/1062-6050-46.4.376?code=nata-site

Jacobs, C. A., Uhl, T. L., Mattacola, C. G., Shapiro, R., & Rayens, W. S. (2007). Hip abductor function of lower extremity landing kinematics: Sex differences. *Journal of Athletic Training,* 41(1), 76-83. Retrieved from https://www.ncbi.nlm.nih.gov/pmc/articles/PMC1896084

Joseph, M. F., Rahl, M., Sheehan, J., MacDougall, B., Horn, E., Denegar, C. R., Trojian, T. H., Anderson, J. M., & Kraemer, W. J. (2011). Timing of lower extremity frontal plane motion differs between female and male athletes during a landing task. *The American Journal of Sports Medicine,* 39(7), 1517-1521. doi:10.1177/0363546510397175

Joseph, M., Tiberio, D., Baird, J. L., Trojian, T. H., Anderson, J. M., Kraemer, W. J., & Maresh, C. M. (2008). Knee valgus during drop jumps in national collegiate athletic association division I female athletes: The effect of a medial post. *The American Journal of Sports Medicine,* 36(2), 285-289. doi:10.1177/0363546507308362

Khayambashi, K., Mohammadkhani, Z., Ghaznavi, K., Lyle, M. A., & Powers, C. M. (2012). The effects of isolated hip abductor and external rotator muscle strengthening on pain, health status, and hip strength in females with patellofemoral pain: A randomized controlled trial. *The Journal of Orthopaedic and Sports Physical Therapy,* 42(1), 22-29. doi:10.2519/jospt.2012.3704

Khayambashi, K., Ghoddosi, N., Straub, R.K., Powers, C.M. (2015). Hip muscle strength predicts noncontact anterior cruciate ligament injury in male and female athletes: A prospective study. *The American Journal of Sports Medicine,* 44(2), 355-361. doi:10.1177/0363546515616237

Khuu, S., Musalem, L. L., & Beach, T. A. (2015). Verbal instructions acutely affect drop vertical jump biomechanics—implications for athletic performance and injury risk assessments. *Journal of Strength and Conditioning Research,* 29(10), 2816-26. doi:10.1519/JSC.0000000000000938

Kristianslund, E., Krosshaug, T., & van den Bogert, A. J. (2012). Effect of low pass filtering on joint moments from inverse dynamics: Implications for injury prevention. *Journal of Biomechanics,* 45, 666-671. doi:10.1016/j.jbiomech.2011.12.011

Levine, J. W., Kiapour, A. M., Quatman, C. E., Wordeman, S. C., Goel, V. K., Hewett, T. E. & Demetropoulos C. K. (2013). Clinically relevant injury patterns after an anterior cruciate ligament injury provide insight into injury mechanisms. *The American Journal of Sports Medicine,* 41(2), 385-395. doi:10.1177/0363546512465167

Miller, A. E. J., MacDougall, M. A., & Sale, D. G. (1993). Gender differences in strength and muscle fiber characteristics. *European Journal of Applied Physiology,* 66, 254-262. doi:10.1007/BF00235103

Myer, G. D., Ford, K. R., Palumbo, J. P., & Hewett, T. E. (2005). Neuromuscular training improves performance and lower-extremity biomechanics in female athletes. *Journal of Strength & Conditioning Research,* 19(1), 51-60. doi:10.1519/13643.1

Myer, G., Ford, K. R., McLean, S. G., & Hewett, T. E. (2006). The effects of plyometric versus dynamic stabilization and balance training on lower extremity biomechanics. *The American Journal of Sports Medicine,* 34(3), 445-455. doi: 10.1177/0363546505281241

Nadler, S. F., Malanga, G. A., Solomona, J. L., Feinberg, J. H., Foyea, P. M., & Park, Y. I. (2002). The relationship between lower extremity injury and the hip abductor to extensor strength ratio in collegiate athletes. *Journal of Back and Musculoskeletal Rehabilitation, 16,* 153–158. doi:10.3233/BMR-2002-16406

Painter, K. B., Haff, G. G., Ramsey, M. W., McBride, J., Triplett, T., Sands, W. A., Lamont, H. S., Stone, M. E., & Stone, M. H. (2012). Strength gains: Block versus daily undulating periodization weight training among track and field athletes. *International Journal of Sports Physiology and Performance,* 7, 161-169. doi:10.1123/ijspp.7.2.161

Powers, C. M. (2010). The influence of abnormal hip mechanics on knee injury: a biomechanical perspective. *Journal of Orthopaedic & Sports Physical Therapy,* 40(2), 42-51. doi:10.2519/jospt.2010.3337

Snyder, K. R., Earl, J. E., O'Connor, K. M., & Ebersole, K. T. (2009). Resistance training is accompanied by increases in hip strength and changes in lower extremity biomechanics during running. *Clinical Biomechanics,* 24(1), 26-34. doi:10.1016/j.clinbiomech.2008.09.009

Tsao, H., Galea, M., & Hodges, P. (2010). Driving plasticity in the motor cortex in recurrent low back pain. *European Journal of Pain,* 14, 832-839. doi:10.1016/j.ejpain.2010.01.001

11

Investigation of Positional Differences in Fitness of Male University Ice Hockey Players and the Frequency, Time Spent and Heart Rate of Movement Patterns During Competition

Joel Jackson[1], Gary Snydmiller[2], Alex Game[1], Pierre Gervais[1], Gordon Bell[1]*

[1]Faculty of Physical Education and Recreation, University of Alberta, Edmonton, Alberta Canada, T6G2H9

[2]Augustana Faculty, University of Alberta, Camrose, Alberta Canada, T4V2R3

Corresponding Author: Gordon Bell, E-mail: bell.gordon@gmail.com

ARTICLE INFO

Conflicts of interest: None
Funding: None

ABSTRACT

Background: Men's university ice hockey has received little scientific attention over the past 30 years, a time in which the traits of the players and the demands of the game have evolved. **Objectives:** This study compared the physiological characteristics of university ice hockey players and examined the frequency and duration of the different movement patterns and heart rate (HR) responses during competition. **Methods:** Twenty male ice hockey players from the same team ($\bar{X}$ age ± SD = 22±2 years) underwent a fitness evaluation and were filmed and HR monitored during regular season games. **Results:** Forwards and defense had similar fitness and only differed on % fatigue index and peak heart during on-ice sprinting (P<0.05). Defense stood, glided and skated backwards more than forwards and forwards skated at a moderate intensity and glided forward more than defense (P<0.05). All players spent the majority of game time gliding forward (60% of the time) followed by skating forward at a moderate intensity (17%) and standing with little movement (9%). Average HR during the game reached 96 and 92 % and peak HR was 100 and 96 % of maximum in forwards and defense, respectively. **Conclusions:** Male university hockey players present with a high level of physical fitness in a variety of categories with few differences between forwards and defense. Movement patterns during games suggest that players are performing low to moderate intensity on-ice activities the majority of the time. Paradoxically, HR continues to climb to near maximum during on ice shifts.

Key words: Time Motion Analysis, Positional Differences, Performance

INTRODUCTION

Ice hockey is a popular team sport primarily played in North America and Europe. It is conducted on ice with skates and full body equipment and includes three, twenty minute periods where players, excluding the goaltender, substitute on and off the ice in shifts of varying lengths (e.g., 45-90s) depending on the flow of the game and coaching decisions (Green, Bishop, Houston, McKillop, Norman & Stothart, 1976; Cox, Miles, Verde & Rhodes, 1995; Jackson, Snydmiller, Game, Gervais & Bell, 2016). Competitive ice hockey requires a high level of skill and tactical awareness and is characterized by repeated bouts of high intensity sprinting (< 5s), directional changes and body contact interspersed with rest periods of low intensity activity such as gliding, standing, struggling with other players, and other movements (Montgomery, 1988; Cox et al, 1995; Bracko, Fellingham, Hall, Fisher & Cryer, 1998; Jackson et al, 2016). Furthermore, there are three primary positions in ice hockey that can be separated into forwards (left wing, right wing and center), defense (right and left) and a goaltender that have different duties and possibly different physiological profiles (Vescovi, Murray, Fiala & Vanbeest, 2006; Burr, Jamnik, Baker, MacPherson, Gledhill & McGuire, 2008; Bell, Snydmiller & Game, 2008). It has been reported that the overall intensity of ice hockey games is high and this requires players to possess exceptional anaerobic, aerobic and musculoskeletal fitness and a mesomorphic body type (Cox et al., 1995; Geithner, Lee, & Bracko, 2006; Stanula & Roczniak, 2014). It is also evident that there has been a significant increase in player size, strength, leanness and aerobic fitness over the past three decades indicating a change has occurred in the characteristics of the player and demands of the game especially at the professional level (Montgomery, 2006; Quinney, Dewart, Game, Snydmiller, Warburton & Bell, 2008). However, whether this has occurred at other levels of ice hockey has not been scientifically documented.

To evaluate the demands of a sport and the physiological requirements of competition, research generally focuses on a fitness evaluation of the players; an analysis of the type, frequency and duration of the different activities featured in the sport; and, measurement of various physiological indicators of the intensity of the movement patterns during the game (Cox et al., 1995; Bracko, 2001; Geithner et al., 2006; Barris & Button, 2008; Bell et al., 2008; Peterson, Fitzgerald, Dietz, Ziegler, Ingraham, Baker & Snyder, 2015; Jackson et al., 2016). This type of research provides a more complete understanding of the sport and can offer insight into fitness components, game performance characteristics, positional differences, coaching tactics and more specific strength and conditioning methods (Barris & Button, 2008; Taylor, 2003). There are some investigations that have reported fitness of ice hockey players as well as time motion characteristics of ice hockey games at a variety of competitive levels, some in combination with physiological measurements in men, women and youth, but research investigating University level players and competition has been limited and dated (Green et al., 1976). Furthermore, this latter research (Green et al., 1976) provided only partial movement analyses. Therefore, the purpose of this study was to measure the physiological characteristics of male university ice hockey players; examine the frequency and time spent performing various movements during ice hockey games; and, to assess the heart rate demands of ice hockey games. Supported by our recent research in female university ice hockey (Jackson et al., 2016), it was hypothesized that ice hockey players will present with high levels of conditioning, especially anaerobic fitness and muscular power parameters. As well, the frequency of and time spent performing movement patterns during games will favor gliding and moderate intensity activity and cardiovascular demands of the game will be intense as indicated by high HR responses. Furthermore, a comparison of these parameters between players in the forward and defense positions were conducted.

METHODS

Participants

The participants were 20 male ice hockey players (13 forwards and 7 defensemen) with a mean age of 22 ± 2 (SD) that belonged to the same University team. Age, anthropometric and fitness results are presented in Table 1. A verbal and written explanation of the study was provided and each volunteer signed a physical activity readiness questionnaire (PAR-Q) and an informed consent form. This study was approved by a University of Alberta Research Ethics Board.

Experimental Approach to the Problem

This study included a convenient sample of players belonging to the same University Hockey Team that were silver medalists at the University Sports National Championships during the same year this study was conducted. Players in the forward (center, right wing, left wing) and defense (right, left) position were examined with the goaltenders being excluded from the present analysis. Each player completed a series of standardized fitness tests (Table 1). A time motion analysis (TMA) was used to determine the frequency and duration that players performed at different movements

Table 1. Participant fitness testing results

Measurement	Forward (n=7)	Defense (n=13)
Age (yrs)	22±1	22±2
Height (cm)	179.2±6.9	180.9±3.9
Weight (kg)	84.4±6.7	84.3±6.3
Body fat (%)	10.7±1.5	10.9±2.1
5s Repeated anaerobic cycle test (RACT)		
Peak 5 s anaerobic PO (w)	1324.0±150.0	1345.3±132.5
Peak 5 s anaerobic PO (w×kg^{-1})	15.6±0.6	15.9±0.9
Mean anaerobic PO (w)	1187.3±126.0	1160.2±97.4
Mean anaerobic PO (w×kg^{-1})	14.1±0.7	13.8±0.9
Fatigue index (%)	23±6	28±4*
15m repeated on ice sprint test (ROIST)		
5m skating sprint time (s)	1.09±0.08	1.13±0.09
15m skating sprint time (s)	2.53±0.11	2.59±0.14
5m skating sprint velocity (m×s^{-1})	4.62±0.33	4.43±0.36
15m skating sprint velocity (m×s^{-1})	5.93±0.26	5.80±0.31
Skating sprint fatigue index (%)	4±2	5±3
Mean HR during ROIST	169±13	161±8
Peak HR during ROIST	179±11	170±6*
Musculo-skeletal fitness		
Maximum curl-ups (#)	41±10	46±16
Maximum push-ups (#)	33±6	29±6
Combined grip strength (kg)	137±17	135±17
Sit and reach flexibility (cm)	40.6±7.2	43.7±6.3
Lower & upper body power		
Vertical jump height (cm)	67.3±10.2	64.2±12.6
Vertical jump leg power (w)	5869.6±716.3	5645.8±801.7
Medicine ball chest throw (cm)	470.8±57.8	502.0±30.3
Aerobic Fitness		
VO$_2$ at VT (L×min^{-1})	3.62±0.49	3.47±0.40
HR at VT (b×min^{-1})	167±7	165±10
VT % of VO2peak	78±4	74±4
VO$_{2peak}$ (L×min^{-1})	4.64±0.54	4.68±0.30
VO$_{2peak}$ (ml×kg-1×min^{-1})	54.9±4.8	55.8±5.0
Maximum heart rate (b×min^{-1})	182±10	186±5

Values are given in $\bar{x}$ ± SD. PO=Power output; HR=Heart rate; VO$_2$ = Oxygen uptake; VT=Ventilatory threshold. *=Significantly different from forwards (p<0.05)

during competitive league ice hockey games played in the same arena. To do this, two digital cameras were affixed to the wall at opposite sides of the arena at the center line and set to record complete games that were later downloaded and analyzed using a computer software program (Dartfish©

Team Pro 5.0, Fribourg, SUI). Three ice hockey games were videotaped at different times in the season (October 1, October 20 and November 19) after several exhibition and four league games were completed. These games were chosen by the investigators after advice from the coaching staff that the opponents would accurately reflect a competitive level of play indicative of Canadian University hockey. In support of this, there was a mean (±SD) of 33 ± 6 versus 26 ± 5 shots on goal, 6 ± 2 versus 3 ± 1 goals scored and 6 ± 4 and 6 ± 5 penalties per game for the team reported in this research versus the opponents, respectively. Heart rate (HR) monitors were worn during each game and exercise testing. A complete rationale for this experimental design has been previously published by our research group (Jackson et al., 2016).

Physiological Measurements.

Each player underwent a series of standardized measurements in an exercise physiology laboratory. Age (years) was recorded, height (cm) measured with a standiometer (Tanita Arlington, IL) and body mass (BM; kg) determined using a balance beam scale (HealthoMeter, Bridgeview, IL). A sum of the mean of 2 repeated skinfolds measurements (required to be within 5 mm of each other) taken at 6 different upper and lower body sites (subscapular, mid tricep, chest, iliac crest, abdomen and mid-thigh) using Harpenden calipers (West Sussex, UK) was calculated and used in a formula [% body fat = ($\sum$of 6 skinfolds × 0.097) + 3.64] to predict body fat percentage (Yuhasz, 1996; Forbes, Bell & Kennedy, 2013).

Anaerobic fitness was measured using a five second repeated anaerobic cycling test (RACT) and a 15m repeated on-ice sprint test (ROIST). The RACT has been previously validated and the reliability determined by our lab for ice hockey players (Wilson, Snydmiller, Game, Quinney & Bell, 2010). Briefly, each player completed a standardized warm-up on a Monark Ergometric 894E Peak Bike (Monark, Vansbro SE) followed by four repeated, maximal sprints for five seconds separated by 10s of active recovery against an individualized resistance setting (0.095 × BM in kg) for a total test time of 60s. The data was captured using a custom designed computer interface and software program (Wilson et al., 2010). Peak (highest 5 s power output; PO), mean (average PO of all 4 sprints and a fatigue index was calculated {(% fatigue index = [(highest 5s PO – lowest 5s PO) ÷ peak 5s PO] × 100}. The ROIST involved seven repeats of maximal skating for a 15m distance set within the neutral zone on the ice. The on ice set up was regularly moved to ensure that ice quality did not influence the test results. Players wore a complete set of equipment excluding their hockey sticks. Each maximal sprint started from a stationary position and continued for 15m, immediately followed by a low intensity skating return to the starting line prior to the start of the subsequent sprint that began exactly every 15s for a total test time of 105s. A verbal count down of time was provided to each skater to ensure they returned to the start line, were completely stopped and ready for each sprint. Timing lights were used and positioned at the start and at 5m and 15m distances (Brower Timing Systems, Draper, and UT). Fast-

est 5m and 15m time and velocity (v) as well as a fatigue index were calculated {(% fatigue index = [(fastest 15m v – slowest 15m v) ÷ fastest 15m v] × 100}. Heart rate was measured during the ROIST test using a Polar® HR monitor set to memory for later analysis. Musculo-skeletal fitness was assessed according to established protocols. Maximum number of abdominal curl-ups was used to indicate abdominal muscular endurance (Quinney, Smith, & Wenger, 1984; Quinney et al., 2008). In addition, maximum number of push-ups for upper body muscular endurance, maximum hand grip of both hands combined for forearm strength and maximum sit and reach forward flexion using a Wells-Dillon flexometer was performed to assess flexibility (Canadian Society for Exercise Physiology, 2013). Lower body muscular power was indicated using a maximal vertical jump test (Canadian Society for Exercise Physiology, 2013) conducted with a Vertec jump height measuring device (Gill Athletics, Champaign, IL). Maximum jump height was recorded and leg power was calculated according to the formula [leg power (w) = (60.7 × jump height in cm) + (45.3 × body mass in kg) – 2055] of Sayers, Harackiewicz, Harman, Frykman & Rosenstein (1999). Upper body muscular power was measured using a 5.5kg seated medicine ball (Champion Sports, Marlboro, NJ) chest press style throw for maximum distance as reported by Gledhill and Jamnik (2007). Aerobic fitness was determined during a graded cycling exercise test to volitional exhaustion according to our protocol (Forbes et al., 2013). Briefly, each participant was provided with a standardized warm-up followed by an incremental protocol on a Monark 818E cycle ergometer until they were unable to continue (volitional fatigue). Respiratory gas exchange measurements were made using a Hans Rudolf valve assembly and headgear (Shawnee Mission, KS) that was attached to a calibrated metabolic measurement system (ParvoMedics, Sandy, UT). Ventilatory threshold was determined using the V-Slope method (Beaver, Wasserman & Whipp, 1986) and peak oxygen uptake (VO_{2peak}) was recorded as the highest VO_2 achieved during the test. Heart rate was measured throughout the test using a Polar® heart rate monitor.

Video Taping and Time Motion Analysis

We have published recent research on the identical camera setup, recording, TMA, and reliability of measurement for all movement patterns during ice hockey games in the same arena (Jackson et al., 2016). In brief, two GoPro HD cameras (set at 720 p and 60 fps) were positioned at the same height (20 m) from the ice surface on opposite walls of the area at center ice to ensure the complete ice surface (59.1 by 25.9 m) was captured. The files associated with each game were downloaded and player movements were analyzed using Dartfish© Team Pro 5.0 software (Fribourg, SUI). The software categorized the number of movement and time spent performing them as determined by a trained user with files exported to Excel for further analysis. The reliability (intra and inter observer, test retest) for coding movements and the frequency and time associated with each player using this technique was high as previously reported by our laboratory (Jackson et al., 2016). As well, the rationale for selection of the 10 primary different movement patterns performed in University ice hockey games has been justified and a complete description with examples have been reported by our lab (Jackson et al., 2016). The primary movements were: standing or little movement; forward accelerating skating start; gliding forward; moderate intensity forward skating; high or maximal intensity forward skating; accelerating backward skating start; gliding backward; moderate intensity backward skating; high or maximal intensity backward skating; and struggling for position or the puck with an opposing player.

Game Heart Rate Measurements

Polar® Team Sport HR monitors were worn by 13 different players (9 forwards and 4 defense) and set to record 5s average HR during each hockey game including the time between periods, as previously reported (Jackson et al., 2016). Seven players did not wear the monitors during the game for personal reasons feeling that it would be a distraction and/or a hindrance which may affect their performance.

Data Analyses

Data is presented as means ± SD. Percentage of total game time for each of the 10 movements was calculated for all players using Microsoft Excel® 2010. Separate one-way analysis of variance (ANOVA) was used to compare the fitness variables between positions. The TMA data and HR responses were collapsed across all three games for each player (see Jackson et al., 2016 for further rationalization). Separate 2 (positions) × 3 (periods) ANOVA with repeated measures was used to compare the frequency of movements, movement time and HR between forwards and defense across each of the three periods of the game. A one-way ANOVA compared the number of movement frequencies, times and HR for the game totals by positions. Alpha was pre-set at P<0.05. Statistica™ software was used for these latter analyses (Palo Alto, California).

RESULTS

A summary of the fitness variables for all players are shown in Table 1. A significantly greater % fatigue index during the RACT test and a lower peak HR during the ROIST was observed in the defensemen compared to forwards with no difference being observed in mean and peak HR's during the ROIST between forwards and defense, with each achieving 91 ± 8 and 96 ± 8 % of HR max combined, respectively.

Players in the defense position stood, glided and skated backwards at a moderate intensity more frequently and for longer time than forwards (P<0.05; Table 2). Forwards skated at a moderate intensity significantly more frequently and for longer periods of time in the forward direction compared to defense. However, both positions struggled more frequently and for longer times in the third period compared to the first two periods with defense struggling more than forwards in periods one and two (P<0.05). There were more sprint starts in the forward direction by both forwards and

defense in the third period and these occurred for longer periods of time for the forwards over the whole game (P<0.05). Forwards also glided for significantly longer periods of time in the forward direction compared to defense. Defense started sprinting backwards more often and for longer times compared to forwards during the whole game (P<0.05).

Figure 1 illustrates that the greatest time spent was associated with forward gliding on the ice for all players followed by forward skating at a moderate intensity, standing and backward gliding, sprint starts in the forward direction, struggling and forward maximal skating. The second greatest percentage of time spent for defense was gliding backwards and skating at a moderate intensity for forwards.

Heart rate responses did not differ between forwards and defense during ice hockey games (Table 3). Mean and peak HR responses during the game reached 94 ± 3 and 99 ± 3 % of HRmax for both positions, respectively. Heart rate recovered to levels significantly lower than mean and peak HR in between shifts. However, during the intermission periods

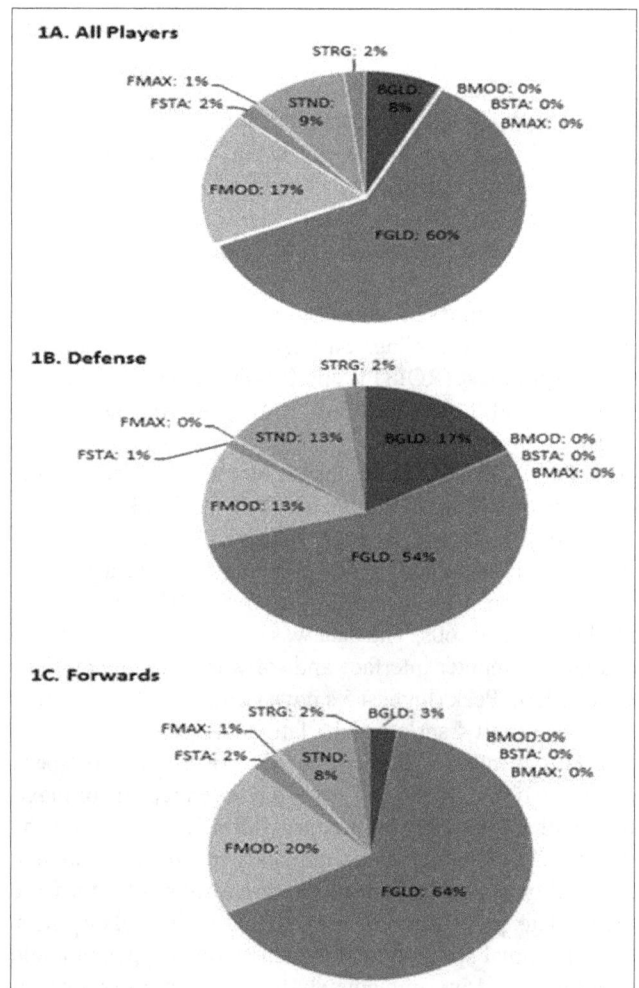

Figure 1. Percentage (%) of time spent in each of the movement categories for all players (A), Defense (B) and Forwards (C) during male ice hockey games. STND = Standing; FSTA = Forward start; FGLD = Gliding/cruising forward; FMOD = Moderate intensity forward skating; FMAX = High/maximal intensity forward skating; BGLD = Gliding/cruising backward; BMOD = Moderate intensity backward skating; STRG = Struggling

Table 2. Mean (±SD) frequency and duration in each of the movement categories for forwards and defense during men's ice hockey games

MC	Position	Frequency				Duration (s)			
		P1	P2	P3	Game total	P1	P2	P3	Game total
STND	D	14±3[a]	13±3[a]	14±4[a]	41±4[a]	32.4±9.8[a]	27.2±9.8[a]	31.5±11.7[a]	91.1±16.3[a]
	F	11±3	15±10	9±2	30±4	19.4±5.5	17.5±6.5	16.7±5.1	53.5±7.0
FSTA	D	3±1	3±1	5±2[b]	11±3	1.5±0.6[a]	1.8±0.8[a]	5.0±3.8[a,b]	8.3±4.1[a]
	F	3±2	3±1	6±4[b]	12±5	3.8±3.0	3.0±1.8	9.0±7.8[b]	15.9±7.9
FGLD	D	35±6	31±6	32±11	98±9	144.1±26.8[a]	124.8±28.4[a]	121.0±35.8[a]	390.0±37.6[a]
	F	35±8	32±5	31±6	98±13	157.1±44.2	145.7±26.4	150.2±45.3	452.9±76.1
FMOD	D	14±4[a]	12±3[a]	23±4[a,b]	49±9[a]	19.9±6.0	15.8±4.5	57.1±32.7[b]	92.7±38.3[a]
	F	21±6	21±4	25±9[b]	66±15	34.5±12.5	39.9±35.6	65.3±32.2[b]	139.7±65.4
FMAX	D	1±1	2±1	2±1	6±2	0.7±0.7	1.0±0.8	1.5±1.3	3.1±1.7
	F	1±1	1±1	2±1	4±2	1.4±1.2	1.2±1.6	1.6±1.2	4.3±2.9
BSTA	D	0±0	0±0	0±0	1±1[a]	0±0	0±0	0±0	0.3±0.4[a]
	F	0±0	0±0	0±0	0±0	0±0	0±0	0±0	0±0
BGLD	D	14±4[a]	21±6[a]	17±4[a,b]	43±12[a]	39.0±12.2[a]	33.8±19.1[a]	49.1±18.1[a,b]	122.0±43.5[a]
	F	4±1	3±1	6±3b	13±4	5.5±3.0	3.9±3.3	8.7±5.3	18.1±8.4
BMOD	D	1±1[a]	0±0	2±4a	3±4a	0.6±0.5[a]	0±0	0.4±0.6[a]	1.8±0.8[a]
	F	0±0	0±0	0±0	0±0	0.6±0.3	0±0	0.1±0.4	0.5±0.8
BMAX	D	0±0	0±0	0±0	0±0	0±0	0±0	0±0	0±0
	F	0±0	0±0	0±0	0±0	0±0	0±0	0±0	0±0
STRG	D	3±1	2±1	8±3[a,b]	12±4	1.8±0.8	1.1±1.1	13.7±8.7[a,b]	16.6±8.9
	F	3±1	2±1	5±3[b]	10±3	2.9±1.9	2.4±2.1	8.2±5.7[b]	13.6±6.6

MC=Movement category; D=Defense; F=Forwards; AP=All players. P=Period; STND=Standing; FSTA=Forward start; FGLD=Gliding/cruising forward; FMOD=Moderate intensity forward skating; FMAX=High/maximal intensity forward skating; BGLD=Gliding/cruising backward; BMOD=Moderate intensity backward skating; STRG=Struggling. Game Total=sum of movements for all three periods; Values given are the Mean±SD. a=significantly different from forwards. b=significantly different from Period 1 and 2

Table 3. Mean (±SD) heart rate measurements for forwards and defense during each period and complete ice hockey games

Variables	Period 1		Period 2		Period 3		Game	
	F	D	F	D	F	D	F	D
Mean shift HR (b×min⁻¹)	172±6	170±1	175±6	169±4	175±7	168±3	174±6	168±3
Peak shift HR (b×min⁻¹)	180±7[a]	177±3[a]	183±6[a]	177±8[a]	183±7[a]	179±3[a]	182±6[a]	178±5[a]
Mean recovery HR between shifts (b×min⁻¹)	139±9[b]	132±4[b]	138±10[b]	136±6[b]	136±8[b]	132±7[b]	137±8[b]	135±4[b]
Lowest HR between shifts (b×min⁻¹)	119±9[b,c]	112±4[b,c]	118±10[b,c]	117±6[b,c]	116±9 [b,c]	114±6 [b,c]	118±9 [b,c]	117±5 [b,c]

HR=heart rate; F=forward; D=defense; b=beats. a=significantly different from mean shift HR within period. b=significantly different from mean and peak shift HR within period. c=significantly different from mean and peak shift HR and mean recovery HR between shifts within period

it decreased significantly below the HR's recorded during game (Table 4).

DISCUSSION

The evaluation of the physical demands of sport are multi-faceted involving physiological assessments, an analysis of the different movement patterns, the time spent performing these activities during competition, including certain physiological measurements during competition to assess the in-tensity requirements of the game. Some early research investigating time motion, HR and fitness of university level ice hockey players was over 30 years ago (Green et al., 1976). Since that research, there has been an increase in both the physical and fitness attributes of players, as well as changes in the demand of the game, which is presently thought to be played at a higher intensity. In addition, different strategies have also emerged. Despite recent research in women's hockey (Jackson et al., 2016), no research has quantified the types and duration of movements performed in men's uni-

Table 4. Mean (±SD) heart rate measurements for forwards and defense during the intermissions between periods of men's ice hockey games

Variables	1st Intermission		2nd Intermission	
	F	D	F	D
Intermission mean HR (b×min^{-1})	109±7[a]	105±6[a]	110±7[a]	104±4[a]
Intermission low HR (b×min^{-1})	97±7[b]	94±5[b]	96±6[b]	93±3[b]

HR=heart rate; F=forward; D=defense; b=beats. a=significantly different from mean and peak shift HR and mean and low recovery HR from Table 3 during the game. b=significantly different from all other game HR's from Table 3.

versity ice hockey. However, various studies have investigated fitness and skating characteristics of players (Geithner et al., 2006; Lafontaine, Lamontagne & Lockwood, 2008; Bracko et al., 1998; Falinger, Kruisselbrink & Fowles, 2007; Gilenstam, Thorsen & Henriksson-Larsen, 2011), performed longitudinal comparisons of fitness (Montgomery, 2006; Quinney et al., 2008), examined position differences (Vescovi et al., 2006) and have investigated different physiological measurements during games (Spiering, Wilson, Judelson, & Rundell, 2003; Jackson et al., 2016) in players of different levels and sex. Our findings indicate that male university ice hockey players present with a high level of fitness in a variety of categories with only a few differences noted between players in the forward and defense positions. Players in both positions spend more than half of the game gliding forward, with positional requirements of playing, either defense or forward, eliciting some differences in movement patterns. The present results indicate that HR rapidly increases to near maximum levels in all players during each shift within competition regardless of position, with this increase in HR response being observed as well during short duration, on-ice sprint testing.

Assessment of hockey player fitness has become a cornerstone of both male and female player evaluation, athlete health and return to play after injury at all levels of hockey (amateur, university, national hockey league (NHL) draftees and professional players) (Montgomery, 1988; Cox et al., 1995; Game, Voaklander, Syrotuik & Bell, 2003; Montgomery 2006; Burr et al., 2008; Quinney et al., 2008; Jackson et al., 2016). Despite the suggestion that ice hockey is an "anaerobic" sport, the physical and fitness demands of the game and the repetition of certain activities, physical contact involved, as well as required positional differences (forwards vs. defense) during the three 20 minute periods suggest this would be an oversimplification (Vescovi et al., 2006; Jackson et al., 2016). The current study completed an extensive evaluation of fitness parameters observing that university hockey players present with high levels of fitness in several different categories (body composition, anaerobic, musculo-skeletal, agility and aerobic) supported by other research in men's (Green et al., 1976; Vescovi et al., 2006; Burr et al., 2008) and women's ice hockey (Bracko, 2001; Geithner et al., 2006; Ransdell & Murray, 2011; Jackson et al., 2016). Our findings revealed more similarities than differences between player positions. For instance, although defense had significantly higher fatigue index on the anaerobic cycle test (RACT) and a lower peak HR during on ice sprinting (ROIST) compared to forwards, no other fitness differences

were noted. In comparison to the research conducted over 30 years ago (Green et al., 1976), the present study observed players to be 2% taller, 11% heavier and achieved 5% higher on relative aerobic fitness. This trend in the differences in height, body mass and anaerobic power was also observed in NHL players over a 26 year period (Quinney et al., 2008). Other research has shown a greater relative aerobic fitness in collegiate forwards compared to defense (Peyer, Pivamik, Eisenmann & Vorkapich, 2001), with defense players being heavier than forwards in NHL draft aged players (Vescovi et al., 2006). As well, defense players in the NHL were taller, heavier and have lower relative aerobic fitness compared to forwards (Quinney et al., 2008) and this is likely somewhat due to NHL teams intentionally drafting larger players into the defense position to accommodate the increased physicality of ice hockey at this level (Montgomery, 2006). Conversely, in an analysis of a similar sample of NHL drafted players reported by Vescovi et al. (2006), and Burr et al (2008) they found eight fitness variables (excluding body composition) that were higher in defense than forwards and one variable (relative aerobic fitness VO2max) that was higher in forwards. Thus, it appears that any differences in the various indices of fitness between player positions may be somewhat dependent on level of play (i.e. University vs. entry draft aged vs. NHL) or related to differences in player selection practices of the type of player recruited to play University hockey versus NHL (Montgomery, 2006; Burr et al., 2008). Regardless, these findings underlie the importance of fitness testing in evaluating players, as well as for player positions in order to best design an athlete preparation training program. Future research should select, design and incorporate fitness testing specific to the goaltender position in ice hockey (Bell et al., 2008).

Research has used video analysis, global position systems, HR, thermoregulatory and various blood parameters to assess the physical demands experienced by athletes during actual sport competition with the validity, reliability and limitations of the various methods being reviewed (Dobson & Keogh, 2007; Barris & Button; 2008). Despite these methods, the ability to accurately quantify all the movement components of athletes during competitive games can be challenging. The combination of videotaping actual competitions and later coding the frequency of movements carried out and the time spent performing them using custom designed or commercially available software applications has been termed TMA of sport (Dobson & Keogh, 2007; Barris & Button, 2008; Forbes et al. 2013; Jackson et al., 2016). Despite recent TMA research of university ice hockey in women (Jackson et al., 2016), there seems to be no research that quantifies the types and duration of movement patterns in men's hockey despite some earlier studies that included some descriptive aspects of the game but did not provide an analysis of movements (Selinger et al., 1972; Thoden & Jette, 1975; Green et al., 1976). Knowing the types of movements, the frequency they are performed, and the time spent performing them is valuable information to the athlete and coach for training preparation, designing sport specific assessments, and the development of game strategies.

The present study revealed that the majority of time spent in the various activities during a University ice hockey game for all players was forward gliding (60%) followed by skating forward at a moderate intensity (17%), standing (9%), gliding backward (8%), struggling (2%), forward sprint starts (2%) and forward maximal sprinting (1%). Backward sprinting or backward skating at a moderate intensity were not frequently observed by any player (all <1%) during competition. Unfortunately, there is a lack of published data to compare these findings. However, the hierarchy of observed movement patterns aligns closely with women university ice hockey with a minor exception (Jackson et al., 2016). Men glided almost twice as long as women (60 vs. 36%, respectively) whereas women skated forward at a moderate intensity for long times than men (31 vs. 17%, respectively) and struggled longer (6 vs. 2%, respectively) during university ice hockey. Despite a similar order of game activities performed, these findings outline some differences in the amount of time spent performing certain activities between male and female university players.

Some expected differences in movement patterns between the two primary positions in ice hockey were observed. Defense stood, glided backwards and skated backwards at a moderate intensity as well as performed backwards sprint starts more frequently and for longer times compared to forwards during games. Forwards skated forward at a moderate intensity more frequently and for a greater duration while gliding and performing forward sprint starts for longer times compared to defense. We hypothesized that there may be differences in movement patterns between the three periods of play due to changes in game strategies which may depend on the score of the game or the possibility of an accumulation of fatigue. Both forwards and defense performed more sprint starts and moderate skating movements in the forward direction and for longer periods of time in the third period compared to first two periods. As well, all players glided backward and struggled for position or for the puck for greater periods of time in the third period. However, no other differences in movement patterns were observed between periods suggesting that the physical and mental fatigue aspects of the game may not have adversely influenced player movement as the game progressed.

In comparison to data reported by Green et al. in 1976, the mean game playing time of University hockey players was 9% shorter (20:08 vs. 22:05, min: s) while mean shift time was 30% shorter (65 vs. 88 s) and the mean number of shifts per game were 18% fewer (15 vs. 18) than observed in the present study. As well, the mean number of play stoppages

by referees was 129% fewer (0.5 vs. 2.3) and the mean time of play stoppages was 18% shorter (11 vs. 26s) with a similar recovery time between shifts (2%, 4:38 vs. 4.30, min: s), respectively. These data suggest that there have been changes in the characteristics of the game supporting the contention that player's shifts are shorter and more intense based on fewer and shorter play stoppages in a shift. Interestingly, Green et al (1976) also measured skating velocities during competition and found that forwards (center + wingers) achieved a mean of 270 $m \times s^{-1}$ while defense averaged 159 $m \times s^{-1}$ during ice hockey games. While the present study did not measure skating velocity during actual games, maximal skating velocities were measured during the ROIST test and showed that forwards and defense reached 356 $m \times s^{-1}$ and 348 $m \times s^{-1}$ over 15 m, respectively. These observations may suggest that current players and the game of University ice hockey is "faster" compared to over 30 years ago (Green et al., 1976).

Cardiovascular fitness is often overlooked in athletes and sports that are thought to be more anaerobic (sprint) in nature such as ice hockey. However, various research has shown a high HR response to repeated sprinting in different exercise modes (Buchheit, Laursen & Ahmaidi, 2007; Little & Williams, 2007; Meckel, Casorla & Eliakim, 2009; Lee, Lin & Cheng, 2011) as well as during men's and women's ice hockey (Green et al., 1976; Spiering et al., 2003; Jackson et al., 2016). Despite the majority of time spent gliding and skating at a moderate intensity during a game, HR continued to increase throughout a player's shift that lasted less than 65s and reached an average of 96 and 90 % and a peak of 100 and 96 % of HRmax for forwards and defense, respectively. Furthermore, our ROIST which included seven repeated skating sprints lasting less than three seconds also resulted in a continual increase in HR throughout the test eliciting HR's that averaged 87 and 93% of HRmax. Given that an ice hockey shift is often less than one minute during which players glide 60% of the time and perform low to moderate intensity activities 36% of the time, it is paradoxical that HR continues to increase to near maximum during a shift. As well, there were consistent increases in HR responses in some players during shifts that did not include sprints at a high intensity. It is possible, that the combination of physiological and psychological (emotional) stress experienced during competition likely contributes to the high heart rate response (Fernandez, et al., 2014). Other possibilities include increased sympathetic neural activity, elevated catecholamines, increased chemoreceptor stimulation (e.g. hydrogen ion), greater afferent neural activity from upper and lower body limb movement, thermoregulatory demands and increased aerobic metabolic demand are other possible factors (Jackson et al., 2016). Heart rates decreased to an average of 73 and 80% of HRmax between shifts for defense and forwards reaching a mean low between 63 and 65 % of HRmax. As well, HR decreased to similar low levels during the intermission between periods (51-59% of HRmax). These findings are similar to Green et al., (1976) and other research in female ice hockey players (Spiering et al., 2003; Jackson et al., 2016). These findings also underscore that ice hockey player's reach near maximum HR levels during most shifts, and although these HR's recover, they remain somewhat elevated in between shifts while sitting on the bench throughout a game. Thus, the role that cardiovascular fitness plays in the performance and health of the players should not be underestimated (Atwal, Porter & MacDonald, 2002) and further research is suggested to investigate the underlying stimuli to this rapid HR response in ice hockey players.

Limitations

The present study used a convenient sample of players from the same team and caution is advised if generalizations are to be made to other CIS teams and comparison should not be made to other levels of ice hockey (e.g., professional or international hockey). The games chosen for observation were in-season (CIS league games) and may not reflect the demands associated with playoff or championship games. As well, the sample sizes were small within each of the player position groups increasing the likelihood of a type II error in the statistical analyses. Visual observation of video-taped sport performance relies on the skill of the observer to accurately judge the different types of movements and the length of time they were performed. Despite our high inter and intra tester reliability, some movements, especially those that occur rapidly, may have been underestimated. Maximal backward skating and backward sprint starts were two categories that were absent or very infrequently observed but this finding was similar to our study in female ice hockey (Jackson et al., 2016). Furthermore, we did not separate movement activities when a player was in possession of the puck or not and that may have influenced the type of activity performed. Finally, there are differences in coach strategy that can influence game play that were beyond the control of the investigators.

Practical Applications

As previously mentioned, physiological assessment of athletes in a sport such as ice hockey consisting of a high level of fitness can be used to assist with player evaluation, selection, training programming, athlete health and player help with decisions for return to play after an injury. The knowledge of the types of movement patterns and the duration that these activities are performed during games can be used to support the selection of appropriate fitness assessments and the design and periodization of sport specific training programs. This would also aid the development of game simulated workouts for team members with limited ice time or are not playing in a particular game based on coaching decisions and would benefit from specific game simulation exercise (Jackson et al., 2016). The lack of difference in the fitness profiles of forwards and defense in the present study would suggest that similar supplementary training prescriptions would be feasible and practical for players in both positions. As well, there was some evidence in the present study that University level players and the game have changed and that players are taller, heavier and faster and the overall intensity of the game has increased over the past few decades.

CONCLUSIONS

Male university ice hockey players present with a high level of fitness in a variety of categories of fitness emphasizing the need for a well-rounded conditioning program. During ice hockey games, players spend the most time gliding forward and performing moderate intensity activity interspersed with shorter and less frequent high intensity movements. There were some differences in movement patterns between forwards and defense since players in the defense position are required to skate backwards and have some different responsibilities than forwards. Finally, despite the majority of the game time spent in low to moderate intensity activities, the intermittent nature of activities in a hockey shift coupled with the psychological stress of competition contributed to near maximal HR responses in all players.

ACKNOWLEDGEMENTS

The authors thank Jessie Gill, Ben Davis, Ciaran O'Flynn, the involved players, coaches and training staff.

REFERENCES

Atwal, S., Porter, J., & MacDonald, P. (2002). Cardiovascular effects of strenuous exercise in adult recreational hockey: the hockey heart study. *Canadian Medical Association Journal, 166*(3), 303-307.

Barris, S. & Button, C. (2008). A review of vision-based motion analysis in sport. *Sports Medicine, 38*(12), 1025-1043. http://dx.doi:10.2165/00007256-200838120-00006.

Beaver, W. L., Wasserman, K., & Whipp, B. J. (1986). A new method for detecting anaerobic threshold by gas exchange. *Journal of Applied Physiology, 60*, 2020-2027.

Bell, G., Snydmiller, G., & Game, A. (2008). An investigation of the type and frequency of movement patterns of national hockey league goaltenders. *International Journal of Sports and Performance, 3*, 80-87. http://dx.doi: org/10.1123/ijspp.3.1.80.

Bracko, M.R. (2001). On-ice performance characteristics of elite and non-elite woman's ice hockey players. *Journal of Strength and Conditioning Research, 15*(1), 42-47.

Bracko, M. R., Fellingham, G. W., Hall, L. T., Fisher, A. G., & Cryer, W. (1998). Performance skating characteristics of professional ice hockey forwards. *Sports Medicine, Training and Rehabilitation, 8*(3), 251-263. http://dx.doi.org/10.1080/15438629809512531.

Buchheit, M., Laursen, P. B., & Ahmaidi, S. (2007). Parasympathetic reactivation after repeated sprint exercise. *American Journal of Physiology – Heart and Circulatory Physiology, 293*, H133-H141. http://dx.doi:10.1152ajpheart.00062.2007.

Burr, J., Jamnik, V., Baker, J., MacPherson, A., Gledhill, N., & McGuire, E. (2008). Relationship of physical fitness test results and hockey playing potential in elite-level ice hockey players. *Journal of Strength and Conditioning Research, 22*(5), 1535-1543. http://dx.doi:10.1519/jsc.0b013e318181ac20.

Canadian Society for Exercise Physiology (2013). CSEP-

PATH Physical Activity Training for Health. Ottawa: Canadian Society for Exercise Physiology.

Cox, M. H., Miles, D. S., Verde, T. J., & Rhodes, E. C. (1995). Applied physiology of ice hockey. *Sports Medicine, 19*(3), 184-201. http://dx.doi: 10.2165/00007256-199519030-00004.

Dobson, B. P. & Keogh, J. W. L. (2007). Methodological issues for the application of time-motion analysis research. *Strength and Conditioning Journal, 29*(2), 48-55.

Falinger, C. M., Kruisselbrink, L.D., & Fowles, J. R. (2007). Relationships to skating performance in competitive hockey players. *Strength and Conditioning Journal, 21*(3), 915-922.

Fernandez-Fernandez, J., Boullosa, D.A., Sanz-Rivas, D., Abreu, L., Filaire, E., & Mendez-Villanueva, A. (2014). Psychophysiological stress response during training and competition young female competitive tennis players. *International Journal of Sports Medicine, 36*(1), 22-28. http://dx.doi: 10.1055/s0034-1384544.

Forbes, S. C., Kennedy, M. D., & Bell, G. J. (2013). Time-motion analysis, heart rate, and physiological characteristics of international canoe polo athletes. *Journal of Strength and Conditioning Research, 27*(10), 2816-2822.

Game, A., Voaklander, D., Syrotuik, D., & Bell, G. (2003). Incidence of exercise-induced bronchospasm and exercise induced hypoxaemia in female varsity hockey players. *Research in Sports Medicine*, 11: 11-21. http://dx.doi: 10.1080/15438620390192971.

Geithner, C. A., Lee, A. M., & Bracko, M. R. (2006). Physical and performance differences among forwards, defensemen, and goalies in elite women's ice hockey. *Journal of Strength and Conditioning Research, 20*(3), 500-505.

Gilenstam, K. M., Thorsen, K., & Henriksson-Larsen. (2011). Physiological correlates of skating performance in women's and men's ice hockey. *Journal of Strength and Conditioning Research, 25*(8), 2133-2142.

Gledhill, N. & Jamnik, V. (2007). Detailed assessment protocols for NHL entry draft players. Toronto: York University.

Green, H., Bishop, P., Houston, M., McKillop, R., Norman, R., & Stothart, P. (1976). Time-motion and physiological assessments of ice hockey performance. *Journal of Applied Physiology, 40*(2), 159-163.

Jackson, J., Snydmiller, G., Game, A., Gervais, P., & Bell, G. (2016). Movement characteristics and heart rate profiles displayed bzy female university ice hockey players. *International Journal of Kinesiology & Sport Science, 4*(1), 43-54. http://dx.doi:10.7575/aiac.ijkss.v.4n.1p.43.

Lafontaine, D., Lamontagne, M., & Lockwood, K. (1998). Time-motion analysis of ice-hockey skills during games. *International Symposium on Biomechanics in Sport, 16*, 481-484.

Lee, C. L., Lin, J. C., & Cheng, C. F. (2011). Effect of caffeine ingestion after creatine supplementation on intermittent high-intensity sprint performance. *European Journal of Applied Physiology, 111*, 1669-1677. http://dx.doi: 10.1070/s00421-010-1792-0.

Little, T., & Williams, A. (2007). Effects of sprint duration and exercise: rest ratio on repeated sprint performance and physiological responses in professional soccer players. *Journal of Strength and Conditioning Research, 21*(2), 646-648.

Meckel, Y., Casorla, T. & Eliakim, A. (2009). The influence of basketball dribbling on repeated sprints. *International Journal of Coaching Science, 3*(2), 43-56.

Montgomery, D. L. (1988). Physiology of ice hockey. *Sports Medicine, 5*, 99-126. http://dx.doi: 10.2165/00007256-198805020-00003.

Montgomery, D. L. (2006). Physiological profile of professional hockey players – a longitudinal comparison. *Applied Physiology, Nutrition and Metabolism, 31*(3), 181-185. http://dx.doi:10.1139/H06-012.

Peterson, B. J., Fitzgerald, J. S. Dietz, C. C., Ziegler, K. S., Ingraham, S. J., Baker, S. E., & Snyder, E. M. (2015). Aerobic capacity is associated with improved repeated shift performance in hockey. *Journal of Strength and Conditioning Research, 29*(6), 1465-1472.

Peyer, K. L., Pivarnik, J. M., Eisenmann, J. C., & Vorkapich, M. (2011). *Journal of Strength and Conditioning Research, 25*(5), 1183-1192.

Quinney, H. A., Smith, D., & Wenger, H. A. (1984). A field test for the assessment of abdominal muscular endurance in professional ice hockey players. *Journal of Orthopeadic and Sports Physical Therapy, 6*, 30-33. http://dx.doi: 10.2519/jospt.1984.6.1.30.

Quinney, H. A., Dewart, R., Game, A., Snydmiller, G., Warburton, D., & Bell, G. (2008). A 26 year physiological description of a National Hockey League team. *Applied Physiology, Nutrition and Metabolism, 33*(4), 753-760. http://dx.doi:10.1139/H08-051.

Ransdell, L. B. & Murray, T. (2011). A physical profile of elite female ice hockey players from the USA. *Journal of Strength and Conditioning Research, 25*(9), 2358-2363.

Sayers, S. P, Harackiewicz, D. V, Harman, E. A., Frykman, P. N, & Rosenstein, M. T. (1999). Cross-validation of three jump power equations. *Medicine and Science in Sport and Exercise, 31*(4): 572-577. http://dx.doi: 10.1097/00005768-199904000-00013.

Seliger, V., Kostka, V., Grusova, D., Kovac, J., Machovcova, J., Pauer, M., & Urbankova, R. (1972). Energy expenditure and physical fitness of ice-hockey players. *European Journal of Applied Physiology, 30*(4), 283-291. http://dx.doi: 10.1007/BF00696119.

Spiering, B. A., Wilson, M. H., Judelson, D. A., & Rundell, K. W. (2003). Evaluation of cardiovascular demands of game play and practice in Women's Ice Hockey. *Journal of Strength and Conditioning Research, 17*(2), 329-333.

Stanula, A. & Roczniok, R. (2014). Game intensity analysis of elite adolescent ice hockey players. *Journal of Human Kinetics, 44*, 211-221. http://dx.doi: 10.2478/hukin-2014-0126.

Taylor, J. Basketball: Applying time motion data to conditioning. (2003). *Strength and Conditioning Journal, 25*(2), 57-64.

Thoden, J. S. & Jette, M. (1975). Aerobic and anaerobic activity patterns in junior and professional hockey. *Movement (Special Hockey), 2*, 145-153.

Vescovi, J. D., Murray, T. M., Fiala, K.A., & Vanheest, J. L. (2006). Off-ice performance and draft status of elite ice hockey players. *International Journal of Sports, Physiology and Performance, 1*, 207-221. http://dx.doi:org/10.1123/ijspp.1.3.207.

Wilson, K., Snydmiller, G., Game, A., Quinney, H. A., & Bell, G. (2010). The development and reliability of a repeated anaerobic cycling test in female ice hockey players. *Journal of Strength and Conditioning Research, 24*(2), 580-584.

Yuhasz, M. (1996). Physical fitness and sports appraisal laboratory manual. London: The University of Western Ontario.

12

Back Squat Potentiates Both Vertical and Horizontal Jump Performance in Collegiate Ice Hockey Players

Cale Bechtel, Joshua A. Cotter, Evan E. Schick*

Physiology of Exercise and Sport (PEXS) Laboratory, Department of Kinesiology, Long Beach State University, 1250 Bellflower Blvd., Long Beach, CA, 90840-4901

Corresponding Author: Evan E. Schick, E-mail: evan.shick@csulb.edu

---

ARTICLE INFO

Conflicts of interest: None
Funding: None

ABSTRACT

Background: Back squats (BSQ) have been shown to transiently improve performance in explosive vertical movements such as the vertical jump (VJ). Still, understanding of this phenomenon, termed post-activation potentiation (PAP), remains nebulous as it relates to explosive horizontal movements. **Objective:** Therefore, the purpose of the present investigation was to assess whether heavy BSQ can potentiate both VJ and horizontal jump (HJ) performance. **Method:** Nine male ice hockey players from the Long Beach State ice hockey team performed five testing sessions separated by 96-hours. The first testing session consisted of a one repetition maximum (1-RM) BSQ to determine subsequent testing loads. The four subsequent testing sessions, which were randomized for order, consisted of five repetitions of BSQ at 87% 1-RM followed by horizontal jump (BSQ-HJ), five repetitions of BSQ at 87% 1-RM followed by vertical jump (BSQ-VJ), horizontal jump only (CT-HJ) and vertical jump only (CT-VJ). During the potentiated conditions, rest intervals were set at five minutes between the BSQ and either VJ or HJ. Alpha-level was set a priori at 0.05. **Results:** The results indicate that both vertical ($p=0.017$) and horizontal ($p=0.003$) jump were significantly increased (VJ= +5.51cm, HJ= +11.55cm) following a BSQ. **Conclusion:** These findings suggest that BSQ may improve both vertical and horizontal jump performance in athletes who participate in sports emphasizing horizontal power, such as ice hockey.

Keywords: Plyometric Exercise, Muscle Strength, Resistance Training, Back Squat, Acute Exercise

---

INTRODUCTION

Heavy-load lifting has been shown to transiently improve muscular power (Hodgson, Docherty and Robbins, 2005, Tillin and Bishop, 2009). This phenomenon, termed post activation potentiation (PAP), is maximized by performing an explosive movement task subsequent to a heavily loaded lift that shares a similar movement pattern (Golas, Maszczyk, Zajac, Mikolajec and Stastny, 2016). PAP is influenced by a combination of factors such as volume and intensity, intraset and intertask rest intervals, participant characteristics and the type of exercise performed (Hodgson, Docherty and Robbins, 2005, Seitz and Haff, 2016, Seitz, Mina and Haff, 2016, Tillin and Bishop, 2009, Tobin and Delahunt, 2014). Used effectively in a training program, PAP may enhance sensitivity to power training such as plyometrics (Docherty and Hodgson, 2007, Tillin and Bishop, 2009). As peak performance in most sports is a function of maximizing muscular power, PAP training may be an important asset to resistance training programs (Docherty and Hodgson, 2007).

Back squats (BSQ), which are ubiquitously used in exercise training, have consistently been shown to potentiate vertical jump (VJ) performance across various populations (Docherty and Hodgson, 2007, Evetovich, Conley and McCawley, 2015, Seitz and Haff, 2016, Seitz, Mina and Haff, 2016, Tillin and Bishop, 2009, Tobin and Delahunt, 2014). VJ height is a measure of lower body power that is commonly used as an indicator of athletic potential since explosive leg power correlates to performance in many sports (Burkett, Phillips and Ziuraitis, 2005, Gourgoulis, Aggeloussis, Kasimatis, Mavromatis and Garas, 2003). Robust VJ potentiation occurs following BSQ performed with loads of up to 87% of the one repetition maximum (1-RM) and four to eight minutes of post-squat rest (Hodgson, Docherty and Robbins, 2005, Kilduff, Owen, Bevan, Bennett, Kingsley and Cunningham, 2008, Nibali, Chapman, Robergs and Drinkwater, 2015, Seitz and Haff, 2016, Tillin and Bishop, 2009). The apparent efficacy of BSQ-VJ potentiation may be due to shared activation patterns in lower body musculature, including: quadriceps, hamstrings, gastrocnemius, gluteus maximus, gluteus medius, plantar flexors, dorsiflexors, abdominals and spinal erectors (Delavier, 2010, Docherty and Hodgson, 2007, Gullett, Tillman, Gutierrez and Chow, 2009,

Seitz and Haff, 2016, Tillin and Bishop, 2009). Although VJ predominates PAP research, it is imperative to explore alternative movement patterns that may be potentiated by BSQ as certain sports do not emphasize vertical movement patterns.

One such sport is ice hockey, which emphasizes horizontal movement patterns instead of vertical. In fact, the musculoskeletal fitness assessment section of the National Ice Hockey League (NHL) combine utilizes standing horizontal jump performance as their primary means of assessing muscular power (Glendhill, 2007). High scores on this assessment indicate a player's ability to skate powerfully, shoot hard, and push opponents out of the way (Glendhill, 2007). Yet, a review of current PAP research reveals a dearth of literature surrounding the sport of ice hockey as well as the nature of horizontal jump potentiation; to date, just one study using rugby players has reported that loaded BSQ can potentiate HJ performance (Seitz, Mina and Haff, 2016). Furthermore, insufficient data exists in support of whether the aforementioned BSQ-VJ potentiation extends to athletes specializing in sports which stress horizontal movement. Therefore, the present study examined collegiate ice hockey players to pursue the following aims: 1) to clarify whether BSQ-VJ potentiation extends to athletes competing in horizontal movement-dominant sports, 2) to assess whether HJ is also sensitive to BSQ-induced potentiation, and 3) to compare levels of VJ and HJ potentiation. The primary hypothesis follows that heavy BSQ will potentiate both VJ and HJ performance.

MATERIALS AND METHODS

Experimental Approach

Participants performed all five testing sessions. The first testing session consisted of a 1-RM BSQ. The four remaining testing sessions, performed in random order, consisted of: 1) back squat followed by horizontal jump (BSQ-HJ), 2) back squat followed by vertical jump (BSQ-VJ), 3) horizontal jump only (CT-HJ) and 4) vertical jump only (CT-VJ). Participants completed five BSQ repetitions at 87% of their 1-RM during the BSQ-HJ and BSQ-VJ testing sessions. Table 1 summarizes the study design.

Participants

Nine male ice hockey players (22 ± 0.47 years) from the Long Beach State University club ice hockey team voluntarily participated for this study (Table 2). Participants were college level athletes with experience in ice hockey (11 ± 1.47 years) and resistance training (4 ± 0.94 years). The Institutional Review Board of Long Beach State University approved the research protocol. Participants signed a Physical Activity Readiness Questionnaire (PAR-Q) and informed consent before participation. Inclusion criteria consisted of: 1) active member of LBSU ice hockey team, 2) free from unresolved orthopedic injuries for the preceding 12 months, 3) free from diagnosed cardiopulmonary or metabolic disease, 4) two or more years of resistance training experience, and 5) five or more years of ice hockey experience.

Instrumentation and Tools

For the BSQ, a 45lb standard Olympic barbell and bumper plates (45, 35, 25, 15, 10 lbs.) were utilized (Rogue® Columbus, OH). Participants performed the BSQ inside a squat rack (Rogue® Columbus, OH). A Vertec® (Sports Imports Inc., OH) jumping apparatus was used to measure vertical jump (VJ) height to the nearest (cm). The horizontal jump (HJ) performance test was assessed on the floor using a cloth tape measure with increments to the nearest (cm) (Jackson, 2017).

Procedures

Testing encompassed five separate sessions, each separated by 96-hours, during which participants refrained from resistance exercise. Past reports confirm robust VJ potentiation following BSQ performed with loads of to 87% 1-RM and four to eight minute post-squat rest periods (Hodgson, Docherty and Robbins, 2005, Kilduff, Owen, Bevan, Bennett, Kingsley and Cunningham, 2008, Seitz and Haff, 2016, Seitz, Mina and Haff, 2016, Tillin and Bishop, 2009). Thus, we chose a BSQ intensity level of 87% 1-RM as well as five minute post-squat rest periods for the BSQ-VJ and BSQ-HJ conditions. The first testing session consisted of a 1-RM BSQ in order to calculate the load corresponding to 87% of the 1-RM load. All participants successfully performed five repetitions of BSQ at 87% 1-RM during the BSQ-VJ and BSQ-HJ testing sessions. The 1-RM BSQ protocol was adopted from the National Strength and Conditioning Association (Baechle, 2008). Briefly, participants first performed five to ten repetitions at a light resistance (<30% projected 1-RM) as part of a squat-specific warm-up. Following a one minute rest period, three to five more repetitions were performed with an additional 30-40lbs. Participants then rested for two minutes before performing two to three repetitions with an additional 30-40lbs. All subsequent sets included two minute rest periods and only single repetitions with incremental increases between 10-40 lbs. until the 1-RM was completed. Load was incrementally added to achieve the 1-RM within 3-5 sets. A general warm up protocol for all five testing sessions (1-RM, BSQ-HJ, BSQ-VJ, CT-HJ, CT-VJ) began with a three to five minute warm up on a stationary bike at a self-selected resistance. A choice was given after the three minute mark whether they wanted to continue until five minutes or began their mandatory athletic drills and ballistic stretches. Next a series of athletic drills (internal/external hip rotations, lateral shuffles, high knees, butt kicks) were performed. Athletic drills were performed twice over the length of the laboratory. Two ballistic stretching exercises (frontal and lateral leg swings) were utilized after the athletic drills prior to beginning the testing session (Delavier, 2010, Ojeda, Rios, Barrilao and Serrano, 2016, Tobin and Delahunt, 2014). Participants performed five repetitions using 87% of their 1-RM load for the BSQ-HJ and BSQ-VJ conditions. Participants were encouraged to use a squat stance width and bar placement that was consistent with their typical technique. Depth of the squat was strictly enforced; terminal range was reached once the inguinal

Table 1. Study Design

Condition	Sets	Reps	S.I. (% 1-RM)	R.I. (min)	HJ (cm)	VJ (cm)
1-RM	3-5	NSCA Protocol	-	-	-	-
BSQ-HJ	1	5	87%	5	HJ	-
BSQ-VJ	1	5	87%	5	-	VJ
CT-HJ	0	0	0%	Warm up	HJ	-
CT-VJ	0	0	0%	Warm up	-	VJ

1-RM=Back Squat Max Test; BSQ=Back Squat; CT=Control; HJ=Horizontal Jump; VJ=Vertical Jump; S.I. = Squat Intensity; R.I. = Rest Interval

crease and proximal portion of the knee were level (Baechle, 2008, Reardon, Hoffman, Mangine, Wells, Gonzalez, Jajtner, Townsend, McCormack, Stout, Fragala and Fukuda, 2014). Squat depth was visually monitored by two certified strength and conditioning specialists (CSCS), one on each side of the lifter. Following the BSQ, participants rested for 5 minutes before performing either the VJ or HJ (Ray, 2017). The NHL Entry Draft protocol was used to assess HJ (Glendhill, 2007). The participants stood with feet slightly apart with their toes behind the jumping line. Using an arm swing the participants jumped as far as possible, and the average of the three trials was used. Distance was recorded to the nearest (cm) from the jumping line to the heel mark utilizing a cloth tape measure. The VJ was assessed using a Vertec® apparatus following the National Strength and Conditioning Association vertical jump protocol (Baechle, 2008) Participants were not required to squat to a certain depth. VJ was recorded to the nearest ¼ inch from the average of three jumps and later converted to (cm).

Statistical Analysis

VJ and HJ potentiation was assessed by paired samples t-tests (SPSS version 24). Effect sizes were determined by Cohen's d for paired samples t-test (Lakens, 2013), which assessed the magnitude of the change in VJ and HJ performance following BSQ. These changes were considered trivial <0.20; small, 0.20–0.50; medium, 0.5–0.8; large, 0.8–1.30; or very large, >1.30 (Hopkins, 2010). Shapiro-Wilk test confirmed normality for all conditions (Sig >0.05). Alpha-level was set a priori at 0.05.

RESULTS

The characteristics of participants are illustrated in table 2. Our primary objective was to examine the effect of BSQ on VJ and HJ performance in athletes participating in horizontal movement-dominant sports. To this end, we subjected nine collegiate ice hockey players to four randomized testing sessions (CT-VJ, BSQ-VJ, CT-HJ, BSQ-HJ). VJ performance was significantly increased (+5.51 cm) following the BSQ (p=0.017). HJ performance was also significantly increased (+11.55 cm) following the BSQ (p=0.003). Additionally, Cohen's d revealed a large effect size for both VJ (1.00) and HJ (1.38). Table 3 summarizes the horizontal and vertical jump distances in both testing conditions.

Table 2. Subject Descriptive Data

Variables	Mean±*SD*
Height (cm)	188.62±2.73
Weight (kg)	87.94±20.49
RT (yrs)	4.02±2.82
HE (yrs)	11.01±4.41
Age (yrs)	22.04±1.41
1-RM	86.22±35.19

SE=Standard Deviation RT=Resistance Training Experience HE=Ice Hockey Experience

Table 3. Horizontal and Vertical Jump Distance (mean±standard error)

Condition	*n*	Jump Distance (cm)	Effect Size
CT-VJ	9	54.45±3.34	1.00
BSQ-VJ	9	59.96±3.20†	
CT-HJ	9	199.35±8.51	1.38
BSQ-HJ	9	210.92±7.98*	

CT-HJ=Horizontal Jump – Control; BSQ-HJ=Back Squat – Horizontal Jump; CT-VJ=Vertical Jump – Control; BSQ-VJ=Back Squat – Vertical Jump; *P<0.05 versus CT-HJ; †P<0.05 versus CT-VJ

DISCUSSION

The present study examined whether loaded BSQ could potentiate VJ and HJ performance in collegiate ice hockey players. Herein, we demonstrate that performing five repetitions of BSQ at 87% 1-RM significantly potentiates both VJ and HJ performance in collegiate ice hockey players. Furthermore, effect size (ES) calculation revealed a large (ES>0.8) magnitude of improvement for each jump following BSQ. The current findings concerning VJ performance have been thoroughly corroborated by past studies which have established that potentiation may occur four to eight minutes following near maximal intensity (>80% 1-RM) dynamic movements or isometric contractions (Evetovich, Conley and McCawley, 2015, Nibali, Chapman, Robergs and Drinkwater, 2015, Seitz, Mina and Haff, 2016, Tillin and Bishop, 2009, Tobin and Delahunt, 2014). Additionally, our data are in-line with past PAP research which has shown significant VJ potentiation following a BSQ at 87% 1-RM (Kilduff, Owen, Bevan, Bennett, Kingsley and Cunningham, 2008, Reardon, Hoffman, Mangine, Wells, Gonzalez,

Jajtner, Townsend, McCormack, Stout, Fragala and Fukuda, 2014). In the present study, BSQ significantly potentiated VJ (p=0.017), and the magnitude of this effect was large (ES = 1.00). These findings are consistent with several other PAP studies using similar procedures (Evetovich, Conley and McCawley, 2015, Nibali, Chapman, Robergs and Drinkwater, 2015, Seitz, Mina and Haff, 2016). Still, to our knowledge, this study is the first to investigate and produce data indicating that BSQ can potentiate VJ performance in collegiate ice hockey players. This suggests that vertical movement patterns can be acutely potentiated in athletes who primarily perform in a horizontal direction. Future research should explore whether vertical potentiation in training can improve an ice hockey player's ability to skate powerfully, shoot hard, and push opponents out of the way.

HJ performance is used as an assessment for lower body power in sports which predominately move in a horizontal direction, such as ice hockey (Glendhill, 2007). This suggests that, 1) improving horizontal power may be advantageous to ice hockey performance, and 2) improving HJ performance may increase the likelihood of being drafted by an ice hockey team. Nevertheless, an overall paucity of data exists regarding HJ potentiation. The current study is the first to explore HJ potentiation in ice hockey players. Our data show that HJ was significantly potentiated by the BSQ (p=0.003) with a mean increase of (+11.55 cm), and, similar to BSQ-VJ, the magnitude of this effect was large (ES= 1.38). These findings are supported by one previous report in which multiple sets of BSQ potentiated HJ in rugby players (Seitz, Mina and Haff, 2016). As noted above, ice hockey movement patterns are primarily in a horizontal direction, thus this finding may suggest that athletes competing predominately in a horizontal direction are sensitive to horizontal movement potentiation. However, future research should explore whether this phenomenon is exclusive to athletes in horizontal movement sports or if athletes who participate in non-horizontal dominant sports experience similar horizontal movement potentiation. A noteworthy limitation of the current study is that of relative BSQ strength. Relative BSQ strength is a key variable in facilitating movement potentiation (Seitz and Haff, 2016, Tillin and Bishop, 2009). Previous reports suggest that PAP training complexes are maximized in male athletes who can BSQ 1.75x their bodyweight (Seitz and Haff, 2016). In the current study, participants back squatted an average of 0.97x their bodyweight. Though the implication of this limitation is unclear, it is possible that greater BSQ performance could have increased effect sizes in both VJ and HJ. Thus, future endeavors should examine the interaction of BSQ strength with both HJ and VJ as well as how this potential interaction compares between the two types of jumps.

CONCLUSION

In conclusion, findings from the present study demonstrate that five repetitions of BSQ, performed at 87% 1-RM, can potentiate VJ and HJ performance. These findings suggest that strength and conditioning practitioners may benefit from incorporating potentiation complexes in order to improve horizontal power in athletes who must excel in a horizontal direction. Future research should explore the extent to which varying levels of relative BSQ strength may influence the magnitude of VJ and HJ potentiation, and whether horizontal potentiation is expressed by athletes who participate in non-horizontal dominant sports.

REFERENCES

Baechle TR, Earle, R.W. (2008) *Essentials of Strength and Conditioning.* Champaign, IL: Human Kinetics.

Burkett LN, Phillips WT, Ziuraitis J. (2005) The best warm-up for the vertical jump in college-age athletic men. *Journal Of Strength And Conditioning Research* 19(3):673-6.

Delavier F. (2010) *Strength Training Anatomy.* 3rd. ed. Champaign, Illinois: Human Kinetics.

Docherty D, Hodgson MJ. (2007) The application of postactivation potentiation to elite sport. *International Journal Of Sports Physiology And Performance* 2(4):439-44.

Evetovich TK, Conley DS, McCawley PF. (2015) Postactivation potentiation enhances upper- and lower-body athletic performance in collegiate male and female athletes. *Journal Of Strength And Conditioning Research* 29(2):336-42.

Glendhill N, & Jannik, V. (2007) *Detailed assessment protocols for NHL entry draft players.* Toronto, ONT: York University.

Golas A, Maszczyk A, Zajac A, Mikolajec K, Stastny P. (2016) Optimizing post activation potentiation for explosive activities in competitive sports. *Journal Of Human Kinetics* 52:95-106.

Gourgoulis V, Aggeloussis N, Kasimatis P, Mavromatis G, Garas A. (2003) Effect of a submaximal half-squats warm-up program on vertical jumping ability. *Journal Of Strength And Conditioning Research* 17(2):342-4.

Gullett JC, Tillman MD, Gutierrez GM, Chow JW. (2009) A biomechanical comparison of back and front squats in healthy trained individuals. *Journal Of Strength And Conditioning Research* 23(1):284-92.

Hodgson M, Docherty D, Robbins D. (2005) Post-activation potentiation: underlying physiology and implications for motor performance. *Sports Medicine* 35(7):585-95.

Hopkins WG. (2010) Linear models and effect magntidues for research, clinical and practical applications. *Sportscience* 14:49-57.

Jackson KM, Beach T.A. and Andrews D.M. (2017) The effect of an isometric hip muscle strength training protocol on valgus angle during a drop vertical jump in competitive female volleyball players. *International Journal of Kinesiology & Sports Science* 5(4):1-9.

Kilduff LP, Owen N, Bevan H, Bennett M, Kingsley MI, Cunningham D. (2008) Influence of recovery time on post-activation potentiation in professional rugby players. *Journal Of Sports Sciences* 26(8):795-802.

Lakens D. (2013) Calculating and reporting effect sizes to facilitate cumulative science: a practical primer for t-tests and ANOVAs. *Frontiers in Psychology* 4:863.

Nibali ML, Chapman DW, Robergs RA, Drinkwater EJ. (2015) Considerations for determining the time course of post-activation potentiation. *Applied Physiology, Nutrition, And Metabolism* 40(11):1163-70.

Ojeda AH, Rios LC, Barrilao RG, Serrano PC. (2016) Acute effect of a complex training protocol of back squats on 30-m sprint times of elite male military athletes. *Journal of Physical Therapy Science* 28(3):752-6.

Ray T, Adams, KJ, DeBeliso, M. (2017) The Relationship Between Core Stability & Squat Ratio in Resistance-Trained Males. *International Journal of Kinesiology & Sports Science* 5(2):7-15.

Reardon D, Hoffman JR, Mangine GT, Wells AJ, Gonzalez AM, Jajtner AR, Townsend JR, McCormack WP, Stout JR, Fragala MS, Fukuda DH. (2014) Do changes in muscle architecture affect post-activation potentiation? *Journal Of Sports Science & Medicine* 13(3):483-92.

Seitz LB, Haff GG. (2016) Factors Modulating Post-Activation Potentiation of Jump, Sprint, Throw, and Upper-Body Ballistic Performances: A Systematic Review with Meta-Analysis. *Sports Medicine* 46(2):231-40.

Seitz LB, Mina MA, Haff GG. (2016) Postactivation Potentiation of Horizontal Jump Performance Across Multiple Sets of a Contrast Protocol. *Journal Of Strength And Conditioning Research* 30(10):2733-40.

Tillin NA, Bishop D. (2009) Factors modulating post-activation potentiation and its effect on performance of subsequent explosive activities. *Sports Medicine* 39(2):147-66.

Tobin DP, Delahunt E. (2014) The acute effect of a plyometric stimulus on jump performance in professional rugby players. *Journal Of Strength And Conditioning Research* 28(2):367-72.

13

Metabolic Response to Four Weeks of Muscular Endurance Resistance Training

John W. Farrell III[1]*, David J. Lantis[1], Carl J. Ade[2], Debra A. Bemben[1], Rebecca D. Larson[1]

[1]Department of Health and Exercise Science, University of Oklahoma, 1401 Asp Ave, Norman, OK, 73019, USA, [2]Department of Kinesiology, Kansas State University, 920 Denison Ave, Manhattan, KS, 66506, USA
Corresponding Author: John W. Farrell III, E-mail: John.W.Farrell-1@ou.edu

ARTICLE INFO

Conflicts of interest: None
Funding: None

ABSTRACT

Background: Previous investigations have shown that muscular endurance resistance training (MERT) is conducive in improving the onset of blood lactate accumulation (OBLA). However, the metabolic response and time course for adaption is still unclear. **Objective:** The aims of the current study were to evaluate and track the metabolic response to an individual session of MERT as well as to assess performance adaptations of supplementing an aerobic exercise training program with four weeks of MERT. **Methods:** Seventeen aerobically active men were randomly assigned to either the experimental (EX) or control group (CON), 9 EX and 8 CON. Baseline measures included a graded exercise test (GXT) and 1-repetition maximum (1RM) testing for leg press (LP), leg curl (LC), and leg extension (LE). CON continued their regular aerobic activity while the EX supplemented their regular aerobic exercise with 4 weeks of MERT. **Results:** No significant group differences were observed for all pre-training variables. Following four weeks of training no significant differences in cardiorespiratory or metabolic variables were observed for either group. However, significant improvements in LC and LE 1-RM were observed in EX compared to CON. Substantial accumulations in blood lactate were observed following each MERT session. **Conclusion:** Four weeks of MERT did not improve cardiorespiratory or metabolic variables, but did significantly improve LC and LE. MERT was also observed to induce a blood lactate response similar to that of HIIT. These findings suggest greater than four weeks is need to see metabolic adaptations conducive for improved aerobic performance using MERT.

Key words: Oxygen Consumption, Physical Endurance, Resistance Training, Lactates, Monocarboxylic Acid Transporters

INTRODUCTION

The development of optimal training methods has been an area of great interest for coaches, athletes and scientists. Current research suggests that blood lactate performance curves provide both reliable and valid information for prescribing exercise intensity due to the strong relationship between various lactate thresholds and performance. Several studies have established a strong correlation between the onset of blood lactate accumulation (OBLA) and aerobic exercise performance (Bergman et al., 1999; Brooks, 2010; Figueira, Caputo, Pelarigo, & Denadai, 2008; Laursen & Jenkins, 2002; Rogatzki, Wright, Mikat, & Brice, 2014; Tanaka & Swensen, 1998). OBLA has been defined as the intensity at which blood lactate reaches a fixed number that is equal to a concentration of 4mmol/L (Figueira et al., 2008; B Sjödin & Jacobs, 1981), and corresponds to the point at which exercise intensity transitions from tolerable to sever (Figueira et al., 2008). Therefore aerobic performance can be improved if the intensity at which OBLA occurs shifts to a higher value, for example running speed, cycling workload, or VO_2.

Recent studies have established a new method for the improvement of OBLA utilizing resistance training with lighter loads and higher repetitions, termed muscular endurance resistance training (MERT). Previous studies have demonstrated that a single bout of resistance training with lighter loads and higher repetitions can induce large accumulations of lactate and a simultaneous drop in pH (Edge, Hill-Haas, Goodman, & Bishop, 2006; Rogatzki et al., 2014; Schott, McCully, & Rutherford, 1995) that are comparable to values seen with high intensity interval training sessions (HIIT) (Edge, Bishop, & Goodman, 2006; Edge, Hill-Haas, et al., 2006), and greater than that of a traditional strength training session (Kraemer et al., 2002; Rogatzki et al., 2014). Researchers have observed improvements in watts and VO_2 at which OBLA occurs during cycling following 8 weeks of MERT (Farrell III, Lantis, Ade, Cantrell, & Larson, 2017; Lantis, Farrell III, Cantrell, & Larson, 2017)). Rightward shifts in blood lactate curves translate into athletes exercising at a higher workload or higher percentage of their VO_2max before experiencing the negative side effects of lactate accumulation. Researchers have speculated that the improvements in lactate kinetics are due to improvements in the metabolic clearance rate of lactate through increases in monocarboxyl transfer proteins (Cruz et al., 2012). Researchers have proposed that the improvements in lactate kinetics observed with HIIT could potentially be the same in MERT. However, the lactate response to several training session throughout a MERT program is unclear. It is not known if the response will decrease over time indicating improvements in lactate kinetics or will continue to be elevated throughout the duration of the program. The tracking of the lactate response could also give insight into the relative metabolic intensity that athletes are training at during each session.

With MERT just recently being utilized to develop improvements in OBLA, proper programming and optimization of this method still needs to be established. Previous studies have reported improvements in OBLA using 8 weeks of muscular endurance training with 1 minute of rest between sets of exercise ((Farrell III et al., 2017; Lantis et al., 2017). However, improvements in OBLA and aerobic power following HIIT and Sprint Interval Training (SIT) have been seen in as little as 4 to 8 sessions over 2 to 4 weeks (Beyranvand, 2017; Burgomaster, Heigenhauser, & Gibala, 2006; Burgomaster, Hughes, Heigenhauser, Bradwell, & Gibala, 2005; Jakeman, Adamson, & Babraj, 2012; Laursen, Shing, Peake, Coombes, & Jenkins, 2005; B. Rønnestad, Hansen, & Ellefsen, 2014; Talanian, Galloway, Heigenhauser, Bonen, & Spriet, 2007). With the proposed mechanisms of adaptations between MERT and HIIT being the same, it can be speculated that similar results can be observed over a similar length of time. The optimal length of rest between sets of exercise is still unclear as well.

Therefore, the purpose of the current study was to examine the cardiorespiratory and metabolic adaptations obtained from the supplementation of an aerobic training program with a 4 week MERT utilizing 30 second rest interval between sets of exercise. Additionally, the purpose of the current study was to evaluate and track the blood lactate response to individual training sessions throughout the course of the training program. It was hypothesized that an aerobic training program supplemented with 4 weeks of MERT with 30 second rest intervals would result in greater improvements in the OBLA and gas exchange threshold (GET) when compared to aerobic training alone. It was also hypothesized that there would be no significant improvements in maximal oxygen uptake (VO_2max) when compared to aerobic training alone.

METHOD

Subjects

Nineteen male participants (18-37 years old) were recruited for the current study. 17 participants completed the study with 2 participants dropping out due to time commitment issues. G*Power software (version 3.1.9.2) (α level = 0.05 and effect size = 0.08) was used to determine proper sample size. Subjects were randomly divided into an experimental (EX) group, whose regular aerobic training was supplemented with a muscular endurance training program, or a control (CON) group who continued their regular aerobic exercise training without the addition of muscular endurance training. All subjects were considered to be aerobically active and had not participated in any resistance training for 6 months prior to start of the study; determined with a self-reported physical activity questionnaire. Aerobically active was defined as having participated in aerobic exercise at least one hour per day for 3 days per week for the past 6 months. All subjects were required to reach a VO_2max of at least 40 ml/kg/min to participate in the study. This threshold has been used previously in similar studies (Farrell III et al., 2017; Lantis et al., 2017), and it indicates an aerobic capacity of good/excellent (Heyward, 1992). This study was approved by the Institutional Review Board at the University of Oklahoma, and each subject gave a verbal and written informed consent before participation. All testing and training was completed in an air-conditioned laboratory at a temperature 20-25°C.

Experimental Protocol

Prior to and following the 4 week training period both groups performed a staged graded exercise test to determine OBLA using the fixed at 4mmol/L method(Bertil Sjödin, Jacobs, & Svedenhag, 1982), GET and, VO_2max. Maximal strength for leg press (LP), leg curl (LC), and Leg extension (LE) was assessed using 1-repetition maximum (1-RM) All subjects were instructed to continue their low-intensity aerobic training without making alterations to volume or intensity. In addition to their current low-intensity aerobic training the EX group returned to the laboratory two times per week for four weeks to perform muscular endurance training under the supervision of the researchers.

Incremental exercise test

A magnetically braked cycle ergometer (Sport Excalibur, Lode; B.V. Medical Technology, Groningen, The Netherlands) along with a metabolic cart (True One 2400, Parvo Medics, Sandy, UT) was utilized to perform an incremental exercise test to determine VO_2max, GET, and OBLA. It was chosen to allow for easy attainment of plasma lactate measurements. Subjects were instructed to abstain from exercise and caffeine twelve hours prior to testing and to fast three to four hours prior to testing. A urine sample was obtained to determine urine specific gravity using a refractometer (model CLX-1, VEE GEE Scientific Inc., Kirkland, WA). Subjects had to have a urine specific gravity between 1.004 and 1.026 to be considered adequately hydrated to perform the incremental exercise test. In the instance a participant was not adequately hydrated they were instructed to consume a glass of water and rest for 30 minutes before collecting a second sample. If at that time they were still under hydrated they were rescheduled for a subsequent day. A resting fingertip capillary blood sample was collected to determine whole blood lactate concentration prior to testing using a commercial lactate meter (Lactate Plus, Nova Biomedical, Waltham,

MA) that was calibrated with known lactate standards (Lactate Plus, Lac Control Level 1, 1.0-1.6 mM) (Lactate Plus, Lac Control Level 2, 4.0-5.4 mM) before each use. Following a one minute rest period and a five minute warm up at 50 watts (W), the staged exercise test was initiated at a work rate of 125 W and increased by 25 W every three minutes until the participant reached their limit of exercise tolerance indicated by a pedal rate dropping below 50 revolutions per minute. At the end of each of the three-minute stage blood lactate and rating of perceived exertion (RPE) based on the Borg Scale (Borg, 1970) was measured. The VO_2 and work rate (W) corresponding to 4.0 mmol/L (OBLA) was calculated by plotting VO_2 and W against blood lactate concentration and using linear interpolation. Metabolic and ventilatory data were continuously measured and averaged over 30 second intervals. The work rate corresponding to the GET was determined by graphing: 1) VCO_2 as a function of VO_2, 2) the factional concentration of end-tidal of O_2 and CO_2 ($FETO_2$ and $FETCO_2$, 3) the ventilatory equivalents for O_2 and CO_2 (VE/VO_2 and VE/VCO_2), and 4) respiratory exchange ratio (RER; VCO_2/VO_2). The vertical alignment of these profiles allows for the verification of the GET via the work rate that aligned with: 1) an increase in VCO_2 out of proportion to VO_2, 2) an increase in VE/VO_2 and no increase in VE/VCO_2, 3) a rise in $FETCO_2$ and $FETO_2$, and 4) no inflection of the RER (can be a result from changes in CO_2 storage dynamics unrelated to blood lactate buffering) (Beaver, Wasserman, & Whipp, 1986).

Repetition maximum (1-RM) testing

1-RM testing was performed to assess maximum strength for leg press (LP), leg curl (LC) and leg extension (LE) based on recommendations of the National Strength and Conditioning Association (Baechle & Earle, 2008). In brief, several sub-maximal repetitions were performed to serve as a warmup. An initial weight was selected to be within 50 to 70 percent of the participant's perceived capacity. The weight was increased incrementally until a weight that could be lifted once but not twice was achieved. Three minutes of rest was given between each attempt. If a participant was able to lift the entire weight stack they were required to complete a full range of motion and immediately attempt additional repetitions through a full range of motion until failure. The number of additional repetitions was then used to calculate their 1-RM (Baechle & Earle, 2008).

Aerobic exercise

Based on previous studies (Farrell III et al., 2017; Lantis et al., 2017) (Karsten, Stevens, Colpus, Larumbe-Zabala, & Naclerio, 2016), subjects were instructed to maintain current aerobic training volume, and intensity throughout the study. If subjects indicated a decrease of > 1/3 or an increase of > 5% in training volume subjects were excluded from the study in order to prevent detraining and additional aerobic adaptations (Baechle & Earle, 2008; Fleck, 1994; Zupan & Petosa, 1995). Also any indications in an increase in aerobic training intensity resulted in exclusion from the study.

Muscular endurance resistance training

The training program consisted of supervised sessions on 2 days*wk^{-1} over a four week period to supplement participants aerobic training program. Participants were instructed to not perform any resistance training outside of the study. Every training session began with the subject arriving to the lab and resting for 10 minutes before a resting blood lactate measurement was taken using a commercial lactate meter (Lactate Plus, Nova Biomedical, Waltham, MA). Each resistance training session included a warmup consisting of 5 to 10 repetitions at 30 to 40 percent of their 1RM followed by four sets of 12 to 15 repetitions at 50% of the subject's established 1-RM for LP, LC, and LE (Cybex Strength Systems) with 30 seconds of rest between sets and 3 minutes of rest between exercises. Immediately after the completion of the final set of exercise a post-training lactate sample was taken. After 2 weeks (4 training sessions) the training weight was increased by 4.54 kilograms (a 2 to 4% increase) if an individual was able to complete four sets of 15 repetitions to compensate for any strength gains (Baechle & Earle, 2008). If participants were unable to complete four sets of 15 repetitions the training weight was kept the same.

Statistical analysis

Data are presented as means ± SD. Delta scores (post-pre) are indicated by Δ. Delta scores were used for data analysis to negate any differences noted in pre measurements due to both groups consisting of individuals that participated in several different aerobic activities (cycling, running, and triathlon). In addition the incremental exercise test was not sport specific for all subjects. Independent t-tests were utilized to determine if significant between group differences existed between the EX and CON groups. Repeated measures ANOVA was utilized to determine if significant differences existed in lactate levels between training visits. All statistical analyses were performed using SigmaPlot (Version 12.5, Systat Software Inc., San Jose, CA). Cohen's d effect sizes (ES) were reported for all significant measures. A value of ≤ 0.20 was considered a weak effect, a value of ≤ 0.50 was considered a moderate effect, and a value of ≥ 0.80 was considered a strong effect (Cohen, 1988). An alpha level of $p ≤ 0.05$ was set for the level of significance.

RESULTS

Subject Characteristics and Training Compliance

Descriptive characteristics are summarized in Table 1. No statistical differences (p>0.05) existed between groups for age, height, and body mass. Of the 9 subjects included in the EX group all participants completed at least 12 repetitions per set for all training sessions. All subjects met the requirements for increasing training load after the 4th training session.

Incremental Exercise Test

The physiological measurements from the incremental exercise test are summarized in Table 2. No significant differences (p>0.05) were observed for any of the physiological variables following the study intervention period between groups.

Maximal Strength Assessment

1-RM strength values are summarized in Table 3. Following the study intervention significant group differences existed for LC (p=0.002; ES=1.79) and LE (p=0.028; ES=1.20) between the EX and CON groups.

Training Session Blood Lactate Response

The average blood lactate response following each MERT session for the EXP group is illustrated in Figure 1. No statistically significant differences were observed in blood lactate levels between training sessions (p>0.05). The average individual blood lactate response across all MERT sessions for the EXP group is summarized in Figure 2.

DISCUSSION

The purposes of the current study were: (1) to examine the physiological and metabolic adaptions from the supplementation of an aerobic training program with 4 weeks of MERT, (2) to evaluate the effects of 30 second rest periods between sets of MERT, and (3) to monitor and track blood lactate responses to MERT sessions. In agreement with the researchers' hypothesis the addition of the MERT did not improve VO_2max. In contrast to the researchers' hypothesis, the addition of the MERT did not improve OBLA or GET.

A large majority of previous studies that have investigated the effects of resistance training on endurance performance have utilized a traditional strength training protocol (high intensity low repetition). Several of these studies indicated improvements in various endurance performance measures but overwhelming majority have reported no improvements in VO_2max when using aerobically trained subjects (Aagaard et al., 2011; Jung, 2003; Losnegard et al., 2011; Mikkola et al., 2011; Millet, Jaouen, Borrani, & Candau, 2002; B. R. Rønnestad, Hansen, & Raastad, 2010; B. R. Rønnestad, Kojedal, Losnegard, Kvamme, & Raastad, 2012). Previous studies that have used a lower intensity higher repetition resistance training program saw similar results. Edge et al.(2006). found no improvements in VO_2max following a high repetition resistance training program for 5 weeks in recreationally active females (Edge, Hill-Haas, et al., 2006). Campos et al. (2002) observed no improvements in VO_2max in untrained males following 8 weeks of high repetition resistance training (20 to 28 reps) training (Campos et al., 2002). Both Lantis et al. (2017). and Farrell et al. (2017) used identical MERT protocols and saw no improvements in VO_2max (Farrell III et al., 2017; Lantis et al., 2017). The findings of the current study in regards to no improvements in VO2max are in agreement with previous studies. The current study also observed no significant improvements in GET or W at GET following the training intervention. This finding is in agreement with Farrell et al. (2017) who also observed no improvements in GET or W at GET (Farrell III et al., 2017). It can be speculated that even with30 second rest intervals MERT does not provide an efficient cardiorespiratory stimulus to see improvements in VO_2max or GET. Although no cardiorespiratory adaptations (VO_2max or GET) have been linked with MERT, metabolic or local muscular

Table 1. Subject characteristics (Mean±(SD))

Variables	Groups			
	Experimental (n=9)		Control (n=8)	
	Pre	Post	Pre	Post
Age (years)	21.4±2.1	21.6±2.1	25.5±6.4	25.6±6.3
Height (cm)	180.2±5.3	180.2±5.3	179.5±3.9	179.5±3.8
Body mass (kg)	75.2±10.0	75.2±8.6	77.2±11.8	76.6±11.4

Differences if present were denoted using *(p<0.05). Standard deviations represent variability

Table 2. Physiological data during incremental exercise test (Mean±SD)

Variable	Groups		Effect size
	Experimental (n=9)	Control (n=8)	
	Δ	Δ	
VO_2 Abs (l/min)	0.019±0.173	0.077±0.139	0.369
VO_2 Rel (ml/kg/min)	0.644±2.91	1.06±2.31	0.158
GET (l/min)	0.10±0.252	0.029±0.150	0.342
Watts @ GET	10.7±19.7	7.14±12.20	0.218
VO_2 (L/min) @ OBLA	0.0±0.357	0.100±0.141	0.368
VO_2 (ml/kg/min) @ OBLA	0.031±4.67	1.72±2.09	0.467
Watts @ OBLA	−7.24±12.09	3.54±9.21	1.00
% of VO_2 max OBLA achieved	−1.01±6.70	2.07±3.15	0.588
Peak Power (W)	8.33±17.68	−3.13±8.84	0.820

Δ denotes gain scores (post – pre). Differences between groups were denoted using *(p<0.05). Standard deviations represent variability. VO_2 Abs: Absolute VO_2; VO_2 Rel: Relative VO_2; GET: Gas Exchange Threshold; OBLA: Onset of Blood Lactate Accumulation at 4mmol/L of lactate.

Table 3. 1-RM measurements (Mean±SD)

Variable	Groups		Effect size
	Experimental (n=9)	Control (n=8)	
	Δ	Δ	
Leg press (kg)	20.5±34.5	1.99±6.58	0.745
Leg Curl (kg)	9.21±5.35*	−0.142±5.08	1.79
Leg extension (kg)	9.93±9.43*	1.00±4.67	1.20

Δ denotes gain scores (post – pre). Differences between groups were denoted using *(p<.05). Standard deviations represent variability

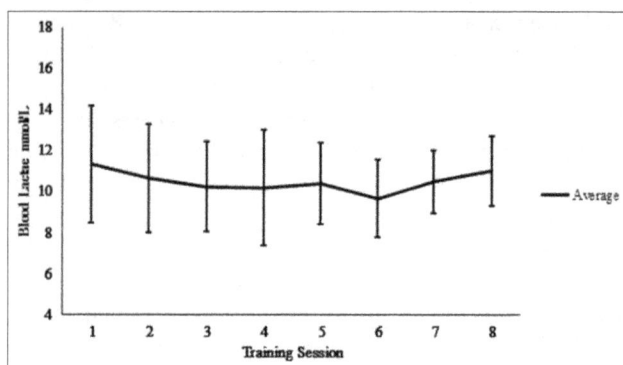

Figure 1. Average blood lactate response (post-pre) to each MERT

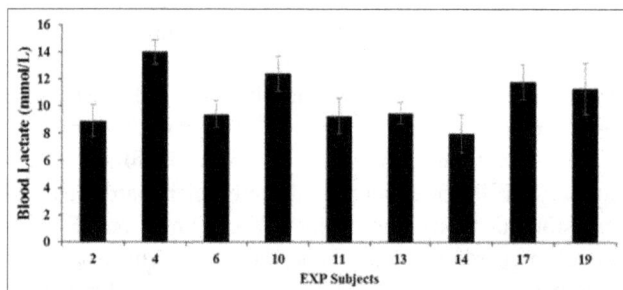

Figure 2. Average individual blood lactate response across all sessions of MERT

adaptations have resulted in improvements in OBLA. Farrell et al. (2017) observed a significant improvement in the VO$_2$ in which OBLA occurred following MERT (Farrell III et al., 2017). As a result, OBLA was achieved at a VO$_2$ 7.2% closer to VO$_2$max following training. Lantis et al. (2017) showed an increase in watts (W) at which OBLA occurred on a cycle ergometer (Lantis et al., 2017). It was speculated that the rightward shift in OBLA observed after 8 weeks of MERT in both studies was due to improvements in the metabolic clearance rate of lactate via increases in MCT proteins (Cruz et al., 2012; Donovan & Brooks, 1983). However, no improvements in lactate kinetics were observed in the current study. The current researchers have speculated that the reduced number of MERT sessions, compared to previous studies, did not allow for proper metabolic adaptations.

Following the MERT intervention the EXP group showed a significant increase in 1RM strength for both LC

and LE. This provides support that the program was effective in eliciting adaptations conducive for improvements in 1RM strength. Due to the lack of resistance training in the subjects' training history and the length of the MERT intervention it can be speculated that the improvements in 1RM strength observed were due to improvements in neural recruitment (Baechle & Earle, 2008). These findings are in agreement with previous research on MERT (Farrell III et al., 2017; Lantis et al., 2017).

Previous studies have shown that resistance training utilizing higher repetitions with lower resistance induces a large accumulation in lactate and a simultaneous drop in pH similar to that observed during HIIT (Edge, Bishop, et al., 2006; Edge, Hill-Haas, et al., 2006; Rogatzki et al., 2014; Schott et al., 1995). Previous investigations examining MERT have speculated that the training protocol also induces a similar lactate response observed with HIIT. However, previous investigations with MERT have not actually measured lactate responses. In the current study, prior to and immediately after each MERT session a blood sample was taken to assess blood lactate concentrations. The average blood lactate response (post-session – pre-session) for each training session is shown in Figure 1. The current study showed an average lactate response of 10.5 ± 1.9 mmol/L to the MERT, indicating a similar lactate response to that of HIIT (Edge, Bishop, et al., 2006). When examining the individual responses to the same relative workload a wide range of responses were observed. Lactate responses for the first four MERT sessions ranged from 7.0 ± 0.716 to 13.8 ± 1.76 while the lactate response to the final four MERT sessions (following the increase in training load) ranged from 8.23 ± 0.956 to 13.8 ± 0.763. This wide range of responses shows that although all subjects were training at the same relative load the training protocol induced very different metabolic responses. The reasoning for this large variation in response is still not clear. The current researchers speculate that differences in muscle fiber composition may partially explain the variation in responses seen. Lactate responses have been used previously to set training intensity zones for endurance training and team sports training as well as monitoring fatigue levels (Billat, 1996; Eniseler, 2005; Faude, Kindermann, & Meyer, 2009; Halson, 2014). It may be more appropriate to utilize an individual's lactate response to prescribe MERT.

The current study observed a similar lactate response following a single session of MERT compared to a single session of HIIT, but did not see similar adaptations even though a similar number of training sessions over a similar length of time was utilized(Burgomaster et al., 2006; Burgomaster et al., 2005; Edge, Bishop, et al., 2006; Jakeman et al., 2012; Laursen et al., 2005; B. Rønnestad et al., 2014). This divergence in the time course of adaptations for the two training methodologies is interesting and remains unclear at the moment. However, it can be speculated the differences in the number of muscular contractions performed during a single session and over the course of the training protocol maybe a reason for differences. A single session of MERT would require between 108 and 135 muscular contractions. Examining the HIIT protocol used by Burgo-master et al. (2006), 4 to 7 30 second sprints, an individual maintaining a cadence between 90 and 100 revolutions per minute could potentially perform up to 315 to 350 muscular contractions per session (Burgomaster et al., 2006). There could potentially be differences in the length of time for exercise between the two protocols. Future studies aiming to immolate the response and adaptions of lactate kinetics associated with HIIT using MERT should take these differences into consideration when designing a training program. Eight sessions of MERT over four weeks was chosen to not only immolate the training program length used in several HIIT studies, but to also coincide with the typical length of a single mesocycle (Baechle & Earle, 2008; Burgomaster et al., 2006; Burgomaster et al., 2005; Jakeman et al., 2012; Laursen et al., 2005; B. Rønnestad et al., 2014). The optimal length of time and the proper implementation of MERT into a macrocycle still needs further research. The current research indicates that at least 2 mesocycles (16 sessions over 8 weeks) is needed for adaptions in lactate kinetics using MERT.

Although the aerobic training of subjects was not directly monitored by the researchers, as it was performed outside the laboratory setting; the researchers do not believe that this aspect of the study negates any of the findings of the current study and provides for a real world application. Additionally, subjects were contacted bi-weekly to ensure that the subjects maintained similar diet and eating habits as well maintaining aerobic training volume within the previously described ranges. The aerobic training was not prescribed as it would have posed a difficult task due to the multitude of aerobic activities the subjects participated in. Also, the goal of the study was to examine the adaptations of the additional resistance training to the current aerobic training of the participants. A similar experimental design was utilized by Hickson et al. (1988) and recently by Karsten et al. (2016), Lantis et al. (2017) (2017), and Farrell et al. (2017) where all strength training was performed under the supervision of the researchers while all aerobic training was performed independently outside the lab when evaluating the potential for simultaneous strength and endurance training to improve endurance performance (Farrell III et al., 2017; Hickson, Dvorak, Gorostiaga, Kurowski, & Foster, 1988; Karsten et al., 2016; Lantis et al., 2017). The current study is not without limitations. All laboratory visits were scheduled for the same time each visit to control for fluctuations in fatigue and nutrient timing. Subjects were instructed to abstain from exercise at least 12 hrs prior to each visit to the laboratory. Subjects were instructed to maintain their current dietary regiment. Diet was not controlled or monitored in the current study and could be considered a limitation. The current study had a small sample size and was thus statistically underpowered, increasing the risk for Type II error. Future studies should aim to have a larger sample size and potentially implant an athlete tracking system to ensure athlete compliance with external training (GPS and/or heart rate monitoring)

CONCLUSION

The current study observed that MERT does indeed induce a lactate accumulation similar to that seen in HIIT, as previously speculated. (Edge, Bishop, et al., 2006; Edge, Hill-Haas, et al., 2006). Although a similar lactate response was observed a similar time course in adaptations for improved lactate kinetics was not observed. Previous research utilizing HIIT and SIT have shown improvements in lactate kinetics and aerobic power in as few as 4 to 8 sessions (Beyranvand, 2017; Burgomaster et al., 2006; Burgomaster et al., 2005; Jakeman et al., 2012; Laursen et al., 2005; B. Rønnestad et al., 2014; Talanian et al., 2007). The current research study found that 4 weeks (8 sessions) of MERT did not provide a sufficient stimulus to result in cardiorespiratory and metabolic adaptions to improve aerobic exercise performance. No improvements in VO$_2$max, GET, or OBLA were observed in the EXP group. However, the EXP group did show a significant improvement in LC and LE 1RM strength. The current study is one of the first to observe lactate kinetics throughout a MERT program. A varied response to the same relative stimulus was observed during the training. Further research is needed to understand the varied responses and how to individualize and prescribe MERT sessions based upon lactate responses. Further research is also needed to understand an optimal length for MERT as the current protocol does not appear sufficient enough to see improvements in aerobic performance.

ACKNOWLEDGMENTS

No external funding was used to support the current study. The authors have no relationships with any companies that who will benefit from the results of the present study.

REFERENCES

Aagaard, P., Andersen, J., Bennekou, M., Larsson, B., Olesen, J., Crameri, R., Kjaer, M. (2011). Effects of resistance training on endurance capacity and muscle fiber composition in young top-level cyclists. *Scandinavian journal of medicine & science in sports, 21*(6), 298-307.

Baechle, T. R., & Earle, R. W. (2008). *Essentials of strength training and conditioning*: Human kinetics.

Beaver, W. L., Wasserman, K., & Whipp, B. J. (1986). A new method for detecting anaerobic threshold by gas exchange. *Journal of applied physiology, 60*(6), 2020-2027.

Bergman, B. C., Wolfel, E. E., Butterfield, G. E., Lopaschuk, G. D., Casazza, G. A., Horning, M. A., & Brooks, G. A. (1999). Active muscle and whole body lactate kinetics after endurance training in men. *Journal of applied physiology, 87*(5), 1684-1696.

Beyranvand, F. (2017). Sprint Interval Training Improves Aerobic and Anaerobic Power in Trained Female Futsal Players. *International Journal of Kinesiology and Sports Science, 5*(2), 43-47.

Billat, L. V. (1996). Use of blood lactate measurements for prediction of exercise performance and for control of training. *Sports Medicine, 22*(3), 157-175.

Borg, G. (1970). Perceived exertion as an indicator of somatic stress. *Scand J Rehabil Med, 2*, 92-98.

Brooks, G. A. (2010). What does glycolysis make and why is it important? *Journal of applied physiology, 108*(6), 1450-1451.

Burgomaster, K. A., Heigenhauser, G. J., & Gibala, M. J. (2006). Effect of short-term sprint interval training on human skeletal muscle carbohydrate metabolism during exercise and time-trial performance. *Journal of applied physiology, 100*(6), 2041-2047.

Burgomaster, K. A., Hughes, S. C., Heigenhauser, G. J., Bradwell, S. N., & Gibala, M. J. (2005). Six sessions of sprint interval training increases muscle oxidative potential and cycle endurance capacity in humans. *Journal of applied physiology, 98*(6), 1985-1990.

Campos, G. E., Luecke, T. J., Wendeln, H. K., Toma, K., Hagerman, F. C., Murray, T. F., Staron, R. S. (2002). Muscular adaptations in response to three different resistance-training regimens: specificity of repetition maximum training zones. *European journal of applied physiology, 88*(1-2), 50-60.

Cohen, J. (1988). *Statistical power analysis for the behavioral sciences (2nd ed.)*. Hillsdale, NJ: Erlbaum.

Cruz, R. S. d. O., de Aguiar, R. A., Turnes, T., Penteado Dos Santos, R., Fernandes Mendes de Oliveira, M., & Caputo, F. (2012). Intracellular shuttle: the lactate aerobic metabolism. *The Scientific World Journal, 2012*.

Donovan, C. M., & Brooks, G. A. (1983). Endurance training affects lactate clearance, not lactate production. *American Journal of Physiology-Endocrinology And Metabolism, 244*(1), E83-E92.

Edge, J., Bishop, D., & Goodman, C. (2006). The effects of training intensity on muscle buffer capacity in females. *European journal of applied physiology, 96*(1), 97-105.

Edge, J., Hill-Haas, S., Goodman, C., & Bishop, D. (2006). Effects of Resistance Training on H$^+$ Regulation, Buffer Capacity, and Repeated Sprints. *Medicine and Science in Sports and Exercise, 38*(11), 2004.

Eniseler, N. (2005). Heart rate and blood lactate concentrations as predictors of physiological load on elite soccer players during various soccer training activities. *The Journal of Strength & Conditioning Research, 19*(4), 799-804.

Farrell III, J. W., Lantis, D. J., Ade, C. J., Cantrell, G. S., & Larson, R. D. (2017). Aerobic exercise supplemented with muscular endurance training improves onset of blood lactate accumulation. *The Journal of Strength & Conditioning Research, (in press)*.

Faude, O., Kindermann, W., & Meyer, T. (2009). Lactate threshold concepts. *Sports Medicine, 39*(6), 469-490.

Figueira, T. R., Caputo, F., Pelarigo, J. G., & Denadai, B. S. (2008). Influence of exercise mode and maximal lactate-steady-state concentration on the validity of OBLA to predict maximal lactate-steady-state in active individuals. *Journal of Science and Medicine in Sport, 11*(3), 280-286.

Fleck, S. J. (1994). Detraining: Its Effects on Endurance and Strength. *Strength & Conditioning Journal, 16*(1), 22-28.

Halson, S. L. (2014). Monitoring training load to understand fatigue in athletes. *Sports Medicine, 44*(2), 139-147.

Heyward, V. H. (1992). Advanced Fitness Assessment and Exercise Prescription. *Medicine & Science in Sports & Exercise, 24*(2), 278.

Hickson, R., Dvorak, B., Gorostiaga, E., Kurowski, T., & Foster, C. (1988). Potential for strength and endurance training to amplify endurance performance. *Journal of applied physiology, 65*(5), 2285-2290.

Jakeman, J., Adamson, S., & Babraj, J. (2012). Extremely short duration high-intensity training substantially improves endurance performance in triathletes. *Applied Physiology, Nutrition, and Metabolism, 37*(5), 976-981.

Jung, A. P. (2003). The impact of resistance training on distance running performance. *Sports Medicine, 33*(7), 539-552.

Karsten, B., Stevens, L., Colpus, M., Larumbe-Zabala, E., & Naclerio, F. (2016). The effects of a sports specific maximal strength and conditioning training on critical velocity, anaerobic running distance and 5-km race performance. *International journal of sports physiology and performance, 11*(1), 80-85.

Kraemer, W., Adams, K., Cafarelli, E., Dudley, G., Dooly, C., Feigenbaum, M., Hoffman, J. (2002). J. Potteiger, MH Stone, NA Ratamess, and T. Triplett-Mcbride. American College of Sports Medicine position stand. *Progression models in resistance training for healthy adults. Medicine & Science in Sports & Exercise, 34*(2), 364-380.

Lantis, D. J., Farrell III, J. W., Cantrell, G. S., & Larson, R. D. (2017). Eight Weeks of High-Volume Resistance Training Improves Onset of Blood Lactate in Trained Individuals. *The Journal of Strength & Conditioning Research, 31*(8), 2176-2182.

Laursen, P. B., & Jenkins, D. G. (2002). The scientific basis for high-intensity interval training. *Sports Medicine, 32*(1), 53-73.

Laursen, P. B., Shing, C. M., Peake, J. M., Coombes, J. S., & Jenkins, D. G. (2005). Influence of high-intensity interval training on adaptations in well-trained cyclists. *Journal of Strength and Conditioning Research, 19*(3), 527.

Losnegard, T., Mikkelsen, K., Rønnestad, B., Hallén, J., Rud, B., & Raastad, T. (2011). The effect of heavy strength training on muscle mass and physical performance in elite cross country skiers. *Scandinavian journal of medicine & science in sports, 21*(3), 389-401.

Mikkola, J., Vesterinen, V., Taipale, R., Capostagno, B., Häkkinen, K., & Nummela, A. (2011). Effect of resistance training regimens on treadmill running and neuromuscular performance in recreational endurance runners. *Journal of Sports Sciences, 29*(13), 1359-1371.

Millet, G. P., Jaouen, B., Borrani, F., & Candau, R. (2002). Effects of concurrent endurance and strength training on running economy and VO~ 2 kinetics. *Medicine and Science in Sports and Exercise, 34*(8), 1351-1359.

Rogatzki, M. J., Wright, G. A., Mikat, R. P., & Brice, A. G. (2014). Blood Ammonium and Lactate Accumulation Response to Different Training Protocols Using the Parallel Squat Exercise. *The Journal of Strength & Conditioning Research, 28*(4), 1113-1118.

Rønnestad, B., Hansen, J., & Ellefsen, S. (2014). Block periodization of high-intensity aerobic intervals provides superior training effects in trained cyclists. *Scandinavian journal of medicine & science in sports, 24*(1), 34-42.

Rønnestad, B. R., Hansen, E. A., & Raastad, T. (2010). Effect of heavy strength training on thigh muscle cross-sectional area, performance determinants, and performance in well-trained cyclists. *European journal of applied physiology, 108*(5), 965-975.

Rønnestad, B. R., Kojedal, Ø., Losnegard, T., Kvamme, B., & Raastad, T. (2012). Effect of heavy strength training on muscle thickness, strength, jump performance, and endurance performance in well-trained Nordic Combined athletes. *European journal of applied physiology, 112*(6), 2341-2352.

Schott, J., McCully, K., & Rutherford, O. (1995). The role of metabolites in strength training. *European journal of applied physiology and occupational physiology, 71*(4), 337-341.

Sjödin, B., & Jacobs, I. (1981). Onset of blood lactate accumulation and marathon running performance. *International journal of sports medicine, 2*(1), 23-26.

Sjödin, B., Jacobs, I., & Svedenhag, J. (1982). Changes in onset of blood lactate accumulation (OBLA) and muscle enzymes after training at OBLA. *European journal of applied physiology and occupational physiology, 49*(1), 45-57.

Talanian, J. L., Galloway, S. D., Heigenhauser, G. J., Bonen, A., & Spriet, L. L. (2007). Two weeks of high-intensity aerobic interval training increases the capacity for fat oxidation during exercise in women. *Journal of applied physiology, 102*(4), 1439-1447.

Tanaka, H., & Swensen, T. (1998). Impact of resistance training on endurance performance. *Sports Medicine, 25*(3), 191-200.

Zupan, M. F., & Petosa, P. S. (1995). Aerobic and Resistance Cross-Training for Peak Triathlon Performance. *Strength & Conditioning Journal, 17*(5), 7-12.

14

Current Evidence of Gait Modification with Real-time Biofeedback to Alter Kinetic, Temporospatial, and Function-Related Outcomes

Oladipo Eddo, Bryndan Lindsey, Shane V. Caswell, Nelson Cortes*
Sports Medicine Assessment, Research & Testing Laboratory, George Mason University, 10900 University Blvd., Manassas, 20110, United States
Corresponding Author: Nelson Cortes, E-mail: ncortes@gmu.edu

ARTICLE INFO

Conflicts of interest: None
Funding: None

ABSTRACT

Background: Gait retraining using real-time biofeedback (RTB) may have positive outcomes in decreasing knee adduction moment (KAM) in healthy individuals and has shown equal likelihood in patients with knee osteoarthritis (OA). Currently, there is no consensus regarding the most effective gait modification strategy, mode of biofeedback or treatment dosage. **Objective:** The purpose of this review was: i) to assess if gait retraining interventions using RTB are valuable to reduce KAM, pain, and improve function in individuals with knee osteoarthritis, ii) to evaluate the effectiveness of different gait modifications and modes of RTB in reducing KAM in healthy individuals, and iii) to assess the impact of gait retraining interventions with RTB on other variables that may affect clinical outcomes. **Methods:** Seven electronic databases were searched using five search terms. Studies that utilized any form of gait retraining with RTB to improve one or a combination of the following measures were included: KAM, knee pain, and function. Twelve studies met the inclusion criteria, evaluating eleven distinctive gait modifications and three modes of RTB. **Results:** All but one study showed positive outcomes. Self-selected and multi-parameter gait modifications showed the greatest reductions in KAM with visual and haptic RTB being more effective than auditory. **Conclusions:** Current evidence suggests that gait modification using RTB can Positively alter KAM in asymptomatic and symptomatic participants. However, the existing literature is limited and of low quality, with the optimal combination strategies remaining unclear (gait and biofeedback mode). Future studies should employ randomized controlled study designs to compare the effects of different gait modification strategies and biofeedback modes on individuals with knee OA.

Key words: Gait Retraining, Real-time Biofeedback, Osteoarthritis, Knee Adduction Moment

INTRODUCTION

Osteoarthritis (OA) is one of the most common joint disorders in the U.S. (Allen & Golightly, 2015; Control & Prevention, 2013; Ma, Chan, & Carruthers, 2014; Neogi & Zhang, 2013). Over the past 20 years the incidence of symptomatic knee OA has risen dramatically (Nguyen et al., 2011), leading to $128 billion in annual healthcare and economic costs (Ma et al., 2014). Knee OA is the predominant form of the disease, with an estimated lifetime risk of developing knee OA of approximately 40% in men and 47% in women (Neogi & Zhang, 2013). The etiology of knee OA is multifactorial, with risk factors such as excessive bodyweight (Sharma, Lou, Cahue, & Dunlop, 2000), aging, varus alignment, and altered joint mechanics (Heijink et al., 2012). Knee OA most commonly occurs in the medial compartment (Dearborn, Eakin, & Skinner, 1996; Thomas, Resnick, Alazraki, Daniel, & Greenfield, 1975), where articular surface damage narrows the medial joint space resulting

in an increased knee adduction moment (KAM) (Andriacchi & Mundermann, 2006; Andriacchi et al., 2004; Simon et al., 2015). Increased KAM has been associated with OA severity (Foroughi, Smith, & Vanwanseele, 2009), cartilage loss (Chang et al., 2015; Chehab, Favre, Erhart-Hledik, & Andriacchi, 2014) and static malalignment (Hurwitz, Ryals, Case, Block, & Andriacchi, 2002), and has been shown to be a reliable indicator of medial knee joint load and alignment (Miyazaki et al., 2002; Sharma et al., 1998; Zhao et al., 2007). Reducing KAM in individuals who have, or who are at elevated risk for knee OA may decrease pain (Amin et al., 2004) and reduce disease severity and progression (Miyazaki et al., 2002).

Numerous treatment and management options for knee OA have been recommended, including the use of orthotic, pharmacologic, and surgical interventions with the goal of reducing symptoms and medial compartment loads (Zhang et al., 2007). Gait retraining using real-time biofeedback is a conservative intervention that has shown positive outcomes in other pathologies (e.g., diabetes, stroke, Parkinson, joint replacement, etc.) (Mayr et al., 2007; Zalecki et al., 2013). It has been suggested that gait modification with RTB results in modest to sizable short-term treatment outcomes when compared to conventional therapy (Tate & Milner, 2010). Recent studies have demonstrated a similar effect of gait retraining and RTB on KAM (Simic, Hinman, Wrigley, Bennell, & Hunt, 2011).

A 6-week gait retraining using haptic RTB exhibited a 20% average reduction of peak KAM and a 30% improvement in pain and function in individuals with knee OA (Shull, Silder, et al., 2013). Reductions in peak KAM were also reported utilizing a medial knee thrust gait with visual RTB in healthy adults with varus malalignment (Barrios, Crossley, & Davis, 2010), while medial weight transfer of the foot resulted in reductions in peak KAM in healthy individuals with normal joint alignment (Dowling, Fisher, & Andriacchi, 2010). Other gait strategies that have been successfully implemented include lateral trunk lean (Simic, Hunt, Bennell, Hinman, & Wrigley, 2012), altered foot progression angle (Shull, Shultz, et al., 2013), multi-parameter (Shull, Lurie, Cutkosky, & Besier, 2011; Shull, Silder, et al., 2013), and self-selected gait strategies (van den Noort, Steenbrink, Roeles, & Harlaar, 2014; Wheeler, Shull, & Besier, 2011). Similarly, a wide variety of biofeedback delivery, including visual (van den Noort et al., 2014), auditory (Ferrigno, Stoller, Shakoor, Thorp, & Wimmer, 2016), and haptic (Shull et al., 2011) have reported positive outcomes.

Limitations of the current literature, however, constrain generalizability and clinical application. Research into the effects of gait retraining using RTB in patients with knee osteoarthritis is lacking. Methodological differences including strategy implemented, training methods, and evaluation of skill acquisition mean there is no clear consensus regarding the most effective gait strategy, mode of feedback, or treatment dosage (Simic et al., 2011). The long-term outcomes of gait modification using RTB are unclear at present. Early results indicate that positive changes can be maintained, at least for a month (Barrios et al., 2010; Shull, Silder, et al., 2013). However, based on current evidence and the limited amount of retention testing, it cannot be determined if motor learning adaptations occur (Tate & Milner, 2010).

A recent systematic review and meta-analysis evaluating the effects of gait retraining with real-time biofeedback on KAM and pain related outcome measures (PROM's) by concluded that despite these limitations, there is sufficient evidence to suggest that gait retraining with real-time biofeedback can be used to reduce KAM in healthy controls (Richards, van den Noort, Dekker, & Harlaar, 2017). However, the effects of gait modification using RTB on kinetic, kinematic, and temporospatial variables other than KAM that may be clinically relevant have largely been ignored (Simic et al., 2011). Unanticipated changes at the knee joint such as increased knee flexion moment (KFM) and KAM impulse may offset the benefits of reduced peak KAM by

increasing joint compression (Manal, Gardinier, Buchanan, & Snyder-Mackler, 2015; Walter, D'Lima, Colwell, & Fregly, 2010), and time under loading (Kean et al., 2012). Additional variables such as stride speed (Browning & Kram, 2007) and length (Russell, Braun, & Hamill, 2010) that may also affect joint loading have not been adequately considered in prior reviews.

Therefore, the purpose of this systematic review was three-fold: (1) to determine if gait retraining interventions using RTB are beneficial to alter KAM, pain, and improve function in patients with knee OA (2) to evaluate the effectiveness of different gait modifications and modes of RTB in reducing KAM in both healthy and asymptomatic individuals. (3) to assess the impact of gait retraining interventions using RTB on other outcome variables that may affect clinical outcomes.

METHODS

The Preferred Reporting Items for Systematic Reviews and Meta-Analyses (PRISMA) guidelines for conducting and reporting on systematic reviews were followed. The search strategy identified all randomized, quasi-randomized, non-randomized controlled, and uncontrolled trials, published in English language, that utilized a form of gait retraining with RTB to improve KAM, pain, and/or function. For randomized, quasi-randomized, and nonrandomized controlled trials, participants in the experimental group were diagnosed with knee OA (Altman, 1991), or self-reported OA based on knee chronic joint pain (Fransen et al., 2015). Gait retraining studies employing any mode of RTB (e.g., video, auditory, etc.) were included. If applicable, a control group was defined as a group not receiving gait retraining or any other type of intervention. Inclusion of uncontrolled trials, primarily focusing on interventions of healthy individuals, was considered relevant due to the information it can provide for future randomized controlled trials. Studies must have included one of the following outcomes: (1) KAM, (2) knee pain, (3) self-reported physical function (Bellamy et al., 1997).

An electronic search was conducted using the following databases: PubMed, EBSCO host (CINAHL, Medline, SPORTDiscus), Embase, PROQuest, and Cochrane [1970 to January 1, 2016]. Searches were limited to full-text accessible, peer-reviewed, and English-language results only. The results were collated and duplicates removed. A CONSORT flow chart depicts the process used (Figure 1). In each database, five search terms were utilized (1."gait AND (training OR retraining OR modification) AND "(feedback OR biofeedback) AND (knee OR tibiofemoral)", 2. "gait AND (training OR retraining OR modification) AND (feedback OR biofeedback) AND (knee OR tibiofemoral) AND osteoarthritis", 3 ."gait AND (training OR retraining OR modification) AND (feedback OR biofeedback) AND (knee OR tibiofemoral) AND (load OR "adduction moment" OR "abduction moment")", 4."gait AND (training OR retraining OR modification) AND (feedback OR biofeedback) AND (knee OR tibiofemoral) AND (pain OR "quality of life")", 5. "gait AND (training OR retraining OR modification) AND

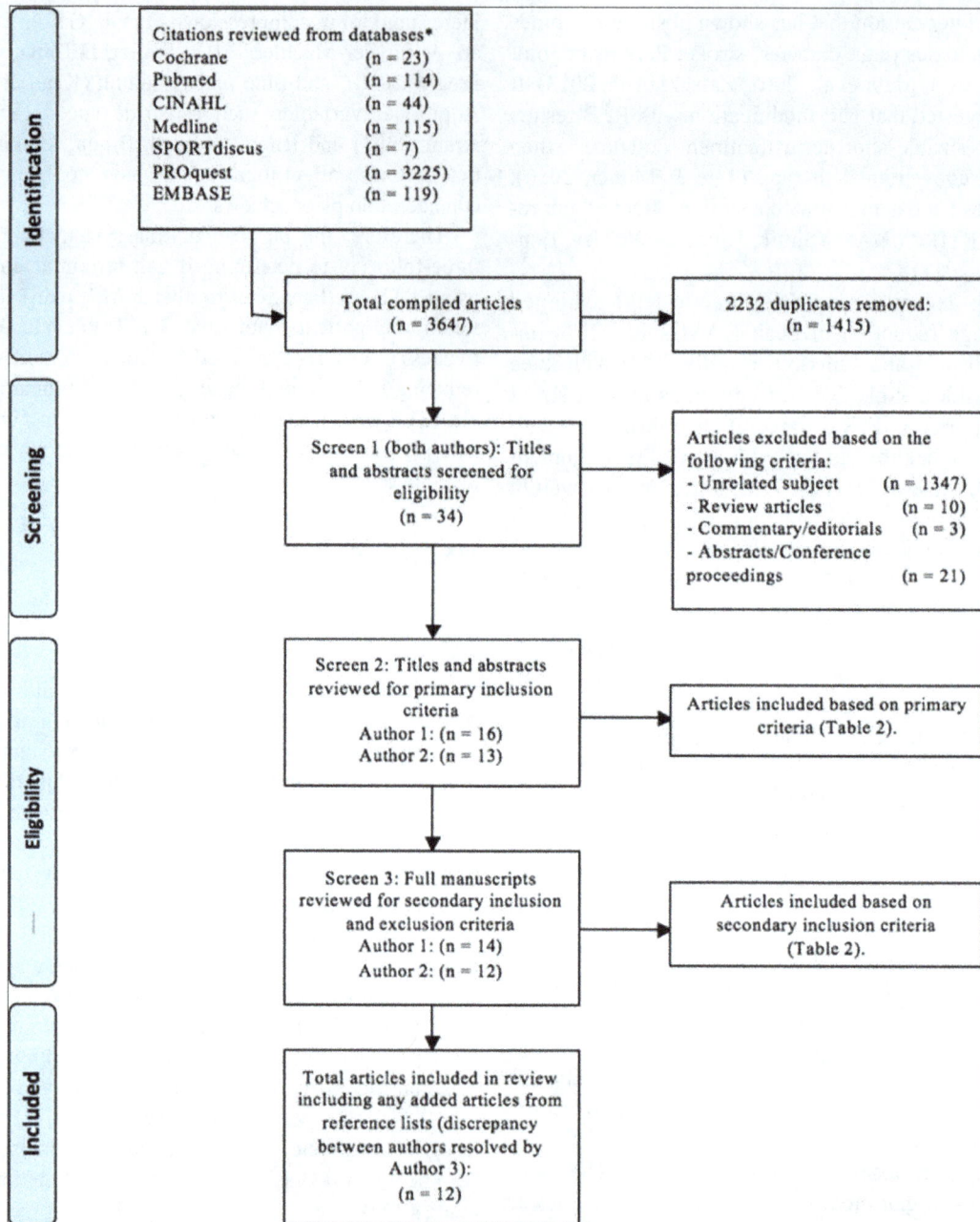

Citations reviewed from databases*
Cochrane   (n = 23)
Pubmed   (n = 114)
CINAHL   (n = 44)
Medline   (n = 115)
SPORTdiscus   (n = 7)
PROquest   (n = 3225)
EMBASE   (n = 119)

Total compiled articles
(n = 3647)

2232 duplicates removed:
(n = 1415)

Screen 1 (both authors): Titles
and abstracts screened for
eligibility
(n = 34)

Articles excluded based on the
following criteria:
- Unrelated subject   (n = 1347)
- Review articles   (n = 10)
- Commentary/editorials   (n = 3)
- Abstracts/Conference
proceedings   (n = 21)

Screen 2: Titles and abstracts
reviewed for primary inclusion
criteria
Author 1: (n = 16)
Author 2: (n = 13)

Articles included based on primary
criteria (Table 2).

Screen 3: Full manuscripts
reviewed for secondary inclusion
and exclusion criteria
Author 1: (n = 14)
Author 2: (n = 12)

Articles included based on
secondary inclusion criteria
(Table 2).

Total articles included in review
including any added articles from
reference lists (discrepancy
between authors resolved by
Author 3):
(n = 12)

Identification / Screening / Eligibility / Included

Figure 1. Preferred Reporting Items for Systematic Reviews and Meta-Analyses (PRISMA) Flow Diagram of search strategy

(feedback OR biofeedback) AND (knee OR tibiofemoral) AND osteoarthritis AND (load OR "knee adduction moment" OR "knee abduction moment") AND (pain OR "quality of life")."

The results of each search term combination were recorded and stored for each database in a bibliographic reference manager software. Duplicates were removed within each database and then across databases. Review articles, commentary/editorials, abstracts/conference proceedings, or articles that were pertaining to an unrelated topic were removed. Two authors independently screened titles and abstracts from the remaining list based on the primary inclusion criteria. Manuscripts of the remaining articles were independently reviewed for secondary inclusion and exclusion criteria. If there was a discrepancy in the articles selected for inclusion, a third author that was blinded from the search

process reviewed the selected articles, and determined those that were appropriate for inclusion. Reference lists of the final selected articles were screened for additional articles that may have been missed in the initial search process but met the inclusion criteria, resulting in the final number included.

Methodological quality was assessed using the PEDro Scale which is a criteria list designed to help identify which of the reviewed experiments are likely to be externally valid (criteria 1), internally valid (criteria 2-9) and have sufficient statistical information to make their results interpretable (criteria 10-11) (Fitzpatrick, 2008). Two authors (BL and OE) independently reviewed and rated each study on both scales. Inter-rater disagreements were discussed and resolved in a consensus meeting. Unresolved items were evaluated by a third author (NC). Data were then extracted for each study.

RESULTS

Study Selection

A total of 3,647 citations were initially retrieved. After removal of duplicates, 1,415 citations were screened for initial eligibility. Of the remaining 34 articles, 12 met both primary and secondary inclusion and exclusion criteria. No additional articles were added from the reference lists of selected articles.

Study Characteristics

Eleven of the twelve studies included were designed to test the effects of a gait retraining intervention using RTB on measures of KAM, pain and/or function (Barrios et al., 2010; Dowling, Fisher, et al., 2010; Ferrigno et al., 2016; Hunt, Simic, Hinman, Bennell, & Wrigley, 2011; Segal et al., 2015; Shull et al., 2011; Shull, Shultz, et al., 2013; Shull, Silder, et al., 2013; Simic et al., 2012; van den Noort et al., 2014; Wheeler et al., 2011). The other study aimed to explore how training with a feedback-providing knee brace affected gait, rate of loading, and proprioception, but was included as KAM was reported as an outcome measure (Riskowski, 2010). Ten studies utilized a quasi-experimental within-subjects design (Barrios et al., 2010; Dowling, Corazza, Chaudhari, & Andriacchi, 2010; Ferrigno et al., 2016; Hunt et al., 2011; Riskowski, 2010; Shull et al., 2011; Shull, Shultz, et al., 2013; Shull, Silder, et al., 2013; Simic et al., 2012; van den Noort et al., 2014), while two employed true experimental designs (Segal et al., 2015; Wheeler et al., 2011), including one randomized controlled trial (Segal et al., 2015). Sample sizes ranged from 8 to 56 participants.

Four tested individuals with knee OA (Segal et al., 2015; Shull, Shultz, et al., 2013; Shull, Silder, et al., 2013; Simic et al., 2012); the remaining eight tested healthy individuals with the goal of developing and informing future studies to be conducted in symptomatic individuals (Barrios et al., 2010; Dowling, Corazza, et al., 2010; Ferrigno et al., 2016; Hunt et al., 2011; Riskowski, 2010; Shull et al., 2011; van den Noort et al., 2014; Wheeler et al., 2011). In studies evaluating symptomatic individuals, radiographic evidence of medial compartment OA was used to confirm the presence and severity of the disease using the Kellgren and Lawrence scale (Shull, Shultz, et al., 2013; Shull, Silder, et al., 2013). A verbal confirmation of knee pain was an additional diagnostic criterion (Segal et al., 2015; Shull, Silder, et al., 2013; Simic et al., 2012). Nine studies employed a single session design (Dowling, Corazza, et al., 2010; Ferrigno et al., 2016; Hunt et al., 2011; Riskowski, 2010; Shull et al., 2011; Shull, Shultz, et al., 2013; Simic et al., 2012; van den Noort et al., 2014; Wheeler et al., 2011) with three performing a single intervention trial (Riskowski, 2010; Shull, Shultz, et al., 2013; Wheeler et al., 2011). Six of these studies tested gait under multiple conditions to compare different types of gait strategies (Ferrigno et al., 2016; Shull et al., 2011) and feedback (Dowling, Fisher, et al., 2010; van den Noort et al., 2014), as well as varying magnitudes (Hunt et al., 2011; Simic et al., 2012). Only three studies were conducted over multiple sessions and included follow-up testing to assess retention (Barrios et al., 2010; Segal et al., 2015; Shull, Silder, et al., 2013).

Gait Retraining Interventions

Eleven gait modification strategies were identified across the twelve studies. Four studies evaluated the effects of modifying trunk position (Hunt et al., 2011; Shull et al., 2011; Shull, Silder, et al., 2013; Simic et al., 2012) with two testing trunk sway (Shull et al., 2011; Shull, Silder, et al., 2013), and two evaluating trunk lean (Hunt et al., 2011; Simic et al., 2012). Three studies investigated reduced foot progression angle (Shull et al., 2011; Shull, Shultz, et al., 2013; Shull, Silder, et al., 2013), two studies utilized a weight shift to the medial side of the foot during the stance portion of gait (Dowling, Corazza, et al., 2010; Ferrigno et al., 2016), and two allowed participants to self-select the kinematic adjustment to reduce KAM (van den Noort et al., 2014; Wheeler et al., 2011).

Other gait modification strategies included medial knee thrust (Barrios et al., 2010); reduced rate of loading through increased knee flexion and decreased vertical acceleration (Riskowski, 2010); gait retraining towards symmetrical and typical displacements of the trunk and pelvis (Segal et al., 2015), and multi-parameter gait retraining through a combination of altered foot progression angle, increased trunk sway, and increased tibia angle (Shull et al., 2011).

Biofeedback

Visual, haptic, and auditory real-time biofeedback or a combination was used to implement gait modification strategies. The two most common biofeedback techniques were visual (Barrios et al., 2010; Hunt et al., 2011; Segal et al., 2015; Shull et al., 2011; Simic et al., 2012; van den Noort et al., 2014; Wheeler et al., 2011) and haptic (Dowling, Corazza, et al., 2010; Shull et al., 2011; Shull, Shultz, et al., 2013; Shull, Silder, et al., 2013; Wheeler et al., 2011). Two studies employed auditory biofeedback (Ferrigno et al., 2016; Riskowski, 2010).

Outcome Assessment

Ten studies reported KAM as the primary outcome measure (Barrios et al., 2010; Dowling, Corazza, et al., 2010; Ferrigno et al., 2016; Hunt et al., 2011; Shull et al., 2011; Shull, Shultz, et al., 2013; Shull, Silder, et al., 2013; Simic et al., 2012; van den Noort et al., 2014; Wheeler et al., 2011). Of these, three studies with OA participants reported measures of pain, and function such as the Western Ontario McMaster Universities OA Index (WOMAC) and visual analog pain scales (VAS) (Hunt et al., 2011; Shull, Silder, et al., 2013; Simic et al., 2012). Seven studies reported additional kinetic and temporospatial variables including KFM (Ferrigno et al., 2016; Riskowski, 2010; Shull, Shultz, et al., 2013; Shull, Silder, et al., 2013), KAM impulse (Simic et al., 2012; van den Noort et al., 2014), stride speed (Ferrigno et al., 2016; Hunt et al., 2014; Riskowski, 2010; Simic et al., 2012), and stride length (Ferrigno et al., 2016; Riskowski, 2010; Simic et al., 2012). Four studies using healthy participants reported numerical ratings (0-10) of awkwardness and difficulty in adopting gait modifications (Barrios et al., 2010; Hunt et al., 2011; van den Noort et al., 2014; Wheeler et al., 2011). Two studies did not report KAM as the primary outcome measure (Riskowski, 2010; Segal et al., 2015). One reported proprioceptive acuity and rate of loading (ROL) as primary outcome measures with KAM being used to determine differences in training gait with and without a feedback based knee brace (Riskowski, 2010). The other did not measure KAM, instead focusing on outcome measures associated with pain and function such as Late-Life Function and Disability Basic Lower Limb Function (LLFDI) score, Knee Injury/Osteoarthritis Outcome (KOOS) score, and mobility tests (Segal et al., 2015). All eleven studies that reported KAM evaluated the overall or first peak during stance. Four studies also reported second peak KAM (Ferrigno et al., 2016; Hunt et al., 2011; Shull, Shultz, et al., 2013; Simic et al., 2012), and one study reported peak KAM at mid-stance in addition to first and second peak KAM (van den Noort et al., 2014).

Quality and Bias Assessment

The mean (±SD) PEDro score was 6.1±0.7 out of a possible 11 (Table 1). While most studies scored well regarding external validity (criterion 1) and statistical information (criteria 10 and 11), internal validity was poor across all studies (criteria 2 through 9). Specifically, all studies scored a zero on blinding of subjects, therapists, and assessors (criteria 5, 6, and 7, respectively). Additionally, eight studies scored a zero on random allocation (criterion 2), while eleven studies scored zeros on allocation concealment (criterion 3).

Definition of criteria as in Fitzpatrick 2008
1. Eligibility criteria were specified
2. Subjects were randomly allocated to groups (in a crossover study, subjects were randomly allocated an order in which treatments were received)
3. Allocation was concealed
4. The groups were similar at baseline regarding the most important prognostic indicators
5. There was blinding of all subjects
6. There was blinding of all therapists who administered the therapy
7. There was blinding of all assessors who measured at least one key outcome
8. Measures of at least one key outcome were obtained

from more than 85% of the subjects initially allocated to groups
9. All subjects for whom outcome measures were available received the treatment or control condition as allocated, or where this was not the case, data for at least one key outcome was analyzed by "intention to treat"
10. The results of between-group statistical comparisons are reported for at least one key outcome
11. The study provides both point measures and measures of variability for at least one key outcome

Synthesis of Results

Benefit of gait retraining using RTB on individuals with knee OA

Three (Shull, Shultz, et al., 2013; Shull, Silder, et al., 2013; Simic et al., 2012) of the four studies conducted on OA patients reported smaller but still significant reductions in KAM compared to healthy individuals, ranging from 9.3% (Simic et al., 2012) to a maximum of 20% (Shull, Silder, et al., 2013) (Table 2). Of these studies, self-selected gait retraining that Allowed participants to choose between using a combination of both altered foot progression and trunk sway angle or only altered foot or trunk sway angle, resulted in the greatest average reduction in KAM (Shull, Silder, et al., 2013). Increased trunk lean resulted in average KAM reductions between 9.3% and 14.9% depending on the magnitude of lean (Simic et al., 2012) while toe-in gait reduced KAM by 13% (Shull, Shultz, et al., 2013). Two studies employed real-time visual feedback (Shull, Shultz, et al., 2013; Shull, Silder, e ., 2013) while the other two used real-time haptic feedback (Segal et al., 2015; Simic et al., 2012) with participants responding equally well to both modes of feedback. All four studies measured pain and function related outcome measures including WOMAC (Shull, Silder, et al., 2013), KOOS (Segal 2015), LLFDI (Segal et al., 2015), and VAS scales (Shull, Silder, et al., 2013; Simic et al., 2012) (Table 3). Ratings of pain and function were significantly improved in all studies but one which was a single session design (Simic et al., 2012). Improvements in WOMAC pain and function were retained at the 1-month

Table 1. PEDro scores of included studies in systematic review (Fitzpatrick, 2008)

	1	2	3	4	5	6	7	8	9	10	11	Total
Barrios et al. (2010)	1	0	0	1	0	0	0	1	1	1	1	6
Dowling et al. (2010)	1	1	0	1	0	0	0	1	1	1	1	7
Ferrigno et al. (2016)	1	1	0	1	0	0	0	1	1	1	1	7
Hunt et al. (2011)	1	0	0	1	0	0	0	1	1	1	1	6
Riskowski (2010)	1	0	0	1	0	0	0	1	1	1	1	6
Segal et al. (2015)	1	1	1	1	0	0	0	0	1	1	1	7
Shull et al. (2011)	0	0	0	1	0	0	0	1	1	1	1	5
Shull et al. (2013a)	1	0	0	1	0	0	0	1	1	1	1	6
Shull et al. (2013b)	1	0	0	1	0	0	0	1	1	1	1	6
Simic et al. (2012)	1	0	0	1	0	0	0	1	1	1	1	6
Van den Noort et al. (2014)	0	0	0	1	0	0	0	1	1	1	1	5
Wheeler et al. (2011)	0	1	0	1	0	0	0	1	1	1	1	6

Table 2. Extracted data from included studies

Author (year)	Gait modification	Natural Gait: Mean value of target parameter	Modified gait: Mean value of target parameter	KAM unit of measure	Biofeedback variable	KAM outcome reported	Natural gait: mean±SD KAM	Modified gait: mean±SD KAM	Calculated % KAM change	Primary Findings
Barrios et al. (2010)	Medial knee thrust	Knee adduction angle: 6.8±2.4°	Post-training: Natural: 6.2±2.2° Modified: 5.0±2.1° 1-month: Natural: 6.6±1.4° Modified: 5.5±2.2°	Nm/kg*Ht	Visual; knee angle	KAM	0.43±0.07	Post-training: Natural: 0.42±0.05 Modified: 0.34±0.07 1-month: Natural: 0.44±0.06 Modified: 0.34±0.07	−2* −20 2* −20	Medial knee thrust significantly reduced KEAM, however at 1-month natural gait remained unchanged although participants could replicate learned gait with similar reductions in KEAM found at post-training.
Dowling et al. (2010)	Weight transfer to medial foot	NR	NR	%BW*Ht	Haptic; lateral foot pressure	KAM 1	Haptic feedback group: 2.54±0.56 Verbal instruction group: 2.48±0.40	2.18±0.57 2.29±0.55	−14.2 −8.3	A slight weight bearing shift to the medial side of the foot during gait using real-time haptic biofeedback reduced first peak KAM.
Ferrigno et al. (2016)	Medial thrust gait and limited lateral foot pressure via pressure based feedback	NR	NR	%BW*Ht	Auditory; lateral foot pressure	KAM, KAM 1, KAM 2	3.03±0.86 1.74±0.76 2.99±0.88	Medial thrust: KAM: 2.66±0.95 KAM 1: 1.08±0.72 KAM 2: 2.64±0.98 Pressure based feedback: KAM: 2.66±0.85 KAM 1: 1.58±0.72 KAM 2: 2.63±0.87	−12 −38 −11.7 −12 −9.2 −12	Pressure-based feedback is equally effective as 'medial thrust gait' in lowering KAM in healthy subjects without the unknown and potentially negative outcomes of other gait modifications.
Hunt et al. (2011)	Lateral trunk lean	Lateral trunk lean 2.6±1.6°	4° lean: 5.0±0.87° 8° lean: 8.34±1.61° 12° lean: 12.88±1.91°	Nm/BW*Ht%	Visual; trunk angle	KAM 1, KAM 2	4.07±1.64 1.89±0.77	KAM 1: 4° lean: 3.82±1.77 8° lean: 3.37±1.72 12° lean: 3.26±1.64 KAM 2: 4° lean: 1.64±0.96 8° lean: 1.64±1.02 12° lean: 1.60±0.90	Average peak KAM: 4° lean: −7 8° lean: −21 12° lean: −25	A gait pattern incorporating at least 8° of lateral trunk lean is successful in lowering early stance peak KAM compared to normal walking and can be achieved quickly by young healthy individuals using real-time visual biofeedback.

(Contd...)

Table 2. (*Continued*)

Author (year)	Gait modification	Natural Gait: Mean value of target parameter	Modified gait: Mean value of target parameter	KAM unit of measure	Biofeedback variable	KAM outcome reported	Natural gait: mean±SD KAM	Modified gait: mean±SD KAM	Calculated % KAM change	Primary Findings
Riskowski (2010)	Reduced rate of loading (ROL)	IC Knee flexion: 1.2±2.2° IC Vertical acceleration: -5.87±1.51°	Training gait (with brace): IC knee flexion: 7.2±1.4° IC vertical acceleration: -4.97±1.29 Post-training (no brace): IC knee flexion: 5.4±1.5° IC vertical acceleration: -4.89±1.05°	BW*Ht	Auditory; knee flexion and vertical acceleration	KAM	0.51±0.07	Training gait (with brace): 0.62±0.05 Post-training (no brace): 0.57±0.07	12.16* 11.18*	Gait retraining with a feedback-based gait monitoring knee brace demonstrated short-term gait and neuromuscular effects while reducing ROL and increasing proprioceptive awareness. However, a concomitant increase in KAM limits the effectiveness of the brace particularly in those with OA.
Segal et al. (2015)	Increased proportioned displacements of the trunk and pelvis for the frontal and transverse axes.	NR	NR	NR	Visual; kinematic measures	NR	NR	NR	NR	In comparison with usual care, three months of individualized physical therapist-supervised gait training reduced self-reported outcomes in older adults with symptomatic knee OA immediately after post-intervention, but it was not retained at 6 or 12-months post-intervention.
Shull et al. (2011)	Foot progression, Trunk sway, Tibia angle using single and multi-parameter models.	Tibia angle: -4.2° Foot progression angle: -5.9° Trunk sway angle: 1.5°	Tibia angle: 3.0° Foot progression angle: 8.4° Trunk sway angle: 9.9°	%BW*Ht	Haptic; trunk, tibia, and foot progression angles	KAM 1	4.1 ± 0.6	2.7±0.6	-36.6*	Data-driven gaits were identified and trained in a single session, lead to a 20-48% reduction in KAM. These findings upkeep the use of localized linear modeling for altered gait identification and real-time haptic feedback.

(*Contd...*)

Table 2. (Continued)

Author (year)	Gait modification	Natural Gait: Mean value of target parameter	Modified gait: Mean value of target parameter	KAM unit of measure	Biofeedback variable	KAM outcome reported	Natural gait: mean±SD KAM	Modified gait: mean±SD KAM	Calculated % KAM change	Primary Findings
										While the change was overall positive, the magnitude of changed varied significantly.
Shull et al. (2013a)	Toe-in gait.	Foot progression angle: KAM 1: 3.3° KAM 2: 3.9°	Foot progression angle: KAM 1: -2.1° KAM 2: -1.4°	%BW*Ht	Haptic; tibia angle	KAM 1, KAM 2	3.28±1.37 1.98±1.14	2.90±1.38 1.94±1.09	-13 -2*	Toe-in gait significantly reduced the first peak of the knee adduction moment, which occurred as the knee joint center shifted medially and the center of pressure shifted laterally. Peak external flexion moment was not increased by toe-in gait modification.
Shull et al. (2013b)	Single and/ or multi-gait parameter data driven gait retraining	Foot progression angle: 2.1±4.0° Trunk sway angle: 1.0±2.1°	Foot progression angle: Post-training: −5.1±5.1° 1-month follow-up: −6.0±4.7° Trunk sway angle: Post-training: 0.7±1.6° 1-month follow-up: 0.7±1.5°	%BW*Ht	Haptic; trunk and foot progression angles	KAM 1	3.11±1.40	Post-training: 2.61±1.47 1-month follow-up: 2.67±1.41	-20 -14.1*	The 20% reduction in KAM achieved post-training and 14.1% reduction at follow up shows that the effects of gait modification can be retained over time. No association was found between KAM decrease and knee flexion moment increase. Generally, increased knee flexion moment may eradicate the potential medial compartment force reduction that derives from the decrease in KAM.

(Contd...)

Table 2. (Continued)

Author (year)	Gait modification	Natural Gait: Mean value of target parameter	Modified gait: Mean value of target parameter	KAM unit of measure	Biofeedback variable	KAM outcome reported	Natural gait: mean±SD KAM	Modified gait: mean±SD KAM	Calculated % KAM change	Primary Findings
Simic et al. (2012)	Trunk lean (a peak of 6° lean, 9° lean, and 12° lean)	Peak lateral trunk lean: 2.0° Early stance trunk lean: 0.9° Late stance trunk lean: 0.8°	Peak trunk lean: 6° lean: 6.1° 9° lean: 8.7° 12° lean: 11.1° Early Stance: 6° lean: 5.1° 9° lean: 7.6° 12° lean: 9.3° Late Stance: 6° lean: 3.0° 9° lean: 4.4° 12° lean: 5.6°	Nm/%BW*Ht	Visual; trunk angle	KAM 1 KAM 2	3.75 2.05	KAM 1: 6° lean: 3.40 9° lean: 3.33 12° lean: 3.19 KAM 2: 6° lean: 1.71 9° lean: 1.69 12° lean: 1.56	KAM 1: 6° lean: −9.3* 9° lean: −11.5* 12° lean: −14.9* KAM 2: 6° lean: −17.1* 9° lean: −18* 12° lean: −23.9*	Increasing lateral trunk lean on the knee OA side can positively reduce the knee load throughout the stance phase of gait.
Van den Noort et al. (2014)	Self-selected gait to reduce KAM and HIR	Early HIR: 1.98±2.69° Mid HIR: 2.52±2.83° Late HIR: 1.92±2.53°	Bar Early: 8.26±2.69° Bar Late: 11.40±2.53° Bar Mid: 10.33±2.83° Polar Early: 10.41±2.78° Polar Late: 12.52±2.61° Polar Mid: 11.27±2.92° Color Early: 8.99±2.78° Color Late: 9.81±2.69° Color Mid: 9.66±3.02° Graph Early: 9.97±2.69° Graph Late: 7.90±2.53° Graph Mid: 9.26±2.83°	%BW*Ht	Visual; KAM and HIR	KAM 1, KAM 2, KAM 3	HIR Feedback: Early: 2.14±0.20 Late: 1.91±0.29 Mid: 1.72±0.22	HIR Feedback: Bar Early: 1.79±0.24 Bar Late: 1.41±0.33 Bar Mid: 1.86±0.25 Polar Early: 1.73±0.24 Polar Late: 1.14±0.32 Polar Mid: 1.54±0.24 Color Early: 1.92±0.25 Color Late: 1.60±0.34 Color Mid: 1.96±0.27 Graph Early: 2.03±0.23 Graph Late: 1.74±0.32 Graph Mid: 1.97±0.24	Bar Early: −16.19 Bar Late: −26.04 Bar Mid: 8.05 Polar Early: −19.22 Polar Late: −40.32 Polar Mid: −10.64 Color Early: −10.07 Color Late: −16.45 Color Mid: 13.75 Graph Early: −4.91 Graph Late: −8.77 Graph Mid: 14.47	Results showed that the gait pattern of healthy subjects can be effectively modified using real-time visual feedback, independently of the type of feedback, however, direct visual feedback of the KAM resulted in greater reductions in peak KAM compared to indirect feedback of HIR. The direction of the gait modifications was also in agreement with the presented modification using visual feedback. Both KAM and HIR were significantly affected during with visual feedback, which decreased KAM by about 50% and the HIR by 6°–10° when compared to baseline

(Contd...)

Table 2. (Continued)

Author (year)	Gait modification	Natural Gait: Mean value of target parameter	Modified gait: Mean value of target parameter	KAM unit of measure	Biofeedback variable	KAM outcome reported	Natural gait: mean±SD KAM	Modified gait: mean±SD KAM	Calculated % KAM change	Primary Findings
							KAM feedback: Early: 2.17±0.25 Late: 2.10±0.16 Mid: 1.91±0.30	KAM feedback: Bar Early: 1.17±0.25 Bar Late: 0.94±0.39 Bar Mid: 0.94±0.30 Polar Early: 0.96±0.26 Polar Late: 0.94±0.34 Polar Mid: 0.94±32 Color Early: 1.20±0.27 Color Late: 0.98±0.36 Color Mid: 0.98±0.33 Graph Early: 1.10±0.26 Graph Late: 1.23±0.30 Graph Mid: 1.23±0.32	Bar Early: −46.08% Bar Late: −55.21% Bar Mid: −50.80% Polar Early: −55.84 Polar Late: −55.00 Polar Mid: −50.57 Color Early: −44.72 Color Late: −53.40 Color Mid: −48.82 Graph Early: −49.48 Graph Late: −41.40 Graph Mid: −35.63	
Wheeler et al. (2011)	Self-selected	NR	NR	%BW*Ht	Visual and haptic; KAM	KAM	All participants: 3.98±0.90 Visual: 4.07±0.89 Haptic: 3.90±0.96	All participants: 3.19 ± 0.93 Visual: 3.29±0.98 Haptic: 3.09±0.94	All participants: −20.67% Visual: −20.24 Haptic: −21.11	The study showed that providing real-time feedback of the KAM and allowing subjects to self-select gait modifications was an effective gait retraining method for reducing the KAM.

(Contd...)

Table 2. (Continued)

Author (year)	Gait modification	Natural Gait: Mean value of target parameter	Modified gait: Mean value of target parameter	Natural gait: mean±SD KAM	Biofeedback variable	Modified gait: mean±SD KAM	Calculated % KAM change	Primary Findings
					KAM unit of measure	KAM outcome reported		

- BW – Body weight
- Ht – Height
- OA – Osteoarthritis
- SD – Standard deviation
- KAM – overall peak knee adduction moment
- KAM 1 – peak knee adduction moment in first half of stance
- KAM 2 – peak knee adduction moment in second half of stance
- KAM 3 – peak knee adduction moment in midstance
- IC – initial contact
- HIR – hip internal rotation angle
- NR – not reported
- * – calculated from data provided

follow up, while improvements in KOOS pain and function and LLFDI scores were retained 12-months post-intervention. Three studies using OA patients measured additional kinetic and temporospatial variables. Two studies reported a reduction in KFM post-training (Shull, Shultz, et al., 2013; Shull, Silder, et al., 2013) that, when tested, was retained at the 1-month follow-up (Shull, Silder, et al., 2013). Lateral trunk lean reduced KAM impulse but did not significantly alter stride speed or length (Simic et al., 2012).

Effects of different gait modifications and modes of biofeedback on healthy individuals

Seven of the eight studies conducted using healthy participants reported a significant reduction in KAM compared to baseline (Barrios et al., 2010; Dowling, Fisher, et al., 2010; Ferrigno et al., 2016; Hunt et al., 2014; Shull et al., 2011; van den Noort et al., 2014; Wheeler et al., 2011). KAM reduction ranged from 7% (Hunt et al., 2014) to 55.8% (van den Noort et al., 2014) with the magnitude of change differing based on gait modification used, mode of biofeedback and study design. Self-selected gait modification showed the greatest reductions in KAM in healthy individuals (van den Noort et al., 2014; Wheeler et al., 2011). Participants who were free to determine their own gait strategy without instruction reduced KAM by an average of 49% (van den Noort et al., 2014), while those who were instructed to select one or any combination of previously studied gait modifications decreased KAM 20.7% (Wheeler et al., 2011). Multi-parameter gait retraining also resulted in a large average reduction in KAM of 36.6% in healthy participants (Shull et al., 2011). Using a data-driven model, Shull et al. (2011) prescribed individual modifications to foot progression, trunk sway, and tibia angle resulting in reductions ranging from 29%-48%. Lateral trunk lean showed increasing reductions in KAM from 7% to 25% based on magnitude of lean (Hunt). Medial knee thrust resulted in an average KAM reduction of 20% which was replicated upon request 1-month post-intervention (Barrios et al., 2010). Gait modifications involving the foot resulted in smaller but still significant reductions in KAM between 9.2% (Ferrigno et al., 2016) and 14.2% (Dowling, Fisher, et al., 2010). An increase in first peak KAM of 12% after training with a feedback-based gait monitoring knee brace was reported (Riskowski, 2010). Of the eight studies investigating healthy participants, three employed visual feedback (Barrios et al., 2010; Hunt et al., 2014; van den Noort et al., 2014), two used haptic (Dowling, Fisher, et al., 2010; Shull et al., 2011), two used auditory (Ferrigno et al., 2016; Riskowski, 2010), and one compared visual and haptic feedback between groups (Wheeler et al., 2011). Participants responded well to both visual and haptic feedback but displayed lesser reductions in KAM with auditory feedback. (Table 2). Only two of the eight studies used direct biofeedback, meaning feedback provided was the dependent variable of interest (KAM) (van den Noort et al., 2014; Wheeler et al., 2011). The remaining studies employed indirect feedback whereby participants were provided feedback based on kinematic measures such as joint angle (Barrios et al., 2010; Hunt et al., 2014; Riskowski, 2010; Shull

Table 3. Extracted data from other outcome measures

Outcome measure	Author (year)	Natural gait: Mean value of target variable	Modified gait: Mean value of target variable	Calculated % change	Findings
Kinetic:					
KFM (%BW*Ht)	Ferrigno et al. (2016)	3.01±1.50	Medial knee thrust: 4.02±1.98 Pressure based feedback: 2.79±1.25	33.55* −7.31*	KFM was reduced concomitantly with peak KAM during toe-in gait, medial weight shift gait, and multi-parameter gait (option of altering foot progression or trunk sway angle). Similar to KAM, KFM showed a continued reduction 1-month post-training following multi-parameter gait retraining. In comparison, medial knee thrust gait, and altered gait using a feedback-based monitoring knee brace increased KFM suggesting that different gait modifications may have different effects on KFM.
	Riskowski (2010)	0.29±0.05	Training gait (with brace): 0.31±0.03 Post-training (no brace): 0.31±0.04	6.9* 6.9*	
	Shull et al. (2013a)	1.48±1.45	1.29±1.39	−12.84*	
	Shull et al. (2013b)	1.95±0.76	Post-training: 1.67±0.75 One-month: 1.43±0.70	−14.36* −26.66*	
KAM impulse (Nm.s/%BW*Ht)	Simic et al. (2012)	1.22	6° lean: 1.05 9° lean: 1.03 12° lean: 0.96	−13.95* −15.57* −21.31*	KAM impulse was reduced when walking with increased lateral trunk lean and during self-selected gait. Like KAM, the reductions in KAM impulse increase with increasing magnitude of trunk lean. During self-selected gait, reductions in KAM impulse were similar to those seen in KAM with direct visual feedback (KAM) providing the greatest reductions in KAM impulse.
	Van den Noort et al. (2014)	KAM feedback: 1.21±0.17 HIR feedback: 1.17±0.13	KAM feedback: Bar: 0.63±0.17 Polar: 0.47±0.18 Color: 0.67±0.19 Graph: 0.62±0.18 HIR feedback: Bar: 0.98±0.15 Polar: 0.90±0.15 Color: 1.10±0.16 Graph: 1.17±0.15	−48.17 −61.02 −44.81 −49.24 −16.77 −23.26 −6.38 −0.34	
Temporospatial:					
Stride speed (m/s)	Ferrigno et al. (2016)	1.31±0.13	Medial knee thrust: 1.17±0.15 Pressure based feedback: 1.26±0.15	−10.69* −3.82*	Stride speed was minimally reduced during all gait modifications apart from a small increase during increased lateral trunk lean of 6° and more significantly during medial knee thrust. The complexity of medial knee thrust suggests that more difficult gait modifications may require a slower speed.
	Hunt et al. (2011)	1.42 ±0.18	4° lean: 1.36±0.19 8° lean: 1.36±0.19 12° lean: 1.40±0.19	−4.23* −4.23* −1.41*	

(Contd...)

Table 3. (Continued)

Outcome measure	Author (year)	Natural gait: Mean value of target variable	Modified gait: Mean value of target variable	Calculated % change	Findings
	Riskowski (2010)	1.28±0.05	Training gait (with brace): 1.26±0.04 / Post-training (no brace): 1.27±0.03	1.56* / -0.78*	
	Simic et al. (2012)	1.24	6° lean: 1.25 / 9° lean: 1.24 / 12° lean: 1.23	0.81* / -0* / -0.81*	
Stride length (m)	Ferrigno et al. (2016)	1.37±0.12	Medial knee thrust: 1.32±0.12 / Pressure based feedback: 1.35±0.12	-3.64* / -1.46*	Stride length was minimally reduced but not significantly altered across all gait modifications studied.
	Riskowski (2010)	1.35±0.12	Training gait (with brace): 1.30±0.08 / Post-training (no brace): 1.30±0.14	-3.70* / -3.70*	
	Simic et al. (2012)	1.35	6° lean: 1.33 / 9° lean: 1.34 / 12° lean: 1.34	-1.48* / -0.74* / -0.74*	
Subjective Rating:					
Difficulty/effort (0/10)	Barrios et al. (2010) 0 – "Effortless" 10 – "Max effort"	Session 1: 6.63±1.83†	Session 8: 2.94±0.94†	-55.66*	Participants reported moderate difficulty adopting medial knee thrust, lateral trunk lean, and self-selected gait. However, by the last session of an 8-week intervention using medial knee thrust, participants reported reduced ratings of difficulty, suggesting that walking with a new gait should become easier with practice.
	Hunt et al. (2011) 0 – "No difficulty" 10 – "Max difficulty"	N/A	4° lean: 3±3 / 8° lean: 3±1 / 12° lean: 4±2	N/A / N/A / N/A	
	Van den Noort et al. (2014) 1 – "Very difficult" 10 – "Very easy"	N/A	KAM feedback: Bar: 6.3±1.5 / Polar: 5.8±2.0 / Color: 6.8±1.8 / Graph: 5.9±2.3	N/A / N/A / N/A / N/A	

(Contd...)

Table 3. (Continued)

Outcome measure	Author (year)	Natural gait: Mean value of target variable	Modified gait: Mean value of target variable	Calculated % change	Findings
Awkwardness/ Intuitive (0/10)	Barrios et al. (2010) 0 – "Natural" 10 – "Maximally unnatural"	Session 1: 7.06±0.78†	HIR feedback: Bar: 6.0±1.7 Polar: 6.1±2.5 Color: 5.9±2.4 Graph: 6.4±1.8	N/A N/A N/A N/A	Participants reported altered gait as moderately awkward during both medial knee thrust and self-selected gait suggesting that adopting a new gait may feel equally as awkward if it is prescribed or chosen by the participant. Similar to ratings of difficulty/effort.
			Last session: 3.88±1.64†	–45.04*	
	Wheeler et al. (2011) 0 – "No different" 10 – "Extremely awkward"	N/A	All participants: 5.31±2.27 Visual: 5.25±1.98 Haptic: 5.38±2.67	N/A N/A N/A	
PROM:					
KOOS pain	Segal et al. (2015)	62.7±10.8	3-month: 70.9 6-month: 68.1 12-month: 72.8	13.07* 8.61* 16.12*	Participant reporting of knee pain, symptoms, and lower extremity function were improved across all conditions. These improvements were retained at 1, 3, 6, and 12-months post-intervention, however, improvements in LLFDI and KOOS symptoms scores were no different between the intervention and control group past 3 months.
KOOS symptoms	Segal et al. (2015)	60.1±16.8	3-month: 71.6 6-month: 68.2 12-month: 68.6	19.13* 13.48* 14.14*	
LLFDI	Segal et al. (2015)	65.8±9.2	3-month: 69.1 6-month: 68.9 12-month: 69.7	5.02* 4.71* 5.93*	These results suggest that gait retraining interventions designed to reduce KAM can translate to improvements in patient reported pain and function. These changes can also be retained over time but may trend back towards baseline values if the new gait is not continually used.
WOMAC pain	Shull et al. (2013b)	70.5†	Post-training: 85.0† One-month: 90.0†	20.57* 27.66*	
WOMAC function	Shull et al. (2013b)	77.4†	Post-training: 91.7† One-month: 91.7†	18.48* 18.48*	

(Contd...)

Table 3. (Continued)

Outcome measure	Author (year)	Natural gait: Mean value of target variable	Modified gait: Mean value of target variable	Calculated % change	Findings
VAS (0/10)	Shull et al. (2013b) 0 – "No hurt" 10 – "Hurts worst"	3.2	Post-training: 1.4 1-month: 1.0	–56.25*	Participant reporting of knee pain and discomfort using visual analogue pain scales were not significantly altered over a single day intervention using increased lateral trunk lean, however, over a 6-week intervention pain ratings were more than halved.
	Simic et al. (2012) 0 – "No pain/ discomfort" 10 – "Worst pain/ discomfort"	2.2	6° lean: 2.3 9° lean: 2.2 12° lean: 2.1	4.54* 0* –4.54*	

- BW – Body weight
- Ht – Height
- KFM – Overall peak knee flexion moment during stance
- KAM – Knee adduction moment
- HIR – Hip internal rotation angle
- ROL – rate of loading
- PROM – Pain related outcome measure
- KOOS – Knee injury and osteoarthritis outcome score (scale from 0-100, a score of 100 indicating no symptoms and a score of 0 indicating extreme symptoms)
- LLFDI – Late-life function and disability instrument (scored on a 0 to 100 scale, with higher scores indicating higher levels of function)
- WOMAC – Western Ontario and McCaster Universities Osteoarthritis Index (scale from 0-100, a score of 100 indicating no symptoms and a score of 0 indicating extreme symptoms)
- VAS – Visual analogue scale
- N/A – not applicable
- ± - standard deviation (if reported)
- * - calculated from data provided
- † – Author contacted for data

et al., 2011) and foot pressure (Dowling, Fisher, et al., 2010; Ferrigno et al., 2016).

Half of the studies involving healthy participants also reported subjective ratings of gait modification using visual analogue scales (0/10) (Barrios et al., 2010; Hunt et al., 2014; van den Noort et al., 2014; Wheeler et al., 2011) (Table 3). Three studies showed moderate ratings of difficulty and effort between 3-6.8/10 when adopting a modified gait (Barrios et al., 2010; Hunt et al., 2014; van den Noort et al., 2014) with a third of healthy participants in one study reporting some form of pain or discomfort during the intervention (Hunt et al., 2014). Participants in two studies rated how awkward and or unnatural adopting a modified gait was with scores ranging from 5.25-7/10 (Barrios et al., 2010; Wheeler et al., 2011). However, participants using medial knee thrust reported that both effort and naturalness of the new gait improved by greater than 3/10 by the end of the 8-week intervention (Barrios et al., 2010).

Four studies using healthy participants measured additional kinetic and temporospatial variables. One study reported an increase in KFM during and after using a feedback providing knee brace designed to reduce rate of loading (ROL) (Riskowski, 2010), while a second study showed a reduction in KFM when using pressure-based feedback to reduce lateral plantar pressure, but an increase in KFM during medial knee thrust gait (Ferrigno et al., 2016). KAM impulse was reduced with both lateral trunk lean (Simic et al., 2012), and self-selected gait (van den Noort et al., 2014). Stride speed and length were minimally reduced, but not significantly changed (Hunt et al., 2014; Riskowski, 2010) except with medial knee thrust which reduced gait speed by an average of 10.69% (Ferrigno et al., 2016).

DISCUSSION

The first aim of this review is to determine if gait retraining using real-time biofeedback are beneficial in reducing KAM, pain, and improving function in patients with knee OA. Analysis of the available literature revealed a lack of high quality evidence, as most studies employed lower level of evidence designs (e.g., quasi-experimental) using young, healthy individuals, with only a few experimental designs studying symptomatic populations. A high degree of heterogeneity was also noted among the studies, with multiple gait modification strategies and real-time feedback modes being employed. Nonetheless, all studies that measured KAM in OA participants (n=4) reported significant reductions post-training (Shull, Shultz, et al., 2013; Shull, Silder, et al., 2013; Simic et al., 2012) suggesting that gait retraining using real-time biofeedback can be beneficial in reducing KAM in some patients with knee OA. There is also limited evidence that gait modification using RTB can reduce pain, and improve function in individuals with knee OA (Segal et al., 2015; Shull, Silder, et al., 2013). The only randomized controlled trial included in the review reported significant improvements in knee pain, symptoms and functional tasks after a 12-week intervention involving intermittent visual RTB designed to make postural adjustment and reinforce correct gait patterns (Segal et al., 2015). WOMAC

pain and function scores showed similar improvements after a 6-week intervention also using visual RTB (Shull, Silder, et al., 2013). These effects lasted up to 12 and 1 months, respectively, suggesting that gait retraining with RTB can have long-term clinical benefits in OA patients. The present evidence is limited to 2 studies and 66 participants, however, and therefore must be interpreted with caution. Future studies should focus on longitudinal designs assessing the short and long-term functional outcomes of OA patients after gait retraining interventions using RTB.

The second aim of this review was to evaluate the effectiveness of different gait modifications and modes of RTB in reducing KAM in healthy individuals. Self-selected gait displayed the greatest change in KAM in healthy individuals. Evidence suggests that reduction in KAM per unit of gait modification is highly variable among participants, signifying that individual dose-response relationships exist (Favre, Erhart-Hledik, Chehab, & Andriacchi, 2016; Gerbrands, Pisters, & Vanwanseele, 2014). As an example, individual reductions in KAM ranged from as little as 3% to more than 50% within the same gait retraining protocol (Wheeler et al., 2011). These results indicate that the optimal gait modification strategy will differ between individuals, meaning interventions may be most effective when adapted to each patient. Entire adaptability to self-select gait modification may not be clinically beneficial, however, as patients may adopt highly variable and inefficient strategies that are not sustainable and increase other biomechanical measures associated with the development of knee OA (Walter et al., 2010). Participants that self-selected their gait modification strategy without further instruction, exhibited 35% of additional modifications such as increased or decreased foot progression angle greater than 15°, increasing step width by greater than 10 cm, and larger knee flexion, hip abduction, and pelvic protraction (van den Noort et al., 2014). Gait modifications to moderate KAM have been shown to have kinematic, kinetic, and spatiotemporal effects across the kinetic chain, yet long-term outcomes due to these changes remain poorly understood (Simic et al., 2011).

Multi-parameter gait modification showed greater reductions in KAM when compared to single parameter and may offer a practical and effective medium between self-selected and single-parameter gait. Recently, it was reported that secondary changes such as increased step width occurred with up to 60% of the amplitude of the instructed modification when using a single parameter strategy (Favre et al., 2016). When participants combined three gait modifications (toe-in, increased step width, and increased trunk sway) a decrease in first peak KAM of approximately 49% was reported, leading the authors to suggest that gait retraining should be addressed as a general scheme as opposed to focusing on a single gait modification (Favre et al., 2016). Multi-parameter strategies may represent an optimum approach to a natural concomitant relationship of the kinetic chain, whereas employing a single variable self-selected strategy appears to lead to unanticipated and unintended outcomes. Single parameter strategies, such as lateral trunk lean, medial knee thrust, and medial weight shift were less effective in reducing KAM than both self-selected and multi-parameter strategies. Employing lateral trunk lean and medial knee thrust, which require substantial and complex adjustments may be less clinically beneficial due to the difficulty of adoption, particularly with OA participants (Barrios et al., 2010; Hunt et al., 2011; Shull et al., 2011; Shull, Silder, et al., 2013). In comparison, medial weight transfer is easier to adopt as it requires only a subtle change in gait and has not been associated with a concomitant increase in KFM unlike other gait modification strategies (Ferrigno et al., 2016; Gerbrands et al., 2014; Walter et al., 2010). Nonetheless, reported reductions in KAM of 9% to 14% when using medial weight transfer is only slightly greater than those observed in orthotic interventions, reducing clinical impact compared to other modification strategies (Hinman, Bowles, Payne, & Bennell, 2008; Kean, Bennell, Wrigley, & Hinman, 2013).

Visual biofeedback provided the greatest reduction in KAM in healthy individuals. Concurrent visual feedback has been effective in rehabilitation of complex motor skills (J. Y. Chang, Chang, Chien, Chung, & Hsu, 2007; Snodgrass, Rivett, Robertson, & Stojanovski, 2010). Yet, the guidance hypothesis states that continued concurrent feedback can be detrimental for long-term retention and that terminal feedback must be introduced to encourage internalization of the new skill (Bernier, Chua, & Franks, 2005; Heuer & Hegele, 2008; Sülzenbrück & Heuer, 2011). Considering this factor, Barrios et al. implemented a fading feedback paradigm and reported no changes in KAM from post-training to 1-month post-training, showing that participants retained the reductions in KAM from gait retraining. For older adults, more susceptible of knee OA, it has been described that they may benefit from receiving only concurrent visual feedback as they remain in an attention-demanding phase of learning longer than their younger counterparts (Wishart, Lee, Cunningham, & Murdoch, 2002). We did not find any studies directly comparing visual, haptic, and auditory feedback, but prior motor learning research suggests that concurrent visual feedback to be preferable for older adults attempting to learn a complex motor skill (Sigrist, Rauter, Riener, & Wolf, 2013). Surprisingly, only two studies used KAM as the biofeedback variable (van den Noort et al., 2014; Wheeler et al., 2011); the majority used kinematic measures (Barrios et al., 2010; Ferrigno et al., 2016; Hunt et al., 2011; Segal et al., 2015; Shull et al., 2011; Shull, Shultz, et al., 2013; Shull, Silder, et al., 2013; Simic et al., 2012). Studies employing KAM as the biofeedback variable resulted in the greatest reductions in KAM, suggesting a better response to biofeedback based on the target kinetic parameter, compared to a surrogate kinematic measure.

The final aim of this review was to assess the impact of gait retraining interventions using RTB on other variables that may affect clinical outcomes. Additional outcome variables that were clinically relevant and were reported in at least more than one study were identified (Table 3). Increased KFM compressive loads at the knee joint (Walter et al., 2010) and is a significant predictor of joint load even after accounting for variance attributed to KAM (Manal et al., 2015). Reductions in KFM were seen with self-selected (Shull, Silder, et al., 2013) and toe-in gait (Shull, Shultz, et al., 2013) in OA participants and with medial weight shift

in healthy individuals (Ferrigno et al., 2016). In contrast, walking with a feedback monitoring knee brace designed to reduce ROL (Riskowski, 2010) and medial knee thrust (Ferrigno et al., 2016) increased KFM. The increase in KFM seen with the use of the feedback monitoring brace may be explained by the fact that the primary purpose of the study was to explore how training with the knee brace affected ROL and proprioceptive acuity, with KAM only being a secondary outcome measure (Riskowski, 2010). However, participants who performed both medial knee thrust and medial weight shift gait in the same study showed opposing effects on KFM despite the fact both interventions were designed to reduce KAM (Ferrigno et al., 2016). This supports the finding that KAM and KFM are not correlated (Manal et al., 2015), suggesting that different gait modifications, regardless of similar effects on KAM, can have varying effects on KFM. It is important that gait retraining interventions do not offset the benefits of reduced KAM with equal or greater increases in KFM. Future research should identify which strategies are most beneficial in terms of both KAM and KFM. KAM impulse integrates the magnitude of KAM and the duration over which KAM acts providing a measure of total mechanical loading during walking as opposed to load only at one instance in time (Creaby et al., 2010; Kean et al., 2012). Similar to KFM, it is important that reduction in KAM does not coincide with increased KAM impulse as it has been associated with the severity and prevalence of cartilage defects (Creaby et al., 2010) as well as knee pain (Robbins et al., 2011). Both increased lateral trunk lean in OA participants (Simic et al., 2012) and self-selected gait in healthy participants (van den Noort et al., 2014) reduced KAM impulse. Though evidence is limited, this suggests that KAM impulse may be more closely correlated with KAM than KFM. More research is needed to determine the relationship between these variables and the impact different gait modifications have on KAM impulse. Stride speed and length remained relatively unchanged across all studied gait modifications (Hunt et al., 2014; Riskowski, 2010; Simic et al., 2012) apart from medial knee thrust (Ferrigno et al., 2016). This can be attributed to the fact that gait speed was controlled to be within 5% of self-selected baseline speeds (Hunt et al., 2014; Riskowski, 2010; Simic et al., 2012). The one study that did not control for gait speed showed a significant reduction during medial knee thrust gait. This may be attributable to the complexity of the gait modification which involves participants to adduct and generate an internal rotation of the hip while concurrently increasing hip, knee, and ankle flexion angles. Reduced stride speed has been argued to be both beneficial and detrimental to patients with knee OA. It has been theorized that slower gait speed may reduce KAM by altering vertical and frontal plane center of mass acceleration, thus reducing the magnitude of the ground reaction force (Browning & Kram, 2007). However, study results do not consistently support this (Simic et al., 2012), as others report that slower gait speeds increase KAM impulse (Robbins & Maly, 2009). Reduced stride length, on the other hand, has been suggested to provide small reductions in KAM impulse due to less time spent during stance in gait (Russell et al., 2010). Similar to gait speed, stride length was not significantly changed as a result of gait retraining. However, future studies should investigate if there is a significant change in these parameters when gait speed is not controlled for, such as the results seen during medial knee thrust, as gait speed is not easily controlled outside of the lab. Limitations of the included studies weakens the clinical applications of these findings. Most studies included in this review provided low quality evidence due to methodological decisions; study design, lack of controls, and small sample sizes. Eight studies recruited young, healthy participants diminishing generalizability to symptomatic individuals (Barrios et al., 2010; Dowling, Corazza, et al., 2010; Ferrigno et al., 2016; Hunt et al., 2011; Riskowski, 2010; Shull et al., 2011; van den Noort et al., 2014; Wheeler et al., 2011). Participant follow-up was limited to three studies, one of which reported the average percentage of time healthy participants spent walking with the modified gait outside of the lab at only 11% (Barrios et al., 2010). Participants reported completing 97% (Shull, Silder, et al., 2013) and 92.4% (Segal et al., 2015) of prescribed at-home gait training in the other two studies, suggesting participant compliance is feasible in long-term interventions. Almost all studies scored poorly regarding internal validity. These scores reflect the quasi-randomized and uncontrolled nature of most of the included studies. The sole RCT included in this review did not require blinding of participants or testers (Segal et al., 2015), and of the four studies to employ random allocation in their study design, none concealed allocation to groups (Dowling, Corazza, et al., 2010; Ferrigno et al., 2016; Segal et al., 2015; Wheeler et al., 2011). Interaction effects make it difficult to separately assess the magnitude of KAM reduction by gait modification type and mode of RTB as the RTB mode may appear to reduce KAM more because of the gait modification it was combined with and vice versa. Publication bias may also have affected the results of this review as studies that report significant or positive results are more likely to be published (Dwan, Gamble, Williamson, & Kirkham, 2013).

CONCLUSION

First peak KAM has been repeatedly associated with knee OA progression, therefore, a non-surgical intervention capable of reducing KAM has profound clinical implications on patients suffering from or at risk of knee OA. Overall, the evidence presented in this review demonstrates that gait modification with RTB may successfully reduce KAM in both symptomatic and asymptomatic participants. However, the existing literature is limited and of low quality, denoting that combination of modification strategy and biofeedback remains uncertain. Future studies should employ randomized, controlled study designs to compare the effects of different gait modification strategies and biofeedback modes across groups (healthy and knee OA) while including additional outcome measures that may affect clinical outcomes. The currently available evidence suggests that self-selected gait modification using multiple gait variables in conjunction with visual RTB may provide the greatest reductions in KAM in healthy individuals.

ACKNOWLEDGEMENTS

Publication of this article was funded in part by the George Mason University Libraries Open Access Publishing Fund.

REFERENCES

Allen, K. D., & Golightly, Y. M. (2015). Epidemiology of osteoarthritis: state of the evidence. *Curr Opin Rheumatol, 27*(3), 276.

Altman, R. D. (1991). Criteria for classification of clinical osteoarthritis. *J Rheumatol Suppl, 27*, 10-12.

Amin, S., Luepongsak, N., McGibbon, C. A., LaValley, M. P., Krebs, D. E., & Felson, D. T. (2004). Knee adduction moment and development of chronic knee pain in elders. *Arthritis Care & Research, 51*(3), 371-376.

Andriacchi, T. P., & Mundermann, A. (2006). The role of ambulatory mechanics in the initiation and progression of knee osteoarthritis. *Curr Opin Rheumatol, 18*(5), 514-518. doi:10.1097/01.bor.0000240365.16842.4e

Andriacchi, T. P., Mündermann, A., Smith, R. L., Alexander, E. J., Dyrby, C. O., & Koo, S. (2004). A framework for the in vivo pathomechanics of osteoarthritis at the knee. *Ann Biomed Eng, 32*(3), 447-457.

Barrios, J. A., Crossley, K. M., & Davis, I. S. (2010). Gait retraining to reduce the knee adduction moment through real-time visual feedback of dynamic knee alignment. *J Biomech, 43*(11), 2208-2213. doi:10.1016/j.jbiomech.2010.03.040

Bellamy, N., Kirwan, J., Boers, M., Brooks, P., Strand, V., Tugwell, P., Lequesne, M. (1997). Recommendations for a core set of outcome measures for future phase III clinical trials in knee, hip, and hand osteoarthritis. Consensus development at OMERACT III. *J Rheumatol, 24*(4), 799-802.

Bernier, P. M., Chua, R., & Franks, I. M. (2005). Is proprioception calibrated during visually guided movements? *Exp Brain Res, 167*(2), 292-296.

Browning, R. C., & Kram, R. (2007). Effects of obesity on the biomechanics of walking at different speeds. *Med Sci Sports Exerc, 39*(9), 1632-1641. doi:10.1249/mss.0b013e318076b54b

Chang, Moisio, K. C., Chmiel, J. S., Eckstein, F., Guermazi, A., Prasad, P. V.,... Sharma, L. (2015). External knee adduction and flexion moments during gait and medial tibiofemoral disease progression in knee osteoarthritis. *Osteoarthr Cartil, 23*(7), 1099-1106. doi:http://dx.doi.org/10.1016/j.joca.2015.02.005

Chang, J. Y., Chang, G. L., Chien, C. J. C., Chung, K. C., & Hsu, A. T. (2007). Effectiveness of two forms of feedback on training of a joint mobilization skill by using a joint translation simulator. *Phys Ther, 87*(4), 418-430.

Chehab, E. F., Favre, J., Erhart-Hledik, J. C., & Andriacchi, T. P. (2014). Baseline knee adduction and flexion moments during walking are both associated with 5 year cartilage changes in patients with medial knee osteoarthritis. *Osteoarthr Cartil, 22*(11), 1833-1839. doi:10.1016/j.joca.2014.08.009

Control, C. f. D., & Prevention. (2013). Prevalence of doctor-diagnosed arthritis and arthritis-attributable activity limitation--United States, 2010-2012. *MMWR. Morbidity and mortality weekly report*, 62(44), 869.

Creaby, M. W., Wang, Y., Bennell, K. L., Hinman, R. S., Metcalf, B. R., Bowles, K. A., & Cicuttini, F. M. (2010). Dynamic knee loading is related to cartilage defects and tibial plateau bone area in medial knee osteoarthritis. *Osteoarthritis Cartilage*, 18(11), 1380-1385. doi:10.1016/j.joca.2010.08.013

Dearborn, J., Eakin, C., & Skinner, H. (1996). Medial compartment arthrosis of the knee. *Am J Orthop (Belle Mead NJ)*, 25(1), 18-26.

Dowling, A. V., Corazza, S., Chaudhari, A. M., & Andriacchi, T. P. (2010). Shoe-surface friction influences movement strategies during a sidestep cutting task: implications for anterior cruciate ligament injury risk. *Am J Sports Med*, 38(3), 478-485. doi:38/3/478 [pii] 10.1177/0363546509348374.

Dowling, A. V., Fisher, D. S., & Andriacchi, T. P. (2010). Gait modification via verbal instruction and an active feedback system to reduce peak knee adduction moment. *J Biomech Eng*, 132(7), 071007. doi:10.1115/1.4001584

Dwan, K., Gamble, C., Williamson, P. R., & Kirkham, J. J. (2013). Systematic review of the empirical evidence of study publication bias and outcome reporting bias - an updated review. *PloS one*, 8(7), e66844. doi:10.1371/journal.pone.0066844

Favre, J., Erhart-Hledik, J. C., Chehab, E. F., & Andriacchi, T. P. (2016). General scheme to reduce the knee adduction moment by modifying a combination of gait variables. *J Orthop Res*, 34(9), 1547-1556. doi:10.1002/jor.23151

Ferrigno, C., Stoller, I. S., Shakoor, N., Thorp, L. E., & Wimmer, M. A. (2016). The Feasibility of Using Augmented Auditory Feedback From a Pressure Detecting Insole to Reduce the Knee Adduction Moment: A Proof of Concept Study. *J Biomech Eng*, 138(2), 021014. doi:10.1115/1.4032123

Fitzpatrick, R. B. (2008). PEDro: a physiotherapy evidence database. *Med Ref Serv* Q, 27(2), 189-198.

Foroughi, N., Smith, R., & Vanwanseele, B. (2009). The association of external knee adduction moment with biomechanical variables in osteoarthritis: a systematic review. *The Knee*, 16(5), 303-309.

Fransen, M., McConnell, S., Harmer, A. R., Van der Esch, M., Simic, M., & Bennell, K. L. (2015). Exercise for osteoarthritis of the knee: a Cochrane systematic review. *Br J Sports Med*, 49(24), 1554-1557. doi:10.1136/bjsports-2015-095424

Gerbrands, T. A., Pisters, M. F., & Vanwanseele, B. (2014). Individual selection of gait retraining strategies is essential to optimally reduce medial knee load during gait. *Clin Biomech*, 29(7), 828-834. doi:10.1016/j.clinbiomech.2014.05.005

Heijink, A., Gomoll, A. H., Madry, H., Drobnič, M., Filardo, G., Espregueira-Mendes, J., & Van Dijk, C. N. (2012). Biomechanical considerations in the pathogenesis of osteoarthritis of the knee. *Knee Surg Sports Traumatol Arthrosc*, 20(3), 423-435.

Heuer, H., & Hegele, M. (2008). Constraints on visuo-motor adaptation depend on the type of visual feedback during practice. *Exp Brain Res*, 185(1), 101-110.

Hinman, R. S., Bowles, K. A., Payne, C., & Bennell, K. L. (2008). Effect of length on laterally-wedged insoles in knee osteoarthritis. *Arthritis Care Res* (Hoboken), 59(1), 144-147.

Hunt, M. A., Simic, M., Hinman, R. S., Bennell, K. L., & Wrigley, T. V. (2011). Feasibility of a gait retraining strategy for reducing knee joint loading: Increased trunk lean guided by real-time biofeedback. *J Biomech*, 44(5), 943-947. doi:S0021-9290(10)00653-6 [pii]. 10.1016/j.jbiomech.2010.11.027

Hunt, M. A., Takacs, J., Hart, K., Massong, E., Fuchko, K., & Biegler, J. (2014). Comparison of mirror, raw video, and real-time visual biofeedback for training toe-out gait in individuals with knee osteoarthritis. *Archives of physical medicine and rehabilitation*, 95(10), 1912-1917.

Hurwitz, D., Ryals, A., Case, J., Block, J., & Andriacchi, T. (2002). The knee adduction moment during gait in subjects with knee osteoarthritis is more closely correlated with static alignment than radiographic disease severity, toe out angle and pain. *J Orthop Res*, 20(1), 101-107.

Kean, C. O., Bennell, K. L., Wrigley, T. V., & Hinman, R. S. (2013). Modified walking shoes for knee osteoarthritis: mechanisms for reductions in the knee adduction moment. J Biomech, 46(12), 2060-2066.

Kean, C. O., Hinman, R. S., Bowles, K. A., Cicuttini, F., Davies-Tuck, M., & Bennell, K. L. (2012). Comparison of peak knee adduction moment and knee adduction moment impulse in distinguishing between severities of knee osteoarthritis. *Clin Biomech (Bristol, Avon)*, 27(5), 520-523. doi:10.1016/j.clinbiomech.2011.12.007

Ma, V. Y., Chan, L., & Carruthers, K. J. (2014). Incidence, prevalence, costs, and impact on disability of common conditions requiring rehabilitation in the United States: stroke, spinal cord injury, traumatic brain injury, multiple sclerosis, osteoarthritis, rheumatoid arthritis, limb loss, and back pain. *Arch Phys Med Rehabil*, 95(5), 986-995. e981.

Manal, K., Gardinier, E., Buchanan, T. S., & Snyder-Mackler, L. (2015). A more informed evaluation of medial compartment loading: the combined use of the knee adduction and flexor moments. *Osteoarthritis Cartilage*, 23(7), 1107-1111. doi:10.1016/j.joca.2015.02.779

Mayr, A., Kofler, M., Quirbach, E., Matzak, H., Fröhlich, K., & Saltuari, L. (2007). Prospective, blinded, randomized crossover study of gait rehabilitation in stroke patients using the Lokomat gait orthosis. *Neurorehabil Neural Repair*, 21(4), 307-314.

Miyazaki, T., Wada, M., Kawahara, H., Sato, M., Baba, H., & Shimada, S. (2002). Dynamic load at baseline can predict radiographic disease progression in medial compartment knee osteoarthritis. *Ann Rheum Dis*, 61(7), 617-622.

Neogi, T., & Zhang, Y. (2013). Epidemiology of osteoarthritis. *Rheum Dis Clin North Am*, 39(1), 1-19.

Nguyen, U.-S. D., Zhang, Y., Zhu, Y., Niu, J., Zhang, B., & Felson, D. T. (2011). Increasing prevalence of knee pain and symptomatic knee osteoarthritis: survey and cohort data. *Ann Intern Med*, 155(11), 725-732.

Richards, R., van den Noort, J. C., Dekker, J., & Harlaar, J. (2017). Gait Retraining With Real-Time Biofeedback to Reduce Knee Adduction Moment: Systematic Review of Effects and Methods Used. *Arch Phys Med Rehabil*, 98(1), 137-150. doi:10.1016/j.apmr.2016.07.006

Riskowski, J. L. (2010). Gait and neuromuscular adaptations after using a feedback-based gait monitoring knee brace. *Gait Posture*, 32(2), 242-247. doi:10.1016/j.gaitpost.2010.05.002

Robbins, S. M., Birmingham, T. B., Callaghan, J. P., Jones, G. R., Chesworth, B. M., & Maly, M. R. (2011). Association of pain with frequency and magnitude of knee loading in knee osteoarthritis. *Arthritis Care Res (Hoboken)*, 63(7), 991-997. doi:10.1002/acr.20476

Robbins, S. M., & Maly, M. R. (2009). The effect of gait speed on the knee adduction moment depends on waveform summary measures. *Gait Posture*, 30(4), 543-546. doi:10.1016/j.gaitpost.2009.08.236

Russell, E. M., Braun, B., & Hamill, J. (2010). Does stride length influence metabolic cost and biomechanical risk factors for knee osteoarthritis in obese women? *Clin Biomech (Bristol, Avon)*, 25(5), 438-443. doi:10.1016/j.clinbiomech.2010.01.016

Segal, N. A., Glass, N. A., Teran-Yengle, P., Singh, B., Wallace, R. B., & Yack, H. J. (2015). Intensive Gait Training for Older Adults with Symptomatic Knee Osteoarthritis. *Am J Phys Med Rehabil*, 94(10 Suppl 1), 848-858. Retrieved from doi:10.1097/PHM.0000000000000264

Sharma, L., Hurwitz, D. E., Thonar, E. J. A., Sum, J. A., Lenz, M. E., & Dunlop, D. D. (1998). Knee adduction moment, serum hyaluronan level, and disease severity in medial tibiofemoral osteoarthritis. Age, 4, 13.

Sharma, L., Lou, C., Cahue, S., & Dunlop, D. D. (2000). The mechanism of the effect of obesity in knee osteoarthritis: the mediating role of malalignment. *Arthritis Rheum*, 43(3), 568-575. doi:10.1002/1529-0131(200003)43:3<568::AID-ANR13>3.0.CO;2-E

Shull, P. B., Lurie, K. L., Cutkosky, M. R., & Besier, T. F. (2011). Training multi-parameter gaits to reduce the knee adduction moment with data-driven models and haptic feedback. *J Biomech*, 44(8), 1605-1609. doi:10.1016/j.jbiomech.2011.03.016

Shull, P. B., Shultz, R., Silder, A., Dragoo, J. L., Besier, T. F., Cutkosky, M. R., & Delp, S. L. (2013). Toe-in gait reduces the first peak knee adduction moment in patients with medial compartment knee osteoarthritis. *J Biomech*, 46(1), 122-128.

Shull, P. B., Silder, A., Shultz, R., Dragoo, J. L., Besier, T. F., Delp, S. L., & Cutkosky, M. R. (2013). Six-Week Gait Retraining Program Reduces Knee Adduction Moment, Reduces Pain, and Improves Function for Individuals with Medial Compartment Knee Osteoarthritis. *J Orthop Res*, 31(7), 1020-1025. doi:10.1002/jor.22340

Sigrist, R., Rauter, G., Riener, R., & Wolf, P. (2013). Augmented visual, auditory, haptic, and multimodal feedback in motor learning: A review. *Psychon Bull Rev*, 20(1), 21-53. doi:10.3758/s13423-012-0333-8

Simic, M., Hinman, R. S., Wrigley, T. V., Bennell, K. L., & Hunt, M. A. (2011). Gait modification strategies for altering medial knee joint load: A systematic review. *Arthritis Care Res (Hoboken)*, 63(3), 405-426. doi:10.1002/acr.20380

Simic, M., Hunt, M. A., Bennell, K. L., Hinman, R. S., & Wrigley, T. V. (2012). Trunk lean gait modification and knee joint load in people with medial knee osteoarthritis: The effect of varying trunk lean angles. *Arthritis Care Res (Hoboken)*, 64(10), 1545-1553. doi:10.1002/acr.21724

Simon, D., Mascarenhas, R., Saltzman, B. M., Rollins, M., Bach, B. R., & MacDonald, P. (2015). The relationship between anterior cruciate ligament injury and osteoarthritis of the knee. *Adv Orthop*, 2015, 928301.

Snodgrass, S. J., Rivett, D. A., Robertson, V. J., & Stojanovski, E. (2010). Real-time feedback improves accuracy of manually applied forces during cervical spine mobilisation. *Manual therapy*, 15(1), 19-25.

Sülzenbrück, S., & Heuer, H. (2011). Type of visual feedback during practice influences the precision of the acquired internal model of a complex visuo-motor transformation. *Ergonomics*, 54(1), 34-46.

Tate, J. J., & Milner, C. E. (2010). Real-time kinematic, temporospatial, and kinetic biofeedback during gait retraining in patients: a systematic review. *Phys Ther*, 90(8), 1123-1134. doi:10.2522/ptj.20080281

Thomas, R. H., Resnick, D., Alazraki, N. P., Daniel, D., & Greenfield, R. (1975). Compartmental Evaluation of Osteoarthritis of the Knee: A Comparative Study of Available Diagnostic Modalities 1. *Radiology*, 116(3), 585-594.

van den Noort, J. C., Steenbrink, F., Roeles, S., & Harlaar, J. (2014). Real-time visual feedback for gait retraining: toward application in knee osteoarthritis. *Med Biol Eng Comput*, 53(3), 275-286.

Walter, J. P., D'Lima, D. D., Colwell, C. W., Jr., & Fregly, B. J. (2010). Decreased knee adduction moment does not guarantee decreased medial contact force during gait. *J Orthop Res*, 28(10), 1348-1354. doi:10.1002/jor.21142

Wheeler, J. W., Shull, P. B., & Besier, T. F. (2011). Real-time knee adduction moment feedback for gait retraining through visual and tactile displays. *J Biomech Eng*, 133(4), 041007. doi:10.1115/1.4003621

Wishart, L. R., Lee, T. D., Cunningham, S. J., & Murdoch, J. E. (2002). Age-related differences and the role of augmented visual feedback in learning a bimanual coordination pattern. *Acta Psychol*, 110(2), 247-263.

Zalecki, T., Gorecka-Mazur, A., Pietraszko, W., Surowka, A. D., Novak, P., Moskala, M., & Krygowska-Wajs, A. (2013). Visual feedback training using WII Fit improves balance in Parkinson's disease. *Folia Med Cracov*, 53(1), 65-78.

Zhang, W., Moskowitz, R. W., Nuki, G., Abramson, S., Altman, R. D., Arden, N.,... Tugwell, P. (2007). OARSI recommendations for the management of hip and knee osteoarthritis, part I: critical appraisal of existing treatment guidelines and systematic review of current research evidence. *Osteoarthr Cartil*, 15(9), 981-1000. doi:10.1016/j.joca.2007.06.014

Zhao, D., Banks, S. A., Mitchell, K. H., D'Lima, D. D., Colwell, C. W., & Fregly, B. J. (2007). Correlation between the knee adduction torque and medial contact force for a variety of gait patterns. *J Orthop Res*, 25(6), 789-797.

15

Effect of Hip Abduction Maximal Voluntary Isometric Contraction on Lumbar Motion and Power Output During the Back Squat

Christopher F. Kelly, Adam M. Gonzalez*, Robert W. Spitz, Katie M. Sell, Jamie J. Ghigiarelli

Department of Health Professions, Hofstra University, 110 Hofstra Dome, 220 Hofstra University, Hempstead, NY 11549, USA

Corresponding Author: Adam M. Gonzalez, E-mail: Adam.gonzalez@hofstra.edu

ARTICLE INFO	ABSTRACT
Conflicts of interest: None Funding: None	**Background:** Post-activation potentiation (PAP) is a neuromuscular phenomenon that has been shown to augment muscular force generating attributes as well as neural and sensory recruitment. While PAP has demonstrated to acutely enhance muscular performance during high-intensity activities, the effect of PAP on lumbopelvic kinematics under load remains unknown. **Objectives:** The purpose of this study was to examine the potential PAP effect of a hip abduction maximal voluntary isometric contraction (MVIC) on lumbar motion and power output during the barbell back squat. **Methods:** Nine resistance-trained men (22.9±2.3 y; 85.0±13.8 kg; 174.3±5.1 cm) performed a set of 5 repetitions of the barbell back squat using 80% one-repetition maximum with and without a hip abduction MVIC prior to performance. Experimental and control trials were randomized and counterbalanced among participants. MVIC was carried out via manual long-lever hip abduction. During the back squat exercise, lumbar motion analysis was performed using wireless motion-sensor technology, and power output was assessed via an accelerometer. **Results:** No significant differences were observed between trials for lumbar flexion range of motion (ROM) (p=0.32), lumbar flexion maximum deviation (p=0.32), lumbar lateral flexion ROM (p=0.81), lumbar lateral flexion maximum deviation (p=0.98), lumbar rotation maximum deviation (p=0.70), average peak power (p=0.98), or average mean power output (p=0.99) during the squat protocol. **Conclusions:** Implementation of a manual long-lever hip abduction MVIC prior to the back squat exercise did not significantly alter lumbar motion or augment power output in resistance trained males. **Key words:** Isometric Contraction, Lumbar Motion, Exercise, Accelerometry, Back Squat

INTRODUCTION

Post-activation potentiation (PAP) is a phenomenon by which muscular performance may be acutely heightened following a previous contraction executed at a relatively high intensity (Tillin and Bishop, 2009). The physiological basis for PAP is not completely understood; however, the mechanism behind this phenomenon is thought to result from increased recruitment of higher order motor units (Xenofondos et al., 2015). While various types of pre-exercise stimuli have been implemented to induce muscle potentiation, there does not appear to be an ideal protocol to consistently provide a potentiating effect (Wilson et al., 2013). Nevertheless, PAP techniques typically involve the use of maximal voluntary contractions. While PAP-based warm-up protocols have demonstrated to augment force exerted by a muscle, it has been hypothesized that the stimulus may also be beneficial for neuromuscular recruitment related to spinal stability and parallel performance (Kibler et al., 2006, McGill, 2001, McGill, 2007, Robbins, 2005, Stevens et al., 2007). A warm-up protocol for the maintenance of dynamic spinal stability under load may have important application for athletes performing resistance

exercise or high-intensity movements. When performing axial-loaded exercises such as the barbell back squat, athletes may experience external forces that exceed the load bearing capacity of an in vivo spinal system. Moreover, subtle departures (e.g. as little as 2 degrees of extension and/or flexion) from neutral alignment increase compressive loads and have been shown to negatively affect internal moment and ensuing performance (Dolan et al., 1995, Schoenfeld, 2010). Instability of this nature may reduce the capacity of the spinal system to disseminate force leading to suboptimal performance and an increased risk for injury (Schoenfeld, 2010, Panjabi, 2003, Panjabi, 1992, Wallden, 2009). A great deal of research has attempted to identify methods to elicit PAP through conditioning activities during warm-up routines (Tillin and Bishop, 2009, Wilson et al., 2013). Furthermore, practical methods with reduced need for specialized equipment are particularly appealing for athletes. A pre-exercise stimulus consisting of a sustained maximal voluntary isometric contraction (MVIC) has demonstrated viable application. MVIC has been shown to produce acute enhancement in variables such as rate of force development, sprint times, and jumping power (French et al., 2003). Furthermore, isometric contraction of lumbar and postural muscles may improve internal stabilization (Kisner et al., 2017). Acute and chronic exposure to isometric contractions may modulate muscle stiffness and augment muscular activity allowing the spine to maintain proximal stability while under load (Kibler et al., 2006, Burgess et al., 2007, Kubo et al., 2001, Lee and McGill, 2017). While MVIC appears to elicit improvements in muscle force-generating attributes, the effect of an MVIC on postural stability and lumbar motion has not been thoroughly investigated (McGill, 2001). Thus, the aim of this investigation was to examine the effect of a hip abduction MVIC on lumbar motion and power output during the back squat exercise. We hypothesized that performing the hip abduction MVIC prior to the barbell back squat would reduce excessive lumbar range of motion, via enhanced muscle stiffness about the lumbopelvic complex, with a potential to augment power output.

METHODS

Participants

Nine resistance-trained men (22.9±2.3; 85.0±13.8 kg; 174.3±5.1 cm) participated in this randomized, counterbalanced, crossover-design research study. Inclusion criteria included being recreationally active and having at least 1 year of resistance training experience. Further inclusion criteria required the participant to be familiar with the barbell back squat exercise. Participants had 5.4±2.2 years of resistance training experience and an average maximum back squat of 145.2±37.6 kg. All participants were free from injury and provided an informed consent prior to participation in this study. The research study was conducted according to the Declaration of Helsinki and approved by the Hofstra University Institutional Review Board prior to participant enrollment.

Maximal Strength Testing

Strength testing occurred at least 72 hours prior to experimental trials. Following a standardized warm-up protocol, participants performed a one-repetition maximum (1RM) strength test for the barbell back squat exercise. The 1RM test was performed using methods previously described (Hoffman, 2006). Participants performed two warm-up sets using a resistance of approximately 40-60% and 60-80% of his perceived maximum, respectively. The 1RM was then determined by applying a prediction formula based on the number of repetitions performed to fatigue using a fixed weight (Brzycki, 1993). All testing was completed under the supervision of a National Strength and Conditioning Association–certified strength and conditioning specialist (CSCS). A successful barbell back squat repetition required the participant to descend to a thigh parallel position defined by the trochanter head of the femur reaching the same horizontal plane as the superior border of the patella.

Experimental Trials

Participants reported to the laboratory for two trials. The experimental trial and control trial were counterbalanced between participants. Prior to each trial, participants were instructed to refrain from resistance training for a minimum of 48 hours and to abstain from the use of stimulants (e.g. caffeine) for a minimum of 4 hours prior to reporting to the HPL. Following the placement of wireless motion-sensors, participants completed a general and specific warm-up. The general warm-up consisted of 10 body weight squats, body weight walking lunges, dynamic walking hamstring stretches, and dynamic walking quadriceps stretches. For the specific warm-up, participants performed one set of 8 repetitions using 40% 1RM and one set of 4 repetitions using 60% 1RM separated by 2 minutes of rest. The participant then rested for 5 minutes. During the control trial, participants began the squat protocol immediately. During the experimental trial, participants performed a hip abduction MVIC prior to the squat protocol. The barbell back squat protocol consisted of a single set of 5 repetitions using 80% 1RM. Proper range of motion (i.e. thigh parallel position) was encouraged and monitored during the squat protocol. By reason of the relatively high-intensity load implemented, cadence of repetitions was not strictly controlled, however participants were instructed not to pause between repetitions.

Hip abduction MVIC

The hip abduction MVIC was carried out through unilateral manual resistance and quantified using a hand-held dynamometer (MicroFET 2, Hoggan Health Industries, Inc, West Jordan, UT). Participants were set up in a standardized, side lying position on a table, and a researcher facilitated a single set of long-lever isometric hip abduction by applying manual resistance following procedures set forth by Hislop et al. (2013) (Figure 1). The participants were instructed to maintain maximal exertion against the resistance for 5 seconds. Subsequently, the participant was immediately instructed to turn over and the same protocol began on the contralateral limb. Hip abduction MVIC peak and mean force were recorded. Participants began the squat protocol immediately following a 1 min rest period.

Movement Analysis

All participants wore a wireless motion-sensor technology that tracks and measures movement in real-time (ViPerform™, DorsaVi, USA). This system consists of two wireless motion-sensors that measure three-dimensional movement and a wireless recording device that captures the sensor data. Data were sent in real time to a computer via bluetooth and recorded for later analysis. One motion-sensor was placed across the posterior superior iliac spine and the second sensor was placed superiorly using a template to allow for consistent sensor placement. Sensors were adhered using disposable adhesive pads. This arrangement allows three-dimensional isolation of the lumbar spine and pelvic components (Figure 2). Prior to the squat exercise, a "baseline" was established with participants standing in their normal upright posture with feet at shoulder width apart. During the squat exercise, range of motion (ROM) and maximum deviation (i.e. maximum value from baseline) data were assessed.

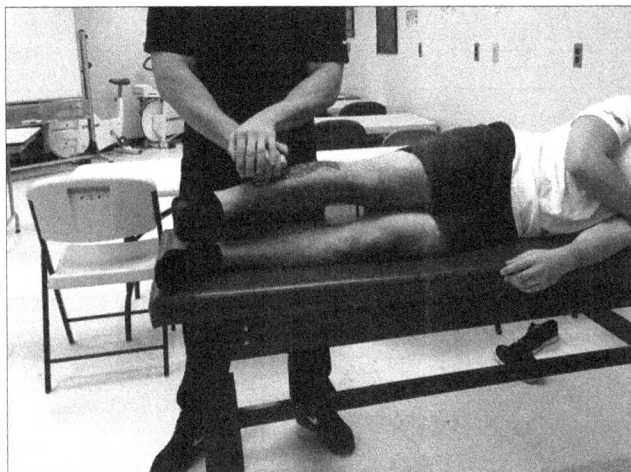

Figure 1. Hip abduction maximal voluntary isometric contraction (MVIC) protocol

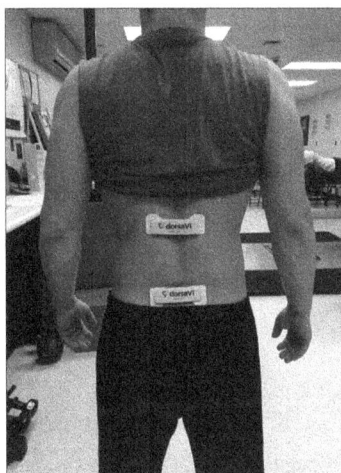

Figure 2. Motion sensor placement

ROM variables assessed the full range of motion throughout the movement (e.g. 10° flexion with 10° extension would yield a ROM of 20°). Data included lumbar flexion ROM and maximum deviation, lumbar lateral flexion ROM and maximum deviation, and lumbar rotation max deviation. The average was calculated for each set of 5 repetitions and used for subsequent analysis. The system software has displayed good inter-tester ($ICC_{2,1}$>0.86) and intra-tester reliability ($ICC_{2,1}$>0.89) for lumbar movements (Ronchi et al., 2008) and excellent concurrent validity with standard errors of measurement of 0.9° [95 % confidence interval (CI)=±1.8°] for the sagittal and 1.8° (95 % CI=±3.6°) coronal planes [46] relative to the "gold standard" Optotrak 3D-motion tracking system (NaturalPoint Inc. Corvallis, Oregon USA) (Charry et al., 2011).

Power Measures

Power output during the barbell bench press exercise was measured for each repetition with a Tendo™ Power Output Unit (Tendo Sports Machines, Trencin, Slovak Republic). The Tendo™ unit consists of a transducer attached to the end of the barbell, which measures linear displacement and time to calculate peak and average barbell velocity. Power was calculated from the barbell load entered into the micro-computer and barbell velocity detected by the unit. Prior to the investigation, intraclass correlation coefficient ($ICC_{3,1}$), standard error of the measurement ($SEM_{3,1}$), and minimal difference (MD) values for barbell velocity values measured by the Tendo™ unit during a single repetition ($ICC_{3,1}$=0.91, $SEM_{3,1}$=0.04 m·sec⁻¹, MD=0.09 m·sec⁻¹) were determined in 10 resistance-trained men (26.8±3.5 years; 92.6±6.5 kg; 180.5±6.6 cm) demonstrating that the Tendo™ unit has high test-retest reliability. Peak and mean power outputs were recorded for each repetition, and average peak and mean power was calculated for each set of 5 repetitions.

Statistical Analysis

Prior to statistical procedures, all data was assessed for normal distribution (Shapiro-Wilk), homogeneity of variance, and sphericity. Paired t-tests were utilized to determine the effect of the hip abduction MVIC on lumbar motion and power output during the back squat. Significance was accepted at an alpha level of $p \leq 0.05$, and all data are reported as mean ± standard deviation.

RESULTS

During the experimental trial, the participants right leg hip abduction MVIC produced a peak and mean force of 25.9±2.0 kg and 20.6±1.9 kg, respectively, while the participants left leg hip abduction MVIC produced a peak and mean force of 23.9±2.8 kg and 19.1±2.3 kg, respectively. No significant differences were noted between right and left leg hip abduction MVIC for peak (p=0.11) or mean force (p=0.15). Lumbar motion analysis and power output during the barbell back squat are depicted in Table 1. No differences were observed between trials in lumbar flexion ROM (p=0.32), lumbar flexion max deviation (p=0.32), lumbar lateral ROM (p=0.81), lumbar lateral max deviation (p=0.98), or lumbar rotation max deviation (p=0.70) during the squat protocol. Additionally, no differences were observed between trials in average peak power (p=0.98) or average mean power output (p=0.99) during the squat protocol.

DISCUSSION

The primary purpose of this study was to investigate the effect of hip abduction MVIC on subsequent lumbar motion and power output during the barbell back squat exercise. To the best of our knowledge, this appears to be the first study to evaluate lumbar motion following the implementation of a long-lever isometric hip abduction with application of manual resistance. Therefore, it was the primary intent of this investigation to implement a practical MVIC protocol and examine the effect through the lumbopelvic complex during the barbell back squat exercise. Our findings indicate that the application of a manual long-lever hip abduction MVIC prior to the back squat exercise did not result in significant alterations in lumbar motion or power output in resistance trained males. A properly functioning spinal system should

Table 1. Lumbar motion analysis and power output during the barbell back squat

	Experimental Trial	Control Trial	p-value
Lumbar flexion ROM (°)	24.7±5.9	21.7±6.4	0.32
Lumbar flexion maximum deviation (°)	21.8±5.2	19.0±6.3	0.32
Lumbar lateral flexion ROM (°)	6.3±1.9	6.0±2.9	0.81
Lumbar lateral flexion maximum deviation (°)	4.4±1.0	4.4±2.5	0.98
Lumbar rotation maximum deviation (°)	3.1±1.1	3.3±1.1	0.70
Average peak power (W)	978.0±341.5	981.1±322.9	0.98
Average mean power (W)	584.6±188.6	585.6±183.4	0.99

ROM=range of motion; W=watts

be capable of managing the instantaneous demand of dy-namic perturbation whilst optimizing muscle force-generating capacity with a relatively low prospect for injury. When an in vivo spinal system is under load and operating outside of neutral zone, instability may exacerbate compressive, shear, and tensile forces (Panjabi, 1992, Wallden, 2009, Adams and Dolan, 1995). Therefore, an effective warm-up strate-gy targeting neuromuscular efficiency prior to axial-loaded exercise may offer application for injury-mitigation, stabil-ity, and performance. A pre-exercise MVIC may modulate muscle stiffness and augment muscular activity allowing the spine to maintain proximal stability while under load (Kibler et al., 2006, Burgess et al., 2007, Kubo et al., 2001, Lee and McGill, 2017). For example, Lee and McGill (2017) recent-ly showed that isometric training exercises could induce immediate changes in core stiffness, which may transiently influence performance and injury resilience. Additionally, core and isometric hip strengthening may improve dynamic postural control (Jackson et al., 2017, Sadeghi et al., 2013). Previous investigations have administered various MVIC protocols prior to assessing an athletic endeavor, however lit-tle is known regarding the value of a simple isometric muscle action for the acute enhancement of spinal stability during dynamic resistance exercise (French et al., 2003, Güllich and Schmidtbleicher, 1996, Hamada et al., 2000, Hodgson et al., 2005). A maximum trunk flexion ROM of 60° has been re-ported during the back squat exercise (Norkin and White, 2016), with a significantly greater degree of hyperextension when subjects lifted at heavier loads (>60% 1RM) attributed to a compensatory action to stabilize the body from falling forward (Walsh et al., 2007). Lumbar deviations have been reported between 5.9-22.1° during the back squat in previ-ous investigations (Walsh et al., 2007, McKean et al., 2010). In the current study, the manual long-lever hip abduction MVIC applied in the current study did not exert significant changes in lumbar flexion, lateral flexion, or rotational ROM during the barbell back squat exercise.

Across the current body of research, the MVIC stimulus has been carried out under several different protocols, differ-ing in contraction type, duration, rest-interval, and specific movement patterns (French et al., 2003, Güllich and Schmidt-bleicher, 1996, Hamada et al., 2000, Hodgson et al., 2005). Findings appear to indicate a strong relationship between the PAP response, fatigue, and pre-load volume (French et al., 2003). In summary, the PAP effect appears to be diminished

if inadequate recovery time is provided between the MVIC stimulus and the subsequent power test. Whereas, when fa-tigue is correctly modulated, the MVIC protocol may confer athletic enhancement. Under conditions where contraction time and fatigue are balanced (i.e., MVIC ≤10-seconds) a heightened neural environment has been shown to augment skeletal muscle force-generating characteristics, along with sensory-related control of short-term muscle action (French et al., 2003, Trimble and Harp, 1998, Vandervoort et al., 1983, Lorenz, 2011). For example, Baudry and Duxhateau (2007) found a large increase in twitch-potentiation follow-ing a 6-second MVIC of the adductor pollicis along with a 9-24% increase in isometric rate of force development within 2 minutes of the intervention. Folland et al. (2008) also demonstrated an augmented twitch-potentiation at the quadriceps femoris following a 10-second MVIC; howev-er, performance measures were not enhanced following the intervention. Rate of force development has shown to either remain unchanged, or decrease, when assessed immediately following a potentiation stimulus (Güllich and Schmidtble-icher, 1996). Similarly, in the current study, the administra-tion of the hip abduction MVIC 1 min prior to performing the back squat exercise did not augment power output during the barbell back squat exercise.

While the results of the current study indicate that the implementation of a manual long-lever hip abduction MVIC prior to the back squat exercise does not significantly alter lumbar motion in resistance trained males, we recognize that our methods are accompanied with limitations and fur-ther research is warranted to determine effective strategies to manage spinal mechanics under load. The ability to draw conclusions from our small sample (n=9) of recreationally trained men using a single load (80% 1RM) may be limit-ed. Additionally, the abduction protocol implemented in the current study does not follow a similar kinematic and kinetic sequence compared to the back squat; therefore its ability to translate to the spinal system during the performance of the back squat remains in question. However, several investiga-tions have highlighted the influence of the dynamic stabi-lizers of the hip on lumbopelvic function, especially during closed-chain exercise (Kibler et al., 2006, Bobbert and Van Zandwijk, 1999, Nadler et al., 2002). While a side-lying iso-metric abduction has shown to activate muscles that facil-itate spinal stability, including the gluteus medius, gluteus minimus, and quadratus lumborum (Cynn et al., 2006), no single muscle has been recognized as most important for the lumbar spine stability (Cholewicki and Vanvliet Iv, 2002). Thus, other practical strategies employing different volume parameters, contractions, and rest times should be investigated. Currently, a 7-12 minute recovery interval has been suggested to optimally enhance the potentiation response to exercise (Wilson et al., 2013, Gouvêa et al., 2013). In the current study, a 1-minute rest was allotted between the pre-conditioning contraction and the performance measure. It is plausible that a greater rest period may be warranted to accommodate the fatigue theory associated with the potentiating mechanisms. Additionally, it has been suggested that the potentiation effect is more sensitive in experienced individuals (Wilson et al., 2013, Gouvêa et al., 2013), therefore MVIC protocols may be more applicable in elite, competitive strength/power athletes (e.g. powerlifters). Further research should also investigate twitch-potentiation and muscle activation, along with spinal mechanics following such MVIC protocols.

CONCLUSION

In conclusion, the application of a manual long-lever hip abduction MVIC prior to the back squat exercise did not significantly alter lumbar motion or augment power output in resistance trained males. Following a maximal exertion hip abduction MVIC against manual resistance for 5 seconds, no significant differences were observed in lumbar flexion ROM and maximum deviation, lumbar lateral flexion ROM and maximum deviation, or lumbar rotation max deviation during a squat protocol consisting of a single set of 5 repetitions using 80% 1RM. Additionally, no significant differences were noted for peak or mean power during the squat protocol. Future research is encouraged to determine practical MVIC protocols to not only improve performance outcomes, but also lumbar kinematics.

REFERENCES

Tillin, N. A. and Bishop, D. (2009). Factors modulating post-activation potentiation and its effect on performance of subsequent explosive activities. *Sports Medicine*, 39(2), 147-166.

Xenofondos, A., Patikas, D., Koceja, D. M., et al. (2015). Post-activation potentiation: The neural effects of post-activation depression. *Muscle & Nerve*, 52(2), 252-259.

Wilson, J. M., Duncan, N. M., Marin, P. J., et al. (2013). Meta-analysis of postactivation potentiation and power: effects of conditioning activity, volume, gender, rest periods, and training status. *The Journal of Strength & Conditioning Research*, 27(3), 854-859.

Kibler, W. B., Press, J. and Sciascia, A. (2006). The role of core stability in athletic function. *Sports Medicine*, 36(3), 189-198.

McGill, S. M. (2001). Low back stability: from formal description to issues for performance and rehabilitation. *Exercise and Sport Sciences Reviews*, 29(1), 26-31.

McGill, S. M. (2007). Lumbar spine stability: mechanism of injury and restabilization. Philadelphia: Lippincott, Williams & Wilkins, 2007.

Robbins, D. W. (2005). Postactivation potentiation and its practical applicability: a brief review. *Journal of Strength and Conditioning Research*, 19(2), 453.

Stevens, V. K., Coorevits, P. L., Bouche, K. G., et al. (2007). The influence of specific training on trunk muscle recruitment patterns in healthy subjects during stabilization exercises. *Manual Therapy*, 12(3), 271-279.

Dolan, P., Adams, M., Aspden, R., et al. (1995). Forces acting on the lumbar spine. Lumbar spine disorders: current concepts. Singapore: World Scientific Publishing Co, 15-25.

Schoenfeld, B. J. (2010). Squatting kinematics and kinetics and their application to exercise performance. *The Journal of Strength & Conditioning Research*, 24(12), 3497-3506.

Panjabi, M. M. (2003). Clinical spinal instability and low back pain. *Journal of Electromyography and Kinesiology*, 13(4), 371-379.

Panjabi, M. M. (1992). The stabilizing system of the spine. Part I. Function, dysfunction, adaptation, and enhancement. *Clinical Spine Surgery*, 5(4), 383-389.

Wallden, M. (2009). The neutral spine principle. *Journal of Bodywork and Movement Therapies*, 13(4), 350-361.

French, D. N., Kraemer, W. J. and Cooke, C. B. (2003). Changes in dynamic exercise performance following a sequence of preconditioning isometric muscle actions. *The Journal of Strength & Conditioning Research*, 17(4), 678-685.

Kisner, C., Colby, L. A. and Borstad, J. (2017). Therapeutic exercise: foundations and techniques (6th ed.). Philladelphia, PA: F.A. Davis Company.

Burgess, K. E., Connick, M. J., Graham-Smith, P., et al. (2007). Plyometric vs. isometric training influences on tendon properties and muscle output. *The Journal of Strength and Conditioning Research*, 21(3), 986.

Kubo, K., Kanehisa, H. and Fukunaga, T. (2001). Effects of different duration isometric contractions on tendon elasticity in human quadriceps muscles. *The Journal of Physiology*, 536(2), 649-655.

Lee, B. and McGill, S. (2017). The effect of short-term isometric training on core/torso stiffness. *Journal of Sports Sciences*, 35(17), 1724-1733.

Hoffman, J. (2006). Norms for fitness, performance, and health. Champaign, IL: Human Kinetics.

Brzycki, M. (1993). Strength testing—predicting a one-rep max from reps-to-fatigue. *Journal of Physical Education, Recreation & Dance*, 64(1), 88-90.

Hislop, H., Avers, D. and Brown, M. (2013). Daniels and Worthingham's muscle testing: Techniques of manual examination and performance testing (9th ed.). Amsterdam, NL: Elsevier Health Sciences.

Ronchi, A. J., Lech, M., Taylor, N., et al. (2008). A reliability study of the new Back Strain Monitor based on clinical trials. Engineering in Medicine and Biology Society, 2008. 30th Annual International Conference, 693-696.

Charry, E., Umer, M. and Taylor, S. (2011). Design and validation of an ambulatory inertial system for 3-D measurements of low back movements. Sensor Networks and Information Processing (ISSNIP), Seventh International Conference, 58-63.

Adams, M. and Dolan, P. (1995). Recent advances in lumbar spinal mechanics and their clinical significance. *Clinical Biomechanics*, 10(1), 3-19.

Jackson, K.M., Beach T.A. and Andrews D.M. (2017). The effect of an isometric hip muscle strength training protocol on valgus angle during a drop vertical jump in competitive female volleyball players. *International Journal of Kinesiology & Sports Science*, 5(4), 1-9.

Sadeghi, H., Shariat, A., Asadmanesh, E. and Mosavat, M. (2013). The effects of core stability exercise on the dynamic balance of volleyball players. *International Journal of Applied Exercise Physiology*, 2(2), 1-10.

Güllich, A. and Schmidtbleicher, D. (1996). MVC-induced short-term potentiation of explosive force. *New Studies in Athletics*, 11(67-84.

Hamada, T., Sale, D. G., MacDougall, J. D., et al. (2000). Postactivation potentiation, fiber type, and twitch contraction time in human knee extensor muscles. *Journal of Applied Physiology*, 88(6), 2131-2137.

Hodgson, M., Docherty, D. and Robbins, D. (2005). Post-activation potentiation. *Sports Medicine*, 35(7), 585-595.

Norkin, C. C. and White, D. J. (2016). Measurement of joint motion: a guide to goniometry. Fa Davis.

Walsh, J. C., Quinlan, J. F., Stapleton, R., et al. (2007). Three-dimensional motion analysis of the lumbar spine during "free squat" weight lift training. *The American Journal of Sports Medicine*, 35(6), 927-932.

McKean, M. R., Dunn, P. K. and Burkett, B. J. (2010). The lumbar and sacrum movement pattern during the back squat exercise. *The Journal of Strength & Conditioning Research*, 24(10), 2731-2741.

Trimble, M. H. and Harp, S. S. (1998). Postexercise potentiation of the H-reflex in humans. *Medicine and Science in Sports and Exercise*, 30(6), 933-941.

Vandervoort, A., Quinlan, J. and McComas, A. (1983). Twitch potentiation after voluntary contraction. *Experimental Neurology*, 81(1), 141-152.

Lorenz, D. (2011). Postactivation potentiation: An introduction. *International Journal of Sports Physical Therapy*, 6(3), 234.

Baudry, S. and Duchateau, J. (2007). Postactivation potentiation in a human muscle: effect on the rate of torque development of tetanic and voluntary isometric contractions. *Journal of Applied Physiology*, 102(4), 1394-1401.

Folland, J. P., Wakamatsu, T. and Fimland, M. S. (2008). The influence of maximal isometric activity on twitch and H-reflex potentiation, and quadriceps femoris performance. *European Journal of Applied Physiology*, 104(4), 739.

Bobbert, M. F. and Van Zandwijk, J. P. (1999). Dynamics of force and muscle stimulation in human vertical jumping. *Medicine and Science in Sports and Exercise*, 99, 303-310.

Nadler, S. F., Malanga, G. A., Bartoli, L. A., et al. (2002). Hip muscle imbalance and low back pain in athletes: influence of core strengthening. *Medicine & Science in Sports & Exercise*, 34(1), 9-16.

Cynn, H.-S., Oh, J.-S., Kwon, O.-Y., et al. (2006). Effects of lumbar stabilization using a pressure biofeedback unit on muscle activity and lateral pelvic tilt during hip abduction in sidelying. *Archives of Physical Medicine and Rehabilitation*, 87(11), 1454-1458.

Cholewicki, J. and Vanvliet Iv, J. J. (2002). Relative contribution of trunk muscles to the stability of the lumbar spine during isometric exertions. *Clinical Biomechanics*, 17(2), 99-105.

Gouvêa, A. L., Fernandes, I. A., César, E. P., et al. (2013). The effects of rest intervals on jumping performance: A meta-analysis on post-activation potentiation studies. *Journal of Sports Sciences*, 31(5), 459-467.

16

Effects of a Physical Exercise Program on the Level of Physical Activity and Energy Expenditure of Obese Workers in Kinshasa in the Democratic Republic of Congo

Godefroid K. Mabele[1]*, Constant N. Ekisawa[1], Christophe DELECLUSE[2], Teddy B.Linkoko[1], Nicaise K. Ngasa[1], Francois L. Bompeka[3]

[1] Department of Physical Medicine and Rehabilitation, University of Kinshasa Faculty of Medicine, Democratic Republic of Congo (DRC) Kinesiology service,

[2] Faculty of movement and Rehabilitation sciences Departement of movement science K.U. Leuven, Belgique,

[3] Department of Internal Medicine, University of Kinshasa Faculty of Medicine, Democratic Republic of Congo (DRC) Nephrology service

Corresponding Author: Godefroid K. Mabele, E-mail : kuswayi.mabele@unikin.ac.cd

ARTICLE INFO

Conflicts of interest: None
Funding: None

ABSTRACT

Background: Obesity has become a public health problem in the world today, especially in the workplace, where workers are subjected to long-term work in a sitting position and in front of computers. The absence of a program of structured physical exercises in our context on obesity in a professional environment in Kinshasa motivated us to carry out this study. **Objective:** To investigate the effect of a structured exercise program on the level of physical activity and energy expenditure of obese workers. **Methods:** In a 6-month follow-up study, 157 obese patients with a mean age of 47 ± 9.54 years were enrolled in a 3-day, one-hour structured exercise program. Day of moderate to high intensity and walking combined with a nutritional education (low calorie, high fiber and vitamins) at the Multimodal Freight Management Office of Kinshasa between January and June 2014. We used the paired Student's T test to compare continuous variables before and after the programs. **Results:** A significant increase was obtained in six months of the structured exercise program combined with nutrition education for most of the studied parameters: number of steps on the working day ($p < 0.0001$); number of steps on the weekend ($p < 0.0001$); energy expenditure on the working day ($p < 0.0001$); energy expenditure on the weekend day ($p < 0.0001$). In contrast, weight, Body Mass Index, Waist circumference and Hip Abdomen Ratio significantly decrease d respectively: weight ($p < 0.0001$); Body Mass Index ($p < 0.0001$); waist circumference ($p < 0.0001$); Hip Abdomen Ratio ($p < 0.0001$).**Conclusion:** Structured exercise combined with nutrition education significantly increases the level of physical activity, energy expenditure and decreases weight, Body Mass Index, waist circumference and morbidity and mortality risk of obese workers.

Key words: Energy Expenditure, Structured Exercises, Obese

INTRODUCTION

Obesity is a dominant current issue. It is considered a major public health problem. Its management is a primary objective, given the growth of this disease and the consequences it has on health, justifying the improvement of therapeutic strategies including the methods of exercise (Karmisholt et al., 2005; Brooke et al.,2014).The level of physical activity of people in developed countries has steadily declined in recent decades to the point that physical inactivity has become a health risk factor along with smoking, and is one of the most important public health concerns (Kesaniemi et al., 2001; Vuori, 2001).It is now recognized that most of the chronic diseases that afflict our society are fundamentally linked to lifestyle (Chakravarthy et al., 2002) and whose

sedentary lifestyle is one of the primary risk factors. The decrease in level of physical activity is therefore responsible for a biological imbalance directed by the hypothalamus, which would lead the person to a situation at risk of obesity (Rowland 1998).For the workers, it is rather the psychosocial and environmental aspects, such as the high grade and function, the level of training, and the accessibility of activities, which determine the decline in the level of physical activity (Dishman et al., 1985). In any case, a more restricted life, partitioned into offices, workshops, industries and mines, promotes lifestyles that are detrimental to health. Every living being subject to the laws of thermodynamics, it responds to the principle of conservation of energy. The body can be considered as a black box and any variation in mass can be explained by the difference between the outputs (total energy expenditure) and the inputs (energy ingested). It is the concept of energy balance according to which any gain in mass can result only from an increase of the caloric contributions and/or a reduction of the total energy expenditure (Bouchard et al., 2005; Serrano et al., 2016). On the other hand, all epidemiological, prospective and longitudinal studies have shown the key role of physical activity in preventing weight gain (Schmitz et al., 2000; Welk et al. 2011). Studies show that active subjects are less likely to gain weight over time than sedentary subjects are. Energy expenditure related to physical exercise can indeed be broken down into structured and spontaneous exercise (Morio et al., 1998).The interrelationships between these components of physical activity are complex and it has been shown that any intervention to improve exercise capacity through participation in a training program results in a parallel reduction of spontaneous exercise. The total energy spent on physical activity is very little changed by the intervention (Schrauwen et al., 1998; David et al., 2016). The importance of spontaneous exercise in weight control has recently been highlighted through the development of complex accelerometers and pedometers able to quantify it. Inter-individual variability in weight gain in response to over nutrition is shown to be related to the modulation of spontaneous exercise (Do Lee et al., 1999). In 2000, the number of deaths related to unhealthy diet and inactivity were increased by 25% compared to the 1990 estimates (Mokdad et al., 2004). The data on inactivity is impressive. From 1950 to 2000, the time spent by day in front of the television almost doubled to reach about 8 hours a day at the beginning of the century. In recent years, there has been a march towards walking, which appears to be an activity with many health benefits in the world (Brownson et al., 2005).However, to our knowledge, no research has verified the effects of a structured exercise program combined with nutrition education on the level of physical activity and energy expenditure specifically designed for obese workers. It is to fill a gap that the present work was undertaken to evaluate the effects of a structured exercise program on the level of physical activity and energy expenditure of obese workers in a city Kinshasa province in the Democratic Republic of Congo.

METHODS

Design of Study and Publication

This is an experimental longitudinal study of 157 randomly selected obese workers from the staff list, including 76 men (48.4%) and 81 women (51.6%), of average age 47 ± 9.54 years old, with a body mass index (BMI) greater than or equal to 30 Kg/m2, submitted during 6 months of combined physical exercise, between January and June 2014, held in a company in the provincial city Kinshasa in the Democratic Republic of Congo, known as the Office of Multimodal Freight Management, specializes in the multimodal transport sector, through appropriate regulatory mechanisms or specific actions, with a constant focus on research efficiency and profitability of any freight operation, from the producer to the consumer. His choice was justified in particular by the rela-

tively better purchasing power of the workers who is characterized by the means of motorized travel and a social life without much trouble. As for the working conditions, they are too intense because most of his workers spend more than 7 hours of time sitting in front of the computer, on workdays and in front of Television, on weekends. All participants had given their informed written consent according to the Helsinki Declarations. They were all obese, aged 25 and over, and had been working regularly in one of the company's management for at least a year. The primary outcome measure being weight loss, all of these obese workers were assessed before (T0) and after 6 months of exercise programs (T6).

Exercise Protocol

We used a structured exercise protocol, combined with spontaneous, high-volume, moderate-to-high-intensity physical exercise at 3 sessions per week of one hour per day. This same program has also been associated with nutrition education. In this study, structured physical exercise includes voluntary physical exercise and supervised by professionals while spontaneous exercise includes all the actions of daily life. The prescribed physical exercises consisted of exercises in aerobic endurance including: jogging, rhythmic gymnastics, basketball, volley ball, swimming, walk of 10.000 not at the rate of three working days and two days of weekend recorded using a pedometer and muscle building exercises: thigh- abdominals-buttocks. These were combined with the spontaneous physical exercises below: walk, climb and go down the stairs instead of taking the elevator, go to the toilet on the upper floor than in his own hall, stretching.). This same program has also been associated with a nutritional education (low calorie, high in fiber and vitamins).

Outcome Measure

The following anthropometric parameters: height in centimeter was measured using the Seca brand portable toe, while waist circumference and hip circumference in a metric rate, the risk morbid-mortal by ratio Abdo-hip, the weight in kilograms by the Omron inpedancemetre BF -511. Overall obesity among workers was defined by BMI ≥ 30 kg/m² calculated by mass (expressed in kilograms) divided by squared person size (in meters) and obesity android or abdominal by the International Diabetes Federation (IDF) criterion measured by waist circumference taken midway between the last rib and the iliac crest defined by the WHO action level 1 thresholds: waist circumference ≥ to 94 cm in men and waist circumference at ≥ 80 cm in women (Alexander et al., 2003; Dekker et al., 2005). The circumferential circumference ≥ 0, 90 cm for men and ≥ 0.85 cm for women (Expert Panel on Detection, 2001, Adams et al., 2009).

The level of physical activity is determined by the number of steps per day and weekend, corresponding to an energy expenditure in the case of an impulse measured by the following values: physical inactivity: less than equal to 4999 steps (less than 300 Kilocalorie) per day, Slightly Active: between 5000 and 7499 steps (300 Kilocalories) per day, Some Active: between 7500 and 9990 steps (300 Kilocal-

Table 1. Number of steps and energy expenditure before the exercise programs structured according to socio-professional status

	Command frameworks (N=75)	Collaborative frameworks (N=52)	Agents execution (N=30)	Total (N=157)
Age (year)	49±10,61	47±9,89	45±6,72	47±9,54
Number of steps per day open	1678±1458	2764±1815	3604±1836	2682±1703,0
Number of steps per day of week-end	1456±1934,6	1603±1050,5	2365±1984,1	1808±1956,4
From the next day (Kcal)	123±40,85	172±68,87	191±89,3	162±66,34
From the days week-end (Kcal)	186±99	234±96,85	288±99,76	236±98,54
Weight (Kg)	95±17,5	92±14	84±7,98	90,4±13,16
Size (cm)	170±7,86	171±8,02	168±7,97	170±7,95
Body mass index (Kg/m^2)	33,9±5,67	31,7±4,52	30±3,55	32±4,58
Waist circumference (cm)	106±84,21	104±82,40	99±80,77	103±82,46
Hip circumference (cm)	112±8,06	114±11,98	113±10,2	113±10,08
Hip abdomen ratio	0,94±6,5	0,91±5,87	0,87±5,03	0,90±5,80

Table 2. Number of steps and energy expenditure after exercise programs structured according to socio-professional status

	Command frameworks (N=75)	collaborative frameworks (N=52)	Agents execution (N=30)	Total (N=157)
Age (year)	49±10,61	47±9,89	45±6,72	47±9,54
Number of steps per day open	11264±2192,8	11350±2591	11424±2546,7	11346±2443,5
Number of steps per day of week-end	11229±2031,7	11991±2731	12138±2876,2	11789±2546,3
From the next day (Kcals)	1748±380,8	1736±399,4	1954±491,2	1812±423,8
From the days week-end (Kcals)	1786±1893,6	1879±2031,2	1982±2176	1881±2033,6
Weight (Kg)	85±8,87	75±8,09	59,5±7,97	70,5±8,31
Size (cm)	170±7,86	171±8,02	168±7,97	170±7,95
Body mass index (Kg/m^2)	30,7±2,79	26,5±2,03	21,6±2,02	26,2±2,28
Waist circumference (cm)	89±5,68	85±5,03	72±4,05	82±4,92
Hip circumference (cm)	109±8,67	110±10,05	111±11,1	110±10,09
Hip Abdomen Ratio	0,82±9,05	0,77±6,99	0,65±4,87	0,74±6,97

ories) per day, Active:> 10000 (greater than or equal to 300 Kilocalories) and Highly Active:> 12000 steps (greater than or equal to 300 Kilocalories) per day (Tudor-Locke et al., 2008a; Tudor-Locke et al., 2000b).

Statistical Analysis

After the quality check for missing or aberrant data, the collected data was captured on a PC, with the EPI INFO software and analyzed using the SPSS 21.0 software. Quantitative variables were expressed as means ± standard deviation. The comparison of the averages of the continuous variables (T0 versus T6) was performed by the paired Student t-test. A value of $p \leq 0.05$ was considered a threshold of statistical significant.

RESULTS

Table 1 Prior to the structured exercise program, the subject parameters were: number of steps per working day 2682 ± 1703.0, number of steps per weekend day 1808 ± 1956.4, energy expenditure on working days 162 ± 66, 34 Kcals, energy expenditure on weekend days 236 ± 98.54 Kcals, weight 90.4 ± 13 kg, Body Mass Index 32 ± 4.58 Kg/m^2, Waist circumference 103 ± 82.46 cm, Hip circumference 113 ± 10.08cm, hip abdomen ratio 0.90 ± 5.80 cm.

After a follow-up of six months of management combined with a nutritional education, the corresponding levels of physical activity and energy activity are as follows in Table 2: number of steps per working day 11346 ± 2443.5, number of steps per day of week -end 11789 ± 2546.3, en-

Table 3. Comparison of step, energy and anthropometric expenditure parameters before and after the structured exercise program combined with nutrition education

	Before (n=157)	After (n=157)	p-value
Number of steps per day open	2682±703,0	11346±2443,5	< 0,0001
Number of steps per day of week-end	1808±1956,4	11789±2546,3	< 0,0001
From the next day (Kcal)	162±66,34	1812±423,8	< 0,0001
From the days week-end (Kcal)	236±98,54	1881±2033,6	< 0,0001
Weight (Kg)	90,4±13,16	70,5±8,31	< 0,0001
Body mass index (Kg/m^2)	32±4,58	26,2±2,28	< 0,0001
Waist circumference (cm)	90,4±13,16	70,5±8,31	< 0,0001
Hip circumference (cm)	103±82,46	82±4,92	< 0,0001
Hip abdomen ratio	0,90±5,80	0,74±6,97	< 0,0001

ergy expenditure on working days 1812 ± 423.8 Kcal, energy expenditure on week-end days 1881 ± 2033.6 Kcal, weight 74.5 ± 8.31 Kg, Body Mass Index 26.2 ± 2.28 Kg/m^2, Waist circumference 82 ± 4.92 cm, Hip circumference 110 ± 10.09 cm, Hip Abdomen Ratio 0.74 ± 6.97 cm.

This Table 3 has shown that a significant increase in the level of physical activity and energy expenditure was observed on weekdays and weekends. The anthropometric parameters were significantly reduced in six months of structured exercises combined with a nutritional education.

DISCUSSION

The present study has shown the effects in six months of a structured exercise program combined with nutrition education on the level of physical activity, energy expenditure and anthropometric parameters of a cohort of 157 obese workers, including 81 women. (51.6%) and 76 men (48.4%).In six months of structured exercises combined with nutritional education, a significant increase was obtained for most of the parameters studied: number of steps on the working day (+8664); number of steps on the day weekend (+ 9981pas); energy expenditure on the working day (+ 1650Kcals); energy expenditure on the weekend (+1645Kcals). On the other hand, weight, Body Mass Index, Waist circumference and Hip Abdomen Ratio significantly decreased respectively: weight (- 19.9 Kg); Body Mass Index (- 5.8 Kg/m^2); waist circumference (- 20.1 cm); Hip Abdomen Ratio (- 0.16 cm). High socioeconomic status, advancement in age, and sedentary lifestyle expose obese employees to cardiovascular and metabolic complications such as high blood pressure, diabetes, stroke, and kidney disease. In this regard, studies have indicated that the increase in the level of physical activity and the decrease in sedentary lifestyles have positive effects on obesity (Ortega et al., 2005).In the presence of obesity, it is recommended to increase the volume of physical activity needed more than the recommended volume for normal weight workers. The practice of walking a good 180 minutes a week would have a positive and protective effect on weight gain and its metabolic consequences (Ortega et al., 2005). In addition, the use of structured exercises combined with nutrition education, increases the level of physical activity and decreases the level of inactivity alone, makes it difficult to reach a negative energy balance that would favor the de-

crease of anthropometric parameters. (Tjonna et al., 2008). Other guidelines are focused more specifically on the maintenance of morphology, in particular that of Tudor-Locke, which recommends that obese persons perform between 7,000 to 10,000 steps per day, 8,000 of which are performed during moderate intensity activity or high (Kim et al. 2009; katzmarzy et al. 2009).Researchers recommend that, in order to manage obesity, encourage activities of a continuous or intermittent aerobic nature and of medium to high intensity (Jago et al., 2006). Adams has suggested that regular physical activity allows for the long-term maintenance and weight loss of an obese person. The promotion of daily physical activity is also encouraged through games, sports, the use of active travel (walking, cycling), active recreation and family exercise (Tudor-Locke.et al., 2008a). Indeed, the new guidelines recommend the practice of a minimum of 60 minutes of moderate to high physical activity per day in addition to physical activities related to daily living In addition, it is recommended to engage in a variety of intensity activities daily, including a minimum of 3 high intensity aerobic sessions and maximize duration to achieve a high volume of weekly physical activity. Activities should include high intensity activities at least 3 days a week and muscle building activities at least 3 days a week (Kino-Québec., 2011; Adams et al., 2009).In obese patients, the use of vigorous physical activity rather than caloric restriction in order to reduce anthropometric parameters seems to be recommended by the literature (Eisenmann et al., 2005; Eliakim et al., 2000).However, in other studies, the decrease in anthropometric parameters was unsuccessful following a treatment that targeted physical activity. These data suggested that physical activity alone is not the best way to reduce the anthropometric parameters of the obese, despite its benefits for different risk factors (Stallmann-Jorgensen et al., 2007) At the global level, WHO has recommended the promotion of health programs through the practice of physical activity in a variety of settings (Gutin et al., 2002). In this sense, it is emphasized that in the area of prevention, businesses represent environments conducive to physical activity initiatives and support for a physically active lifestyle. Several researchers have shown that the combined practice of regular physical activity significantly reduces abdominal obesity and morbidity-mortality risks (Tjonna et al., 2009; brooke et al.,2014). At present, there was little scientific evidence for an appreciable effect of physical exercise on body weight reduction. The challenge was therefore to combine a nutritional education and a structured physical activity supervised by professionals (Atlantis et al., 2006). The major limitation of our study is simple random sampling as the socio-professional status effect where the cadres constituted the majority of subjects studied compared to the executing agents. A major strength of this study lies in the fact that it represents the first longitudinal interventional study in the workplace in Kinshasa where it has implemented a combined physical activity program and sought on the one hand, the effect non-pharmacological measures on the level of physical activity and, on the other hand, on energy expenditure among obese employees. Future research is encouraged to investigate the effect of this structured and spontaneous exercise program on body composition, muscle strength, cardiac fitness, and cardiovascular risk factors related to the metabolic syndrome in obese workers from Kinshasa.

CONCLUSION

The structured exercise program combined with a nutrition education (low calorie, high in fiber and vitamins) and associated with active lifestyle exercises every two hours; significantly increases the level of physical activity, energy expenditure and improves weight, waist circumference, morbi-mortal risks related to the sedentariness of obese Kinshasa workers. It can be considered as an effective non-pharmacological strategy for treating the risk generated by obesity.

REFERENCES

Adams, J. B., Edwards, D., Serviette, D., Bedient, A. M., Huntsman, E., Jacobs, K. A., & Signorile, J. F. (2009). Optimal frequency, displacement, duration, and recovery patterns to maximize power output following acute whole-body vibration. *The Journal of Strength & Conditioning Research,* 23(1), 237-245. doi: 10.1519/JSC.0b013e3181876830.

Atlantis E, Barnes EH and Singh MAF. (2006). Efficacy of exercise for treating overweight in children and adolescents: a systematic review. *International Journal of Obesity,* 30(7), 1027-1040.

Bouchard, C. (2005). Aerobic fitness, body mass index, and CVD risk factors among adolescents: the Quebec family study. *International Journal of Obesity*, 29(9), 1077-1083.

Brooke E. Starkoff, Inhuman U. Eneli, Andrea E. Bonny, Robert P. Hoffman Steven T. Devor. (2014). Estimated Aerobic Capacity Changes in Adolescents with Obesity Following High Intensity Interval Exercise. *International Journal of Kinesiology & Sports Science,* 2(3), 1-8.

Brownson R. C., Boehmer T. K. & Luke D.A. (2005). Declining rates of physical activity in the United States: what are the contributors? *Annual Revue Public Health,* 26, 421-443.

Chakravarthy MV, Joyner MJ, and Booth FW (2002).An obligation for primary care physicians to prescribe physical activity to sedentary patients to reduce the risk of chronic health conditions. *Mayo Clinic Processes*, 77, 165-173.

David C. Archer, Lee E. Brown, Jared W. Coburn, Andrew J. Galpin, Phillip C. Drouet, Whitney D. Leyva, Cameron N. Munger, Megan A. Wong. (2016). Effects of Short-Term Jump Squat Training With and Without Chains on Strength and Power in Recreational Lifters. *International Journal of Kinesiology & Sports Science*, 4(4), 24-31.

Dekker, J.M. (2005). Metabolic syndrome and 10-year cardiovascular disease risk in the Hoorn Study. *Circulation*, 112, 666-673.

Dishman RK, Sallis JF, and Orenstein DR. (1985).The determinants of physical activity and exercise. *Public Health Republic,* 100, 158-171.

Do Lee, C., Blair, S. N., & Jackson, A. S. (1999). Cardio respiratory fitness, body composition, and all-cause and cardiovascular disease mortality in men. The American journal of clinical nutrition, 69(3), 373-380.

Dwyer, T., Magnussen, C. G., Schmidt, M. D., Ukoumunne, O. C., Ponsonby, A.-L., Raitakari, O. T., Cleland, V. J. (2009). Decline in physical fitness from childhood to adulthood associated with increased obesity and insulin resistance in adults. *Diabetes Care*, 32(4), 683-687.

Eisenmann, J. C., Katzmarzyk, P., Perusse, L., Tremblay, A., Despres, J., & Bouchard, C. (2005). Aerobic fitness, body mass index, and CVD risk factors among adolescents: the Quebec family study. *International Journal of Obesity*, 29(9), 1077-1083.

Eliakim A, Makowski GS, Brasel JA and Cooper DM. (2000). Adiposity, lipid levels, and brief endurance training in non-obese adolescent males. *International Journal of Sports Medicine,* 21(6), 332-337.

Expert Panel on Detection E. (2001).Treatment of High Blood Cholesterol in A. Executive Summary of The Third Report of The National Cholesterol Education Program (NCEP) Expert Panel on Detection, Evaluation, And Treatment of High Blood Cholesterol In Adults (Adult Treatment Panel III). *JAMA: The Journal of the American Medical Association*, 285(23), 2486-97.

Gutin, B., Barbeau, P., Owens, S., Lemmon, C. R., Bauman, M., Allison, J., Litaker, M. S. (2002). Effects of exercise intensity on cardiovascular fitness, total body composition, and visceral adiposity of obese adolescents. *The American journal of clinical nutrition*, 75(5), 818-826.

Jago R, Watson K, Baranowski T, Zakeri I, Yoo S, Baranowski J and Conry K. (2006). Pedometer reliability, validity and daily activity targets among 10- to 15-year-old boys. *Journal of Sports Sciences,* 24(5), 241-251.

Karmisholt K, Gyntelberg F, and Gotzche PC. (2005). Physical activity for primary prevention of disease. *Systematic reviews of randomized clinical trials,* 52, 86-89.

Katzmarzyk, P. T., Church, T. S., Janssen, I., Ross, R., & Blair, S. N. (2005). Metabolic Syndrome, Obesity, and Mortality Impact of cardiorespiratory fitness. *Diabetes Care,* 28(2), 391-397.

Kesaniemi YA, Danforth E, Jensen MD, Kopelman PG, Lefebvre P, and Reeder BA. (2001). Dose-response issues concerning physical activity and health: an evidence-based symposium. *Medicine Science Sports Exercise,*4(4), S351-S358.

Kim Y and Lee S. (2009). Physical activity and abdominal obesity in youth. Applied Physiology, Nutrition, And Metabolism, Physiologie Appliquée, *Nutrition et Métabolisme*, 34, 571-581.

Kino-Québec Csd. (2011). L'activité physique, le sport et les jeunes – Savoir et agir. Québec: Secrétariat au loisir et au sport, ministère de l'Éducation, du Loisir et du Sport. Gouvernement du Québec.

Mokdad A. H., Marks J. S., Stroup D. F., Gerberding J. L. (2004). Actual causes of death in the United States, 2000. *The Journal of the American Medical Association*, 291(23), 1238-1245.

Morio B., Montaurier C., Pickering G., Ritz P., Fellmann N., Coudert J., Beaufrere B. &Vermorel M. (1998). Effects of 14 weeks of progressive endurance training on energy expenditure in elderly people. *British Journal of Nutrition*, 80, 511-519.

Ortega, F. B., Ruiz, J. R., Castillo, M. J., Moreno, L. A., González-Gross, M., Wärnberg, J., & Gutiérrez, Á. (2005). Low level of physical fitness in Spanish adolescents. Relevance for future cardiovascular health (AVENA study). *Revista Española de Cardiología (English Edition), 58*(8), 898-909.

Rowland TW. (1998). The biological basis of physical activity. *Medicine Science Sports Exercise, 30*(5), 392-399.

Schmitz K. H., Jacobs D. R. Jr., Leon A. S., Schreiner P. J., Sternfeld B. (2000). Physical activity and body weight: associations over ten years in the CARDIA study. Coronary Artery Risk Development in Young Adults. *International Journal of Obesity,* 4(9), 1475-1487.

Schrauwen P., Lichtenbelt W. D., Saris W. H. &Westerterp K. R. (1998). Fat balance in obese subjects: role of glycogen stores. *American Journal of Physiology,* 74, E1027-E1033.

Serrano-Huete, V., Latorre-Román, P. A., García-Pinillos, F., MorcilloLosa, J. A., Moreno-Del Castillo, R., &Párra-ga-Montilla, J. A. (2016). Acute effect of a judo contest on muscular performance parameters and physiological response. *International Journal of Kinesiology & Sports Science*, 4(3), 24-31.

Stallmann-Jorgensen IS,Gutin B, Hatfield-Laube JL, Humphries MC, Johnson MH and Barbeau P. (2007). General and visceral adiposity in black and white adolescents and their relation with reported physical activity and diet. *International Journal of Obesity*, 31(7), 622-629.

Tjonna, A. E., Lee, S. J., Rognmo, O., Stolen, T. O., Bye, A., Haram, P. M., Wisloff, U. (2008). Aerobic interval training versus continuous moderate exercise as a treatment for the metabolic syndrome: a pilot study. *Circulation, 118*(4), 346-354. doi: 10.1161/CIRCULATION AHA. 108.772822

Tjonna, A. E., Stolen, T. O., Bye, A., Volden, M., Slordahl, S. A., Odegard, R., Wisloff, U. (2009). Aerobic interval training reduces cardiovascular risk factors more than a multitreatment approach in overweight adolescents. *Clinical Science, 116*(4), 317-326. doi: 10.1042/CS20080249.

Tudor-Locke C, Hatano Y, Pangrazi RP and Kang M. (2008a). Revisiting "how many steps are enough. *Medicine and Science in Sports and Exercise*, 40(4), S537-S543.

Tudor-Locke CE, Myers AM. (2000b). Methodological Considerations for Researchers and Practitioners using Pedometers to Measure Physical (Ambulatory) Activity. *Research Questionnaire Exercise Sports*, 2, 1-12.

Vuori IM. (2001). Dose-response of physical activity and low back pain, osteoarthritis, and osteoporosis. *Medicine and Science in Sports and Exercise*, 3(4), S551-586.

Welk, G. J., Laurson, K. R., Eisenmann, J. C., & Cureton, K. J. (2011). Development of youth aerobic-capacity standards using receiver operating characteristic curves. *American Journal of Preventive Medicine*, 41(4 Suppl 2), S111-116. doi: 10.1016/j.amepre.2011.07.007

17

Effects of Point of Aim on the Accuracy and Eye Movement Behavior in Bowling

Jongil Lim[1], Seung Ho Chang[2]*, Adriane Cris Tomimbang[2]

[1]Department of Counseling, Health and Kinesiology, Texas A&M University - San Antonio, One University Way, San Antonio, TX, USA

[2]Department of Kinesiology, San Jose State University, 1 Washington Square, San Jose, CA, USA

Corresponding Author: Seung Ho Chang, E-mail: seungho.chang@sjsu.edu

---

ARTICLE INFO

Conflicts of interest: None
Funding: None

ABSTRACT

Background: A common research question in far-target aiming has been the importance and significance of the final visual fixation before movement initiation. In rolling tasks, such as 10-pin bowling, location of point of aim needs not be at the final target, the pins, but may be located at any point along the trajectory of the ball. **Objective:** Specific interest in the present experiment has focused on the relationship between visual point of aim and performance accuracy, and the relationship of visual control strategies utilized by expert performers. **Methods:** Skilled bowlers (N=7) performed 20 trials per condition concentrating on visual targets in different distances along the bowling lane (20, 40, 60 feet, and self-selected). Ball trajectory was tracked using a video based system and eye movement was measured using an eye tracking system. **Results:** Deviation of the ball from the visual target increased with visual target distance, while deviation of the ball from the pins was the lowest in the self-selected visual targets, followed by aiming at the pins. The final fixation duration before movement initiation was not associated with ball accuracy regardless of visual target locations. However, results demonstrated the association between final fixation duration task difficulty, that is, longer final fixation duration with increased visual target distance. **Conclusion:** The results indicate that visual fixations before movement initiation are uncharacteristically long while visual fixations just before the completion of the movement are relatively short.

Key words: Motor Skill, Attention, Accuracy, Vision, Fixation

---

INTRODUCTION

Bowling is a sport that competes the spatial accuracy of a projectile object, in order to aim a bowling ball correctly towards an intended target. The objective of the sport is to knock down as many pins as possible. The public generally enjoys ten-pin bowling, as a recreational league sport or an entertaining weekend activity, but there are competitive bowlers that train themselves to attain accurate and consistent bowling form (Razman, Abas, Osman, & Cheong, 2011; Young, Sherk, & Bemben, 2011). The projectile motion of a ball is typically divided into 5 sequences: targeting, push-off, down swing, back swing, and ball release, while the whole body is in forward propulsion parallel to the floor. Throughout the projectile motion of the ball, bowlers are instructed to focus on a target (or mark) to which they will project the ball (Taylor, 1979). A common strategy known as spot bowling is a technique in which the target arrows, embedded in the lane about 15 feet down from the foul line, are typically used as locations for aiming. Utilizing these seven arrows as a spatial reference increases the chance of consistently hitting the target pin and achieving the desired outcome. Studies examining the influence of visual behavior in far-target aiming

consistently show that accurate performance is dependent on how vision and focus of visual attention is regulated in order to acquire task-relevant visual information (Vickers, 2011).

The pick-up of essential visual parameters during response preparation was particularly important and characterized by the final visual fixation before movement initiation. An earlier onset of the final eye fixation and longer final eye fixation duration are characteristics distinguishing skill differences in higher versus lower skilled performers and accurate versus inaccurate trial performance. However, in previous studies the location of visual focus and the target location were always coincident (e.g., basketball free-throw, golf putting, billiards, archery, and dart). In a rolling task such as 10-pin bowling, the point of aim need not be at the final target, the pins, but may be located at any point along the trajectory of the ball (Vickers, 2007). The advantages of paying attention on an external source of information have been demonstrated in many motor behavior studies (Wulf, 2007). In a variety of motor skills, age groups, and skill levels, focusing on the external cues such as intended movement effect showed benefits in performance outcome and learning than attending to internal cues such as one's body movements. Tasks demonstrating these effects include balancing (Wulf, McNevin, & Shea, 2001), vertical jumping (Wulf, Dufek, Lozano, & Pettigrew, 2010), golf chipping shot (Wulf & Su, 2007), and dart throwing (Lohse, Sherwood, & Healy, 2010; Marchant, Clough, & Crawshaw, 2007). Advantages of externally focused attention were addressed in regards to reducing consciousness in controlling the movement and enhancing the smooth execution of movements (Wulf & Lewthwaite, 2010). A few studies replicated the effectiveness of an external focus and further demonstrated that the performance and learning of motor skills was improved when attention was located to the external source of information further away from the body (Bell & Hardy, 2009; Porter, Anton, Wikoff, & Ostrowski, 2013). Particularly, for studies in which the far-target aiming task was employed (e.g., golf pitching shot; dart throwing), the group with a distal external cues (flight of the golf ball and bull's eye, respectively) displayed better accuracy compared to the internal cue group (own body movements) (Bell & Hardy, 2009; McKay & Wulf, 2012). However, in both studies participants were novice performers and one of the instructional cues used to focus the attention was difficult to visually focus on. That is, the imaginary attention was emphasized in external focus group (e.g., flight of the golf ball and flight of the dart, respectively).

While the beneficial effects of directing attention externally at a greater distance from the body have been demonstrated, studies that directly controlled the distance of visual focus of attention (e.g., focusing on the ball versus focusing on the hole throughout the entire stroke in golf putting) consistently showed no significant effect on distal attention of focus in performance (Cockerill, 1979) and learning (Mackenzie, Foley, & Adamczyk, 2011). Moreover, after practicing the movements, the performance variability such as face angle, stroke path, and impact spot became equivalent between the two visual attention groups. Putter speed variability, indicating the golfer's ability to correctly estimate the required impulse, however, was further reduced in the distal focus group. This reduction in putter speed variability suggests the benefits of practicing, while visually focusing on the hole, can be amplified (Mackenzie et al., 2011). However, as authors discussed, different head positions might be associated with different levels of anxiety, more specifically "looking up" too soon during the stroke, particularly, when focus is on the ball. A stream of research in golf putting consistently demonstrated that use of characterized gaze control on the ball is an important strategy (Vickers, 1992, 2007, 2011; Vine, Moore, & Wilson, 2011), which facilitates the brain to process task relevant attention for precise ball-club contact (Vickers, 2011). The intermediate spatial location between the performer and the target is frequently used as the location of aim. This location of aim is visually focused on if a projected object is required to travel along a curved path (e.g. breaking putts in golf and delivery of the curling stone), a technique also practiced in bowling. However, no studies have examined the effect of the distance of visual focus of attention, including intermediate targets, on the performance of far-target aiming. The purpose of this study, therefore, was to examine the robustness of the distance effect on visual focus of attention, more specifically

through the direct manipulation of visual focus of attention in distance. Of particular interest in the present experiment were the relationship between the visual point of aim and performance accuracy, and the visual control strategies used by expert performers.

METHOD

Participants and Design of Study

Seven right-handed individuals volunteered for the study. Mean age was 21.14 ± 1.06 years and 3 participants were female and 4 were male. All subjects were skilled bowlers (average score 194.3 ± 17.5), as indicated by national collegiate competitive experience and also by Thomas, Schlinker, and Over (1996) (current average of 170 pins of more). Participants had normal or corrected-to-normal vision, were healthy, without any known oculomotor abnormalities, and signed an Institutional Review Board approved consent form. A descriptive research design (field observation) was utilized to examine the effect of visual target distance on spatial accuracy and fixation duration.

Apparatus

A standard 60-foot long, 40-inch wide, oiled synthetic lane was used for testing. Participants were allowed to use their own shoes and bowling balls. The bowling balls used in the study were regulated to be 8.59 inches in diameter, with a mass between 6 to 16 pounds. Two video cameras (Sony, Japan, Model DCR-TRV520) were positioned in the middle of the lane, facing down, to track ball trajectory from the transverse plane (Figure 1). One camera was directed at the pins (final target) the entire time and the second camera was focused at one of the intermediate targets. The position of the second camera was adjusted according to the order of intermediate target sequence. A third camera synced with the eye tracking system was positioned at the right side of the participants, in order to record the projectile motion of the ball from the sagittal plane (side-view).

Eye tracker (Applied Science Laboratories Series 5000 Head Mounted Eye Tracker) mounted on a helmet worn by the participant was used to record gaze movements. The line of gaze measured by a pupil and corneal reflection system was superimposed on the scene image recorded by an external scene camera. The point of gaze from the participant's view was recorded by the video recorder (JVC, Japan, Model SR-VS30). The sampling frequency was set at 60 Hz, and the gaze position data was exported to the manufacturer provided software (ASL Eye-Trac 6000) for analysis.

Procedures

Participants were given six practice shots prior to the testing session. After completing the practice, the eye-tracking system helmet was put on the participant. Calibration was performed using a nine-point grid on the board placed directly in front of the participant. The participant took a four- or five-step approach and threw the ball underhand at the head pin (Figure 1). Participants were instructed to attempt to get the ball to hit the pins between the 17th and 18th boards, which is considered to be the optimal placement for bowling strikes (Taylor, 1979). Four distances of visual focus of attention were tested using a visual target at 20-, 40-, and 60-feet down the lane, in addition to the participant's preferred location. The importance of examining these locations in the target process has been addressed; one at the end of the lane (pins), one at the end of the oil pattern (typically 40 feet down the lane), and one 15 to 25 feet down the lane (Slowinski, 2007). Participants chose the lateral position of their target for each condition (i.e. which board to aim for). Twenty trials were performed in each condition and three minutes rest between each condition was given. The order of condition was counterbalanced across participants. During each trial, the experimenter monitored each participant's gaze location and determined if location was indeed at the designated visual target location throughout ball projection.

Data Analysis

Temporal components of the bowling swing. For the sake of analyzing the fixation characteristics with respect to the movement execution phases (Figure 2), movement initiation time and release time were analyzed from images taken by the side-view camera (sagittal plane).

Performance

Spatial errors at the visual target and at the end of the lane were measured using frame-by-frame video analysis. Constant error, the signed horizontal deviation of the ball center relative to the visual targets (20-, 40-, and self-selected location) and relative to the pins (60 feet down the lane), was measured in inch of board. Absolute error and variable error were then computed.

Eye movement

A fixation is defined as an eye movement of less than $1°$ of visual angle for 100 ms or longer. The average fixation duration and final fixation duration per trial were calculated. Fixations, which occurred between the push-off and ball release phases, were of specific interest. The last fixation in the preparation phase (e.g., before push-off) and the last fixation in the execution phase (e.g., before ball release) were analyzed and compared to average fixation.

Statistical Analysis

The effect of visual target distance on spatial accuracy and fixation duration was analyzed using one-way ANOVA with repeated measures (SPSS 16.0, Chicago, IL, USA). Data distributions were checked for normality and homogeneity of variances using the Shapiro–Wilk test and the Mauchly's test, respectively. In the case of violations of the sphericity assumption, F values were adjusted with the Greenhouse-Geisser procedures. A post-hoc analysis of the Bonferroni test was used to detect significant pairwise differences of means among visual target distances. A paired t-test (two-tailed) was used to determine if differences existed in absolute and variable error at the visual and final target in each visual target distance. Final fixation durations were

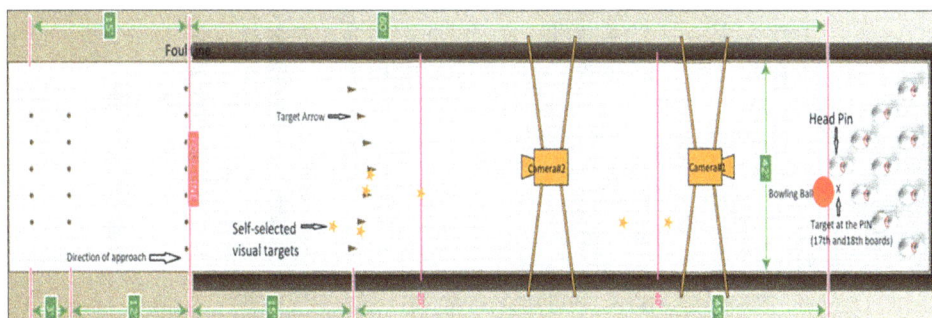

Figure 1. Experimental setup. Stars indicate the visual target locations selected by each participant. Two video cameras were positioned in the middle of lane facing towards the pins (Camera#1) and the foul line (Camera#2)

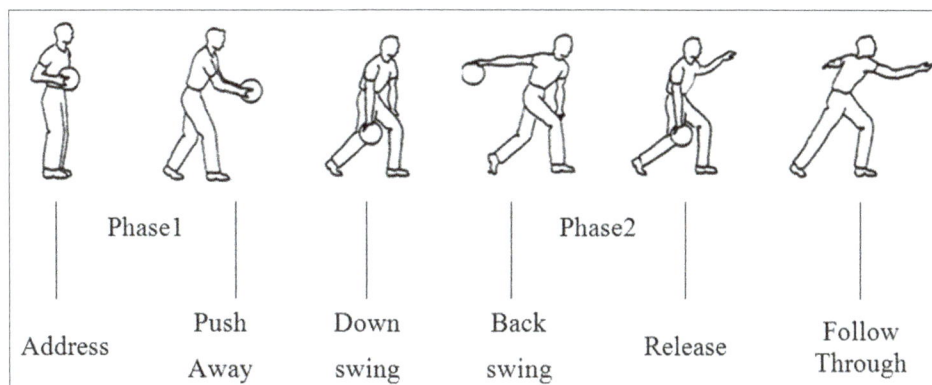

Figure 2. Bowling approach steps and events for eye movement analysis

compared for accurate and inaccurate trials using a paired t-test (two-tailed). The alpha level for all statistical tests was set at.05.

RESULTS

Performance

Most participants preferred to target somewhere near the arrows, located 15 feet down the lane. One participant noted that she focused either 15 or 41 feet down the lane, depending on the oil pattern on the lane. This participant elected to look at 41 feet for the experiment. Absolute and variable error at the visual target and final target were summarized in Table 1.

Visual target error

In general, visual target error increased as target distance increased (Figure 3). The main effect of visual target distance on absolute error at preliminary visual target was significant [$F(3,18)=4.228, p<.05$], and a post hoc pairwise comparison showed that absolute error at 20-foot condition was significantly lower than absolute error at 60-foot condition ($p<.05$). The main effect of visual target distance on spatial variability at visual target was statistically significant [$F(3,18)=11.248, p<.01$]. Post hoc comparisons indicated that variable error was significantly lower at the 20-foot and self-selected condition as compared to the 40-foot and 60-foot condition ($ps<.01$).

Final target error

The main effect of visual target distance on absolute error at final target was statistically significant [$F(3,18)=4.079, p<.05$], however, its effect on variable error did not reach statistical significance [$F(3,18)=3.040, p=.056$] (Figure 4). A post hoc comparison showed that self-selected condition was more accurate at pins compared to the 40-foot intermediate target condition ($p<.05$). In detail, absolute and variable error at final target was the least in the participants' preferred target distance condition and second lowest in 60-foot condition, in comparison to the other two intermediate target distance conditions.

Eye Fixations

Due to device malfunction eye movement data was only available for 6 participants. The duration of the last fixation before the initiation of push-off, the last fixation before ball release, and the average fixation from push-off to ball release were compared (Table 2).

The main effect of visual target distance on fixation duration before initiation of push off was statistically significant [$F(3,18)=5.121, p<.01$]. Fixation duration before push-away

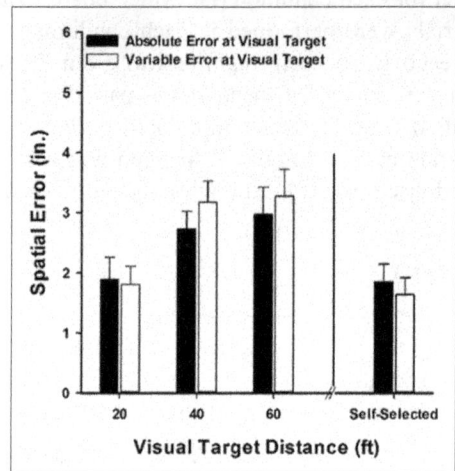

Figure 3. Absolute error and Variable error at visual target.

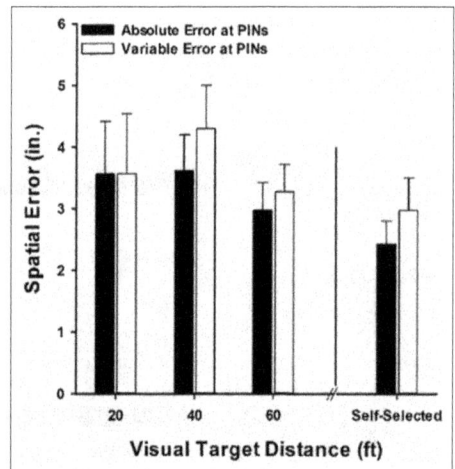

Figure 4. Absolute error and Variable error at PINs.

Table 1. Performance accuracy at visual target and PINs (inch)

Location	Error	Visual target distance (ft)			
		20	**40**	**60**	**Self- selected**
Visual target	AE				
	Mean±SD	1.89±0.97	2.73±0.76	2.96±1.19	1.85±0.77
	VE				
	Mean±SD	1.80±0.80	3.17±0.92	3.27±1.18	1.64±0.72
Target (PINs)	AE				
	Mean±SD	3.55±2.27	3.62±1.53	2.96±1.19	2.42±0.99
	VE				
	Mean±SD	3.56±2.59	4.30±1.85	3.27±1.18	2.97±1.39

AE=Absolute error. VE=Variable error.

Table 2. Fixation duration and frequency (sec)

Fixation		Visual target distance (ft)			
		20	40	60	Self -selected
Duration	Before movement initiation (push-away) Mean±SD	0.325±0.141	0.339±0.102	0.413±0.152	0.299±0.076
	Before ball release Mean±SD	0.127±0.021	0.130±0.020	0.131±0.021	0.125±0.026
	Average Mean±SD	0.196±0.026	0.190±0.016	0.195±0.031	0.203±0.035
Frequency	Average Mean±SD	6.683±0.907	6.825±0.446	6.208±0.890	6.716±1.305

was longer at the 60-foot condition compared to 20-foot condition ($p < .05$). However, fixation duration before ball release showed no differences relative to visual target distance conditions. Fixation frequency was not influenced by visual target distance. The final fixation before movement initiation was significantly longer than the average fixation (for example, $p = 0.03$ for the 60-foot condition), which was in turn significantly longer than the last fixation before ball release ($ps < .01$) (Figure 5). Average fixation duration was longer than fixation duration before ball release in all visual target distance conditions ($ps < .01$).

Fixations and accuracy

Final fixation duration was no longer on accurate trials compared to those of inaccurate trials. Final fixation duration was compared in accurate and inaccurate trials, which were defined as shots either within 1 inch of the preliminary target or within 1 inch of the final target (the 17.5th board 60 feet down the lane). Final fixation duration was almost identical in all cases, as shown in Figure 6.

DISCUSSION

Spatial Accuracy of Aiming

The magnitude and variability of ball deviation from the visual point of aim increased as visual aim point was located closer to the pins. Though practice time was limited at each of the visual target distances, participants in this study presented intermediate skill level and were successful in projecting the bowling ball towards the location of aim with minimal variability. Under these assumptions, increases in spatial error at the visual point of aim may be associated with task difficulty, which increases with target distance. While spatial error at the visual target increased with aiming distance, final target error (i.e., deviation from the head pin) was greater at 20-foot and 40-foot conditions than 60-foot condition. Moreover, similarities in final target error between the 60-foot condition and the self-selected condition have been determined. These findings indicate that placing aim location directly on the pin could reduce the final target error and suggest an alternative strategy compared to aiming at an intermediate space. If more than one visuo-motor task space is available, such as in bowling, directing visual fo-

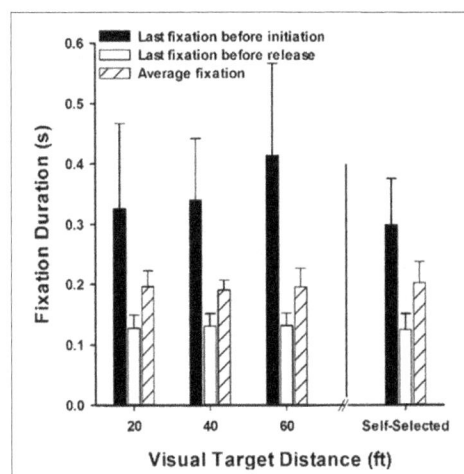

Figure 5. Final fixation duration at two movement events and Average fixation duration.

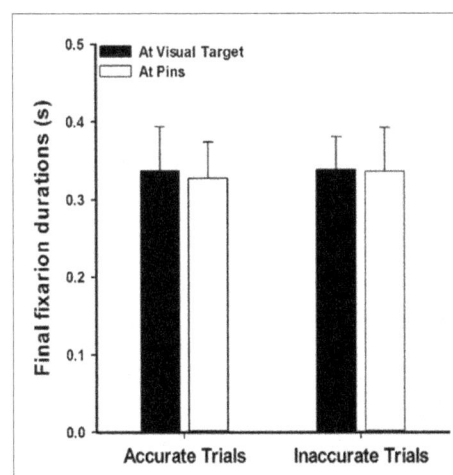

Figure 6. Fixation duration with ball accuracy at visual target and at pins.

cus on the target rather than the intermediate space would be beneficial in terms of accuracy, unless deliberate practice has been provided to aim at a fixed reference spot (e.g., aim spot on the lane). Mackenzie et al. (2011) reported no significant differences in success rate as well as putter speed variability between visually focusing on the hole and looking at the ball in golf putting. Such findings suggest that visual point of aim on the target played a crucial role in focusing the golfer's attention to the outcome of movement execution such as "rolling the ball toward the hole". Given that the variable error at the final target (i.e., pin) was smaller in the 60-foot condition, additional research is necessary, across all levels of expertise, in order to understand the effect of visual focus training on a far-target aiming task.

Gaze Control Characteristics

Gaze fixation duration before the initiation of push-off was longer compared to before ball release and average fixation duration, regardless of the distance of visual aim point. A longer visual target distance (i.e., 60-foot condition) caused constrained gaze control, which is indicated by increased fixation duration. In the current study, this increased fixation duration is consistent with previous research on far-target aiming (Behan & Wilson, 2008; Henry & Rogers, 1960; Vickers, 1996, 2009; Williams, Singer, & Frehlich, 2002), where longer fixation duration has been shown to be associated with increased task difficulty and anxiety level. The findings herein agree with Vickers (2007), who demonstrated the importance of acquired visual information during the movement preparation period. However, the task-specific nature of this gaze control characteristic, has been reported, with limitations exposed, particularly when visual occlusion is accompanied or continuous control of movement is required in aiming tasks (De Oliveira, Oudejans, & Beek, 2006; Glöckner, Heinen, Johnson, & Raab, 2012; Oudejans, van de Langenberg, & Hutter, 2002). Gaze fixation duration during the movement preparation period was not different in terms of aiming accuracy (i.e. accurate trials vs. inaccurate trials). This finding is inconsistent with observations seen in studies on other aiming tasks, where a significant relationship between performance accuracy and gaze fixation duration was found (Causer, Bennett, Holmes, Janelle, & Williams, 2010; Vickers, 1992; Williams et al., 2002; Wilson & Pearcy, 2009). This disparity between such findings may have resulted from the amount of visual information and number of necessary parameters to be controlled during movement execution, and consequences on performance outcome. Future studies should examine gaze fixation duration-performance accuracy relationship, with the consideration of the performers skill level and the number of visuo-motor task space. An alternative view on gaze fixation (occurs before movement initiation) emphasized its significance as a reflection of the efficient processing and anticipation of object location and object characteristics, as well as the acceleration of transitioning focus of attention facilitating the transition (Horn, Okumura, Alexander, Gardin, & Sylvester, 2012). This notion is supported through studies showing that the role of a longer gaze fixation during movement preparation could be limited to tasks requiring high demands of information processing and/or re-parameterization of movement, in order to maintain trial-to-trial consistency (Horn et al., 2012; Klostermann, Kredel, & Hossner, 2013).

This pilot study has several limitations, including limited sample size and differences in preferred visual aiming points between participants. The generalizability of this pilot study is also limited by the skill-based sample of bowlers. Skilled bowlers were recruited in this study to minimize the source of variation originating from throwing motion, and therefore the potential influence on the aiming accuracy. Therefore, different pattern of gaze control may appear, especially, in the people in the lower skill level, who has to allocate a significant amount of attention to the delivery itself (Shank & Lajoie, 2013). Consequently, future research is needed in order to replicate the present findings with different individual as well as task context.

CONCLUSION

The aim of the current study was to directly manipulate the distance of visual focus of attention in a far-target aiming task with experienced bowlers. The present study examined gaze fixation duration and aiming accuracy as a function of the distance of visual focus of attention in far-target aiming. Our results failed to demonstrate the effect of task difficulty (e.g., visual target distance) and performance accuracy on the gaze fixation duration in the movement preparation period. However, the results provided further evidence on the critical role of processing visual information before the execution of movement. The preliminary results of this study imply that visual focus on a far-distance target, instead of an intermediate space, could result in an advantageous effect on performance outcome, especially, with the presence of more than one visuo-motor task space. Future studies should seek to elucidate whether this relationship is consistent across various skill levels, as well as context of aiming tasks.

REFERENCES

Behan, M., & Wilson, M. (2008). State anxiety and visual attention: The role of the quiet eye period in aiming to a far target. *Journal of Sports Sciences, 26*(2), 207-215.

Bell, J. J., & Hardy, J. (2009). Effects of attentional focus on skilled performance in golf. *Journal of Applied Sport Psychology, 21*(2), 163-177.

Causer, J., Bennett, S. J., Holmes, P. S., Janelle, C. M., & Williams, A. M. (2010). Quiet eye duration and gun motion in elite shotgun shooting. *Medicine & Science in Sports & Exercise, 42*(8), 1599-1608.

Cockerill, I. M. (1979). Visual control in golf putting. In C. H. Nadeau, W. R. Halliwell, K. M. Newell, & G. C. Roberts (Eds.), *Psychology of motor behavior and sport* (pp. 377–384). Champaign, IL: Human Kinetics.

De Oliveira, R. F., Oudejans, R. R., & Beek, P. J. (2006). Late information pick-up is preferred in basketball jump shooting. *Journal of Sports Sciences, 24*(9), 933-940.

Glöckner, A., Heinen, T., Johnson, J. G., & Raab, M. (2012). Network approaches for expert decisions in sports. *Human Movement Science, 31*(2), 318-333.

Henry, F. M., & Rogers, D. E. (1960). Increased response latency for complicated movements and a "memory drum" theory of neuromotor reaction. *Research Quarterly. American Association for Health, Physical Education and Recreation, 31*(3), 448-458.

Horn, R. R., Okumura, M. S., Alexander, M. G., Gardin, F. A., & Sylvester, C. T. (2012). Quiet eye duration is responsive to variability of practice and to the axis of target changes. *Research quarterly for exercise and sport, 83*(2), 204-211.

Klostermann, A., Kredel, R., & Hossner, E.-J. (2013). The "quiet eye" and motor performance: Task demands matter! *Journal of Experimental Psychology: Human Perception and Performance, 39*(5), 1270-1278.

Lohse, K. R., Sherwood, D. E., & Healy, A. F. (2010). How changing the focus of attention affects performance, kinematics, and electromyography in dart throwing. *Human Movement Science, 29*(4), 542-555.

Mackenzie, S. J., Foley, S. M., & Adamczyk, A. P. (2011). Visually focusing on the far versus the near target during the putting stroke. *Journal of Sports Sciences, 29*(12), 1243-1251.

Marchant, D. C., Clough, P. J., & Crawshaw, M. (2007). The effects of attentional focusing strategies on novice dart throwing performance and their task experiences. *International Journal of Sport and Exercise Psychology, 5*(3), 291-303.

McKay, B., & Wulf, G. (2012). A distal external focus enhances novice dart throwing performance. *International Journal of Sport and Exercise Psychology, 10*(2), 149-156.

Oudejans, R. R., van de Langenberg, R. W., & Hutter, R. V. (2002). Aiming at a far target under different viewing conditions: Visual control in basketball jump shooting. *Human Movement Science, 21*(4), 457-480.

Porter, J. M., Anton, P. M., Wikoff, N. M., & Ostrowski, J. B. (2013). Instructing skilled athletes to focus their attention externally at greater distances enhances jumping performance. *The Journal of Strength & Conditioning Research, 27*(8), 2073-2078.

Razman R., Abas W.A.B.W., Osman N.A.A., Cheong J.P.G. (2011). Temporal Characteristics of the Final Delivery Phase and Its Relation to Tenpin Bowling Performance. In: Osman N.A.A., Abas W.A.B.W., Wahab A.K.A., Ting HN. (eds) *5th Kuala Lumpur International Conference on Biomedical Engineering 2011*. IFMBE Proceedings, vol 35. Springer, Berlin, Heidelberg.

Shank, V. & Lajoie, Y. (2013). Attentional demands in the execution phase of curling in novices and experts. *International Journal of Kinesiology & Sports Science, 1*(1), 1-8.

Slowinski, J. (2007, June). 3-Point targeting for advanced lane play. [Online forum post]. Retrieved from https://www.bowlingthismonth.com/bowling-tips/lane-play-alignment

Taylor, D. (1979). *Secret of Bowling Strikes*: Wilshire Book Company.

Thomas, P. R., Schlinker, P. J., & Over, R. (1996). Psychological and psychomotor skills associated with prowess at ten-pin bowling. *Journal of Sports Sciences, 14*(3), 255-268.

Vickers, J. N. (1992). Gaze control in putting. *Perception, 21*(1), 117-132.

Vickers, J. N. (1996). Visual control when aiming at a far target. *Journal of Experimental Psychology: Human Perception and Performance, 22*(2), 342-354.

Vickers, J. N. (2007). *Perception, cognition, and decision training: The quiet eye in action*: Champaign, IL: Human Kinetics.

Vickers, J. N. (2009). Advances in coupling perception and action: the quiet eye as a bidirectional link between gaze, attention, and action. *Progress in brain research, 174*, 279-288.

Vickers, J. N. (2011). Mind over muscle: The role of gaze control, spatial cognition, and the quiet eye in motor expertise: Springer.

Vine, S. J., Moore, L. J., & Wilson, M. R. (2011). Quiet eye training facilitates competitive putting performance in elite golfers. *Frontiers in psychology, 2*(8), 1-9.

Williams, A. M., Singer, R. N., & Frehlich, S. G. (2002). Quiet eye duration, expertise, and task complexity in near and far aiming tasks. *Journal of Motor Behavior, 34*(2), 197-207.

Wilson, M. R., & Pearcy, R. C. (2009). Visuomotor control of straight and breaking golf putts. *Perceptual and Motor Skills, 109*(2), 555-562.

Wulf, G. (2007). Attentional focus and motor learning: A review of 10 years of research. *E-journal Bewegung und Training, 1*(2-3), 1-11.

Wulf, G., Dufek, J. S., Lozano, L., & Pettigrew, C. (2010). Increased jump height and reduced EMG activity with an external focus. *Human Movement Science, 29*(3), 440-448.

Wulf, G., & Lewthwaite, R. (2010). Effortless motor learning? An external focus of attention enhances movement effectiveness and efficiency. In B. Bruya (Ed.), *Effortless attention: A new perspective in attention and action* (p. 75-101). Cambridge, MA: MIT Press.

Wulf, G., McNevin, N., & Shea, C. H. (2001). The automaticity of complex motor skill learning as a function of attentional focus. *The Quarterly Journal of Experimental Psychology: Section A, 54*(4), 1143-1154.

Wulf, G., & Su, J. (2007). An external focus of attention enhances golf shot accuracy in beginners and experts. *Research quarterly for exercise and sport, 78*(4), 384-389.

Young, K. C., Sherk, V. D., & Bemben, D. A. (2011). Inter-limb musculoskeletal differences in competitive tenpin bowlers: A preliminary analysis. *Journal of Musculoskeletal Neuronal Interact, 11*(1), 21-26.

18

Influences of Athletic Footwear on Ground Reaction Forces During A Sidestep Cutting Maneuver on Artificial Turf

Jacob R. Gdovin[1*], Charles C. Williams[2,3], Samuel J. Wilson[3,4], Vanessa L. Cazas-Moreno[5], Lauren A. Luginsland[3], Charles R. Allen[6], Harish Chander[7], Chip Wade[8], John C. Garner III[9]

[1]Department of Kinesiology; Missouri State University 901 S. National Ave., Springfield, MO 65897 USA

[2]Department of of Exercise Science; LaGrange College , 601 Broad Street, LaGrange, GA 30240 USA

[3]Department of Health, Exercise Science and Recreation Management; The University of Mississippi 215 Turner Center, P.O. Box 1848, University, MS 38677 USA

[4]Department of Health Sciences and Kinesiology; Georgia Southern University P.O. Box 8076, Statesboro, GA 30460 USA

[5]Department of Human Performance and Sport Sciences; Tennessee State University 3500 John A. Merritt Blvd., Nashville, TN 37209 USA

[6]Department of Exercise Science; Florida Southern College 111 Lake Hollingsworth Dr., Lakeland, FL 33801 USA

[7]Neuromechanics Laboratory, Department of Kinesiology; Mississippi State University PO Box 6186, Mississippi State, MS 39762 USA

[8]Department of Industrial and Systems Engineering; Auburn University Auburn, AL 36849 USA

[9]Department of Kinesiology and Health Promotion; Troy University 112G Wright Hall, Troy, AL 36082 USA

Corresponding Author: Jacob R. Gdovin, E-mail: JacobGdovin@missouristate.edu

ARTICLE INFO

Conflicts of interest: None
Funding: None

ABSTRACT

Background: Recreational athletes can select their desired footwear based on personal preferences of shoe properties such as comfort and weight. Commonly worn running shoes and cleated footwear with similar stud geometry and distribution are worn when performing sport-specific tasks such as a side-step cutting maneuver (SCM) in soccer and American football (hereafter, referred to as football). The effects of such footwear on injury mechanics have been documented with less being known regarding their effect on performance. **Objective:** The purpose of this study was to examine performance differences including peak ground reaction forces (pGRF), time-to-peak ground reaction forces (tpGRF) and the rate of force development (RFD) between football cleats (FB), soccer cleats (SOC), and traditional running sneakers (RUN) during the braking and propulsive phases of a SCM. **Methodology:** Eleven recreationally active males who participated in football and/or soccer-related activities at the time of testing completed the study. A 1 x 3 [1 Condition (SCM) x 3 Footwear (RUN, FB, SOC)] repeated measures ANOVA was utilized to analyze the aforementioned variables. **Results:** There were no significant differences (p > 0.05) between footwear conditions when comparing pGRF, tpGRF, or RFD in either the braking or propulsive phases. **Conclusion:** The results suggest that the studded and non-studded footwear allowed athletes to generate similar forces over a given time frame when performing a SCM.

Key words: Shoes, Football, Soccer, Athletes, Running

INTRODUCTION

The shoe-surface interface defines how an athlete's footwear interacts with the underlying playing surface assisting with the implementation of sport-specific movements such as sprinting, cutting, and stopping. The mechanism allowing this interaction lies in the understanding of vertical and horizontal resistive forces. Vertical resistive forces determine a cleats ability to penetrate a playing surface (Driscoll, Kelley, Kirk, Koerger, & Haake, 2015) which can be influenced by surface hardness as well as cleat design (i.e., stud geometry) (Clarke & Carré, 2010). Surface hardness is the ability of a surface to absorb impact energy upon it being struck by an object (SportsTurf Managers Associations [STMA], 2008). When the energy is created by an athlete's foot, the reactionary force can be referred to as a ground reaction force (GRF). Traction, which comprises the horizontal resistive force and can be referred to as grip-ability, describes how cleated footwear resists the motion of the body relative to the surface (McNitt, Middour, & Waddington, 1997).

Cleats are frequently worn in soccer and football as they play a vital role in an athlete's performance during these sports. Approximately 265 million athletes participate in soccer globally (Fédération Internationale de Football Association [FIFA], 2007); it is accepted to be the most popular sport in the world. Football also maintains its popularity with over one million reported male high school football athletes in the United States (National Federation of State High School Associations, 2017). The increase in participation within both sports has provided shoe manufacturers incentive to develop various cleat designs exclusively for tasks related to a specific sport and position in attempt to improve performance. Cleat differences vary between models and manufacturers with stud geometry (i.e. cylindrical, conical, prismatic, and bladed) and distribution (i.e. turf, artificial grass, hard ground, firm ground, and soft ground) being the differentiating variables (Sterzing, 2016). However, recreational athletes can select their own footwear and are not limited to footwear specific to their sport.

Cleated footwear is designed to assist with foot and ankle stabilization while simultaneously improving an individuals ability to perform sport-specific movements, such as a side-step cutting maneuver (SCM), by allowing for a strong push-off in any direction without slipping (Sterzing, 2016). The SCM is utilized in both sports and is described as a high-speed evasive movement with a sudden change in direction, often at an angle of approximately 45° relative to the running direction (Havens & Siward, 2015; McLean, Neal, Myers, & Walters, 1999; Vanrenterghem, Venables, Pataky, & Robinson, 2012). Within the SCM, two phases exist which enable the change in direction to occur: the braking and propulsion phases. The braking phase occurs from the instance of foot contact until the pGRF and is responsible for assisting with the body's negative acceleration to prepare for a rapid change in direction. The subsequent propulsion phase allows the athlete to generate velocity in the newly intended direction, which occurs in the time between the braking pGRF and foot toe-off. Numerous variables have been associated with effecting lower extremity mechanics and performance during a SCM such as footwear design, cleat arrangements, shoe-surface interaction (Kent, Forman, Lessley, & Crandall, 2015b), cutting angle (Havens & Sigward, 2015), and approach speed (Vanrenterghem et al. 2012). Previous literature has shown that prolonged activity may also effect performance due to the decrease in the neuromuscular response and/or control as the duration of playing time may increase (McGovern et al., 2015).

Injuries within both sports arise due to several factors with a common mechanism stemming from the increasing size, speed, and strength of the athletes. This may indirectly alter the traction developed from cutting with a foot planted while the upper body rotates. Among male high school athletes, game and practice injury rates were highest for football and soccer to the foot and ankle, representing 15.9% and 33.5% of all reported injuries, respectively (Powell & Barber-Foss, 1999). In 2005, the rate of lower limb injuries among high school male athletes was the highest in football while soccer had the highest rate among females with common injuries including sprains (50%), strains (17%), contusions (12%), and fractures (5%) (Fernandez, Yard, Comstock, 2007). Within the sport of soccer, 42% of all injuries are due to intrinsic player-controlled factors such as muscle weakness, while 24% of injuries were due to poor playing surfaces combined with "inferior shoes" (Nigg,

1989). These injuries can arise due to intrinsic risk factors, such as lack of experience, position within the sport, biological age, and joint flexibility combined with extrinsic factors such as shoe-surface interaction, field conditions, and equipment (Dvorak & Junge, 2000; Iacovelli et al., 2013).

While previous research has examined how a SCM and cleated footwear alters injury possibilities, the effect they have on performance variables have not been as widely analyzed, with the exception of a few studies (Brock et al., 2014; Durá, Hoyos, Martinez, & Lozano, 1999; McGhie & Ettema, 2008; Meijer, Dethmers, Savelberg, Willems, & Wijers, 2006; Queen et al. 2008). The GRFs exerted against a cleats sole is vital for understanding how quickly and forcefully an athlete can run and change direction. Previous research on artificial turf analyzing GRFs is scarce with (Saggini & Vecchiet, 1994) evaluating soccer footwear on natural turf at a speed of 2.8 m s^{-1}. However, the latter study did not report footwear characteristics, data filtering techniques, surface thickness, nor how the surface was attached to the force platforms. Similarly, it has also been found that studded cleats produce significantly larger peak impact values compared to bladed cleats and turf shoes during sport-specific movements (McGhie & Ettema, 2013), while GRFs were found to be equal in magnitude on different types of turf with the same fourteen studded cleat (Verhelst et al., 2008). Ultimately, past studies have failed to investigate the GRFs produced while wearing cleated footwear with similar stud configurations designed for different sports. Therefore, the purpose of this study was to examine the performance differences in mediolateral and vertical peak GRF (pGRF), time-to-peak GRF (tpGRF), and the rate of force development (RFD) in football cleats (FB), soccer cleats (SOC), and traditional running shoes (RUN) during the braking and propulsive phases of a SCM on artificial turf. It was hypothesized that the FB cleats would produce larger pGRF, tpGRF, and RFD in the mediolateral direction due to the position of bladed cleats at the medio-lateral surface of the outsole while SOC would produce larger values in the vertical direction. Athletes had previously perceived bladed cleats to increase the interaction between the footwear and the surface during the SCM due to a larger contact area (Sterzing, 2016).

METHODOLOGY

Participants

An a-priori analysis using data from the male subjects in Butler et al. (2014) estimated twelve participants were needed based off the following input parameters: ß=.20, α=.05, effect size =.38, and non-sphericity correction of 1.0 while including 9 different measures of 3 groups with an estimated correlation of 0.3 across the measurements. Twelve participants were recruited and completed the study; however, eleven healthy male participants (Age: 21.8 ± 1.5 years; Height: 1.81 ± 0.05 m; Weight: 87.8 ± 14.4 kg) were used for analysis due to equipment malfunction. All participants were actively engaged in football and/or soccer-related activities such as practices, drills, or games at a competitive recreational level while wearing cleats for a minimum of 1 hour per week within the last year. All participants were Exercise

Science students recruited from various classes. Participants were excluded if they had a history of any lower extremity musculoskeletal injury within the past six months or a lower extremity reconstructive surgery within the past three years. The study was approved by the Institutional Review Board (IRB) at The University of Mississippi. Prior to collection, participants were screened for musculoskeletal, orthopedic, and cardiovascular anomalies using the Physical Activity Readiness Questionnaire (PAR-Q) by the American College of Sports Medicine (2013).

Procedures

Participants were tested in all three types of footwear (FB, SOC, RUN) with the order determined by a counterbalanced design. All participants completed a dynamic warm-up (Cazás-Moreno et al., 2015) with additional self-directed stretching of the trunk and lower extermity, if desired. Upon conclusion of the warm-up and prior to testing in each footwear, participants were allowed as many warm-up repetitions of the SCM as necessary. This allowed the participants to adapt to the shoe-surface interaction in order to mimic game-like speed and technique. Participants began in an upright standing start position and were instructed to run towards the force platform at full speed from a distance of 4.57m away to mimic the initial start in a pro-agility drill. An orange cone was placed on the opposite side of the force platform to indicate the location in which they were supposed to plant their foot and perform the SCM. Within each type of footwear, participants were instructed to complete a SCM on their dominant (kicking) leg. The dominant foot made contact with the force platform while they cut and pushed-off in the opposite direction (i.e., right leg dominance: right foot contacts the force platform while participants cut to the left). Similar to previous studies (Smith, Dyson, & Janaway, 2004; Queen et al., 2008), the testing protocol had participants perform between 5-10 SCM in all three footwear conditions until three successful trials occurred. If numerous trials were deemed successful, the first three were used for analysis. A successful trial was defined as when the participant's entire foot made contact with the force platform. To avoid fatigue, a 30-second rest between SCM trials was allotted as well as a 10-minute break between shoe conditions where participants were instructed to sit down without shoes to act as a washout period.

Instrumentation

A 0.4m x 0.4m AMTI OR6-6 (AMTI, Inc., Watertown, MA, USA) force platform embedded into the floor captured GRFs during foot contact at 1000 Hz. Data were filtered using a fourth-order Butterworth with a cutoff frequency set at 15Hz. Vinyl tile covered the force platform matching the rest of the capture volume to reduce targeting. Similar to previous studies (Bennett, Brock, Brosnan, Sorochan, & Zhang, 2015; Brock et al., 2014; Durá, Hoyos, Martinez, & Lozano, 1999), a 1.83m x 8.54m strip of synthetic turf (AstroTurf, Dalton, GA) with a Styrene-Butadiene Rubber (SBR) infill was securely attached to the force platform and runway via Industrial Strength Extreme VELCRO® (Manchester, NH, USA) (Figure 1). Another 1.83m x 8.54m strip of synthetic turf, comprised of the same material, was cut into two 1.83m x 4.27m strips and was placed parallel to the primary runway.

Footwear

The procedures carried out by each participant were completed in a traditional runnning shoe [Nike Dart], soccer cleat [Nike Tiempo Rio II FG], and football cleat [Nike Alpha Strike 2 TD] (Figure 2). Running shoes acted as a control between the cleated footwear conditions while also imitating recreational athletes not utilizing cleated footwear during competition. The footwear for this study was selected based on the popularity of use with local Division-I National Collegiate Athletic Association (NCAA) athletes. Footwear characteristics are listed in Table 1 with the average shoe size worn by the participants being eleven (U.S. sizing). All cleats utilized were new at the time of testing and were properly fitted and laced by the researchers to minimize variability in lacing techniques. No mechanical data were available on footwear differences.

Data Analysis

The first three successful trials collected were averaged to calculate pGRF, tpGRF, and RFD for each participant in all three footwear conditions. All variables of interest were calculated in both the braking and propulsion phases of the SCM in the mediolateral and vertical directions. pGRF was the largest magnitude along the mediolateral and vertical axes. tpGRF depicts the total length of time it takes a participant to reach their peak magnitude. This variable during the braking phase

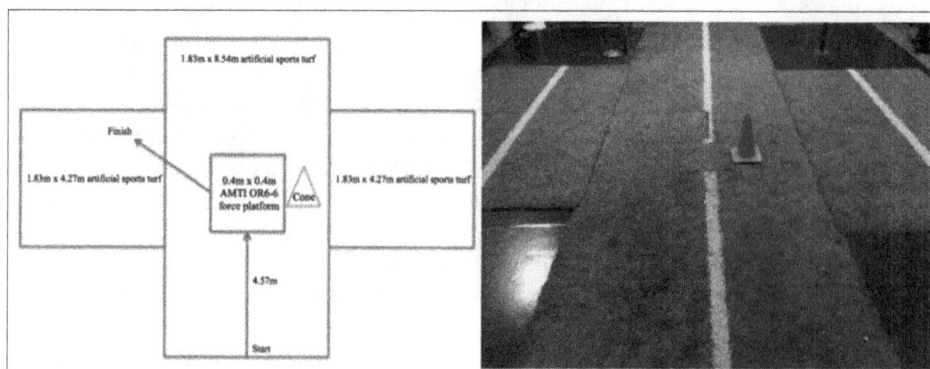

Figure 1. Experimental Setup

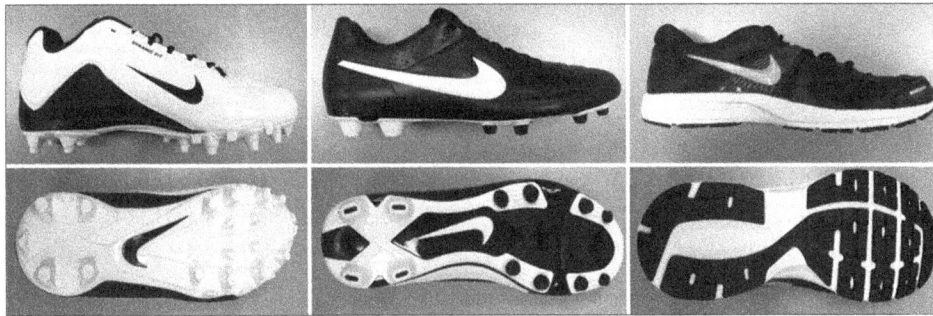

Figure 2. Footwear: Nike Alpha Strike 2 TD Football Cleat (FB); Nike Tiempo Rio II FG Soccer Cleat (SOC); Nike Dart Running Shoe (RUN)

Table 1. Footwear characteristics

	Football cleat (FB)	Soccer cleat (SOC)	Running shoe (RUN)
Mass (kg)	0.318	0.213	0.289
Total # of studs	12	12	n/a
Mid-forefoot stud height (cm)	1.6	1.7	n/a
Medial/lateral forefoot stud height (cm)	2.1	2	n/a
Rearfoot stud height (cm)	2.1	2.4	n/a

looked at the time from initial foot contact (defined as when force increased 1N above body weight) to peak brake, while the propulsion phase was estimated from the time it took from the peak brake time to the peak propulsion time. RFD was determined by the amount of force produced over the change in time within each direction and phase of the SCM (Cazás-Moreno et al., 2015; Haff, Ruben, Lider, Twine, & Cormie, 2015). All kinetic data were normalized to each participant's body weight (N) to allow for comparative analysis.

Statistical Analysis

A 1x3 [1 Condition (SCM) x 3 Footwear (RUN, FB, SOC)] repeated-measures analysis of variance (ANOVA) with an alpha level set at 0.05 was used to measure the effects of the three types of footwear on pGRF, tpGRF, and RFD. If a significant main effect of footwear was found, a Bonferroni post-hoc adjustment was used. Intra-class correlation coefficients (ICC) were then calculated as a reliability measure due to the presence of artificial turf on the force platforms. All analyses were conducted using the SPSS 21 statistical software package (IBM SPSS® Statistics V21.0, Armonk, NY, USA).

RESULTS

There were no statistically significant differences ($p > 0.05$) between footwear when comparing mediolateral and vertical pGRF, tpGRF, or RFD in either the braking or propulsive phases of a SCM (Table 2). However, significant ICCs were present for pGRF in the mediolateral and vertical directions during the braking and propulsion phase as well as RFD in both directions during the braking phase (Table 3).

DISCUSSION

The purpose of this study was to examine the performance differences in mediolateral and vertical pGRF, tpGRF, and

RFD in FB cleats, SOC cleats, and running shoes during the braking and propulsive phases of a SCM on artificial turf. It was hypothesized that the FB cleat would produce larger pGRF, tpGRF, and RFD in the mediolateral direction while the SOC cleat would produce larger values in the vertical direction. The results from this study indicate that there were no statistical differences in any of the kinetic variables of interest between footwear in both the braking and propulsion phases of a SCM. This suggests that footwear, with or without studs, allowed athletes to generate comparable GRFs in a similar time frame. More specifically, football and soccer cleats with similar stud characteristics allow individuals to generate similar forces over a given time frame when performing a SCM. Although no significant differences were present, SOC cleats allowed participants to produce greater forces in the braking and propulsion phase within the mediolateral and vertical directions, respectively. Similarly, SOC cleats had allowed participants to generate faster tpGRF in both directions and phases except for the propulsion phase in the mediolateral direction. This may be explained by the fact the SOC cleat had longer mid-forefoot studs and a lighter mass compared to the FB cleat. Footwear that is lighter with longer studs may provide a greater depth of penetration allowing for a greater shoe-surface interaction; therefore, eliciting greater force production in a shorter time period.

In regard to surfaces, previous literature has shown that artificial turf generates greater peak horizontal forces in translational movements, peak torques in rotation movements, and peak vertical forces in translation/drop tests relative to natural turf (Kent, Forman, Crandall, & Lessley, 2015a). However, since artificial turf has been shown not to tear or divot, the maximum force measured is limited to the maximum force produced by an individual (Kent et al., 2015a). This indicates that varying results may be due to participants' lower extremity strength and experience performing the SCM. Similarly, the exact depth of the infill

Table 2. Kinetic variables of a SCM

Variable (units)	Football cleat (FB)	Soccer cleat (SOC)	Running shoe (RUN)	F-value	η_p^2
Mediolateral braking					
pGRF (BW)	1.55 (0.03)	1.68 (0.24)	1.55 (0.41)	(F (1.447, 14.467)=1.374, P=0.275)	0.121
tpGRF (s)	0.237 (0.052)	0.217 (0.019)	0.214 (0.008)	(F (1.166, 11.661)=1.557, P=0.241)	0.135
RFD (BW/s)	6.81 (1.88)	7.74 (0.98)	7.26 (1.93)	(F (1.393, 13.932)=1.640, P=0.228)	0.141
Vertical braking					
pGRF (BW)	3.86 (0.7)	3.82 (0.7)	3.5 (1.3)	(F (1.368, 13.684)=1.439, P=0.262)	0.126
tpGRF (s)	0.249 (0.052)	0.225 (0.019)	0.224 (0.006)	(F (1.210, 12.096)=2.268, P=0.156)	0.185
RFD (BW/s)	16.04 (4.25)	17.09 (3.43)	15.75 (6.07)	(F (1.734, 17.340)=0.682, P=0.499)	0.064
Mediolateral propulsion					
pGRF (BW)	1.66 (0.24)	1.65 (0.25)	1.57 (0.28)	(F (1.464, 14.638)=1.225, P=0.308)	0.109
tpGRF (s)	0.025 (0.012)	0.033 (0.024)	0.037 (0.012)	(F (1.657, 16.572)=1.148, P=0.331)	0.103
RFD (BW/s)	78.97 (48.7)	59.62 (40.66)	46.2 (12.86)	(F (1.584, 12.673)=1.558, P=0.246)	0.163
Vertical propulsion					
pGRF (BW)	2.45 (0.42)	2.52 (0.45)	2.57 (0.81)	(F (1.903, 19.026)=1.198, P=0.198)	0.019
tpGRF (s)	0.078 (0.024)	0.065 (0.035)	0.066 (0.03)	(F (1.838, 18.380)=0.820, P=0.446)	0.076
RFD (BW/s)	31.15 (10.51)	54.49 (48.83)	36.62 (19.52)	(F (1.309, 11.783)=1.476, P=0.258)	0.141

Data are expressed as means (± SD). Variables: peak ground reaction force (pGRF); time-to-peak ground reaction force (tpGRF); rate of force development (RFD). Units: Body weight (BW), Seconds (s). No significant differences were found between footwear (p>0.05).

Table 3. Intraclass correlation coefficients (ICC)

Variable (units)	ICC	p-value	Confidence intervals	
			Lower bound	Upper bound
Mediolateral braking				
pGRF (BW)	0.801*	0.001	0.448	0.942
tpGRF (s)	−0.063	0.519	−1.948	0.689
RFD (BW/s)	0.727*	0.007	0.243	0.920
Vertical braking				
pGRF (BW)	0.865*	<0.001	0.626	0.961
tpGRF (s)	0.227	0.298	−1.143	0.774
RFD (BW/s)	0.841*	<0.001	0.559	0.954
Mediolateral propulsion				
pGRF (BW)	0.888*	<0.001	0.689	0.967
tpGRF (s)	−0.453	0.724	−3.031	0.575
RFD (BW/s)	−0.484	0.708	−3.637	0.636
Vertical propulsion				
pGRF (BW)	0.722*	0.007	0.228	0.919
tpGRF (s)	0.408	0.153	−0.642	0.827
RFD (BW/s)	−0.177	0.583	−2.448	0.682

Variables: peak ground reaction force (pGRF); time-to-peak ground reaction force (tpGRF); rate of force development (RFD). Units: Body weight (BW), Seconds (s). *Denotes $P<0.05$

and extraneous components that help create the turf construct could alter results. Results from this study are consistent with previous findings (Bennett et al., 2015; Brock et al., 2014; Gehring, Rott, Stapelfeldt, Gollhofer, 2007; Smith et al., 2004) when looking at GRF for various cleats and sport-specific movements. Results showed no differences in vertical pGRF between footwear conditions in this

study. This is supported by Brock et al. (2014) who found no significant differences among peak vertical ground reaction forces and loading rates between natural and synthetic turf cleats, while values were significantly larger when performing a 90° cut versus a 180° cut. Brock et al. (2014) reported values of 5.0 body weight (BW), 5.0 BW, and 4.8 BW for peak vertical GRF in a synthetic turf cleat, natural turf cleat, and running shoe, respectively. Similarly, mediolateral GRF were consistent with 1.4 BW, 1.3 BW, and 1.3 BW, while time-to-peak GRF measured 0.050 s, 0.047 s, and 0.048 s within the same footwear conditions. Values are consistent with, yet slightly higher than the current study; however, the protocol carried out by Brock et al. (2014) had participants complete a single jump followed by a 90° SCM immediately upon landing, potentially accounting for the discrepancies in GRF measurements and impact forces compared to straight-line running.

Differences in RFD were not found between footwear conditions; however, this was expected due to its two calculating variables, force and time, not exhibiting significance. Normalized RFD values have shown to be nearly 103.0 BW/s in running shoes, synthetic turf cleats, and natural turf cleats (Brock et al., 2014) and as low as 21.32 BW/s while wearing a six-studded soccer cleat (Smith et al., 2004). Results match closely with those of the latter study (Smith et al., 2004) taking into account the various phases of the SCM. Smith et al. (2004) reported a loading rate of 21.32 BW/s and 26.09 BW/s for training shoes and soccer cleats, respectively; whereas the current study reports values of 15.75 BW/s and 17.09 BW/s. Utilizing a mechanical device to measure the coefficient of friction of various surfaces and comparing the forces from a 180° turning movement, Dura et al. (1999) concluded that surfaces do not influence maximum GRF, impulse, or total time. However, more time was ultimately spent in the braking phase, similar to the current study, when the frictional force was higher between the cleat and playing surface, while less time was needed to propel the athlete in the desired direction (Durá et al., 1999). During a SCM, a greater frictional force leads to an increase in joint torque; however, while an increase in torque may cause injuries at a joint, added time in the braking phase allows the knee to flex to a greater degree acting as a protective mechanism (Durá et al.,1999). This may indicate that athletes alter their movement based on the shoe-surface interaction.

Often critiqued, placing artificial turf over a force platform will not compromise data. Written in *FIFA Quality Concept for Football Turf: Handbook of Test* Methods (2009) and reported in McGhie et al. (2013), force platform data averaged a mean peak impact which was 98.7% ± 1.2% (range, 98.0-99.8%) of the average recorded by a mechanical apparatus across all artificial turf meeting Fédération Internationale de Football Association (FIFA) standards. It should be noted that this study was limited to a small sample size and it did not control for the participants' approach/running speed and cutting angle to reflect natural on-field SCM mechanics of each participant. However, it has been shown that technique is more important than running speed or cutting angle in regards to preventing injury since it alters posture, muscle activation, and preparation time when it is controlled (Besier, Lloyd, Cochrane, & Ackland, 2001). Future studies should consider the stresses placed on lower extremity joints during a SCM through a kinematic analysis to determine if cleated footwear designed for different sports alter force production. This, in combination with the current study, could poten-

tially provide athletes information to select appropriate and desired footwear without compromising functional comfort for performance or injury risk.

CONCLUSION

To our knowledge, this is the first study to break down the SCM into two distinct phases and analyze how athletic cleats designed for different sports affect kinetic variables in a vertical and mediolateral direction. The SCM is one of many common techniques that allows an athlete to excel on the playing field. It is critical to understand the affect different footwear may have on vertical and mediolateral force generation to assist athletes, parents, and coaches to choose footwear that provides traction to perform the sport movement effectively. The current study suggests commonly worn cleated and non-cleated footwear produce similar GRFs, tpGRFs, and RFD during the braking and propulsion phase of a SCM. While all three types of footwear are providing traction, the similarities between kinetic variables indicate no one footwear analyzed provided specific performance advantages to an athlete in order to rapidly slow down or "brake" and accelerate during a SCM. Future research should examine various cleats with different stud variations to understand how the GRF affect kinematics at the lower extremity.

ACKNOWLEDGEMENTS

The authors would like to thank all of the participants for their time and efforts. The results of the present study do not constitute endorsement of any product and there are no conflicts of interests or affiliations with any of the manufacturers of equipment used.

REFERENCES

American College of Sports Medicine (ACSM). (2017). *ACSM's guidelines for exercise testing and prescription* (10th ed.). Philadelphia, PA: Lippincott, Williams, & Wilkins.

Bennett, H. J., Brock, E., Brosnan, J.T., Sorochan, J.C., & Zhang, S. (2015). Effects of two football stud types on knee- and ankle kinetics of single-leg land-cut and 180° cut movements on infilled synthetic turf. *Journal of Applied Biomechanics, 31*(5). https://doi.org/10.1123/jab.2014-0203

Besier, T. F., Lloyd, D.G., Cochrane, J.L., & Ackland, T.R. (2001). External loading of the knee joint during running and cutting maneuvers. *Medicine and Science in Sports and Exercise, 33*(7), 1168-1175. doi: 10.1097/00005768-200107000-00014

Brock, E., Zhang, S., Milner, C., Liu, X., Brosnan, J.T., & Sorochan, J.C. (2014). Effects of two football stud-configurations on biomechanical characteristics of single-leg landing and cutting movements on infilled synthetic turf. *Sports Biomechanics, 13*(4), 362-379. doi: 10.1080/14763141.2014.965727

Cazás-Moreno, V. L., Gdovin, J.R., Williams, C.C., Allen, C.R., Fu, Y.-C., Brown, L.E., & Garner, J.C. (2015). Influence of whole body vibration and specific warm-ups on force during an isometric mid-thigh pull. *International al Journal of Kinesiology and Sports Science, 3*(4), 31-39. doi: 10.7575/aiac.ijkss.v.3n.4p.31

Clarke, J. & Carré, M. (2010). Improving the performance of soccer boots on artificial and natural soccer surfaces. *Procedia Engineering, 2*(2), 2775-2781. doi: 10.1016/j.proeng.2010.04.065

Driscoll, H., Kelley, J., Kirk, B., Koerger, H., & Haake, S. (2015). Measurement of studded shoe–surface interaction metrics during in situ performance analysis. *Sports Engineering, 18*(2), 105-113. doi: 10.1007/s12283-014-0163-1

Durá, J. V., Hoyos, J., Martinez, A., & Lozano, L. (1999). The influence of friction on sports surfaces in turning movements. *Sports Engineering, 2*, 97-102. doi: 10.1046/j.1460-2687.1999.00024.x

Dvorak, J. & Junge, A. (2000). Football injuries and physical symptoms. A review of the literature. *American Journal of Sports Medicine, 28*(5), S3-9. doi: 10.1177/28.suppl_5.S-3

Fernandez, W. G., Yard, E.E., & Comstock, R.D. (2007). Epidemiology of lower extremity injuries among US high-school athletes. *Academic Emergency Medicine, 14*(7), 641-645. doi: 10.1197/j.aem.2007.03.1354

Fédération Internationale de Football Association (FIFA). (2007). FIFA big count 2006: 270 million people active infootball. *FIFA Communications Division, Information Services, 31*. Available from: www.fifa.com

Gehring, D., Rott, F., Stapelfeldt, B., & Gollhofer, A. (2007). Effect of soccer shoe cleats on knee joint loads. *International Journal of Sports Medicine, 28*(12), 1030-1034. doi: 10.1055/s-2007-965000

Haff, G. G., Ruben, R.P., Lider, J., Twine, C., & Cormie, P. (2015). A comparison of methods for determining the rate of force development during isometric midthigh clean pulls. *The Journal of Strength & Conditioning Research, 29*(2), 386-395. doi: 10.1519/JSC.0000000000000705

Havens, K. L. & Sigward, S.M. (2015). Joint and segmental mechanics differ between cutting maneuvers in skilled athletes. *Gait & Posture, 41*(1), 33-38. doi: 10.1016/j.gaitpost.2014.08.005

Iacovelli, J. N., Yang, J., Thomas, G., Wu, H., Schiltz, T., & Foster, D.T. (2013). The effect of field condition and shoe type on lower extremity injuries in American football. *British Journal of Sports Medicine, 47*(12), 789-793.doi: 10.1136/bjsports-2012-092113

Kent, R., Forman, J.L., Crandall, J., & Lessley, D. (2015a). The mechanical interactions between an American football cleat and playing surfaces in-situ at loads and rates generated by elite athletes: A comparison of playing surfaces. *Sports Biomechanics, 14*(1), 1-17. doi: 10.1080/14763141.2015.1024277

Kent, R., Forman, J.L., Lessley, D., & Crandall, J. (2015b). The mechanics of American football cleats on natural grass and infill-type artificial playing surfaces with loads relevant to elite athletes. *Sports Biomechanics, 14*(2), 246- 257. doi: 10.1080/14763141.2015.1052749

McGhie, D. & Ettema, G. (2013). Biomechanical analysis of surface-athlete impacts on third-generation artificial turf. *The American Journal of Sports Medicine, 41*(1), 177-185. doi: 10.1177/0363546512464697

McGovern, A., Dude, C., Munkley, D., Martin, T., Wallace, D., Feinn, R., Dione, D., & Garbalosa, J.C. (2015). Lower limb kinematics of male and female soccer players during a self-selected cutting maneuver: Effects of prolonged activity. *The Knee, 22*(6), 510-516. Retrieved from https://spts.org

McLean, S. G., Neal, R.J., Myers, P.T., & Walters, M.R. (1999). Knee joint kinematics during the sidestep cutting maneuver: Potential for injury in women. *Medicine and Science in Sports and Exercise, 31*(7), 959-968. doi: 10.1097/00005768-199907000-00007

McNitt, A., Middour, R. & Waddington, D. (1997). Development and evaluation of a method to measure traction on turfgrass surfaces. *Journal of Testing and Evaluation, 25*(1), 99-107. Retrieved from www.astm.org

Meijer, K., Dethmers, J., Savelberg, H., Willems, P., & Wijers, B. (2006). Biomechanical analysis of running on third generation artificial soccer turf. *The Engineering of Sport 6*, 29-34. doi: 10.1007/978-0-387-46051-2_6

National Federation of State High School Associations. (2017). *2016-17 high school athletics participation survey.* Available at: http://www.nfhs.org/ParticipationStatistics/PDF/2016-17_Participation_Survey_Results.pdf

Nigg, B. M. (1989). Surface-related injuries in soccer. *Sports Medicine, 8*(1), 56-62. doi: 10.2165/00007256-198908010-00006

Powell, J. W. & Barber-Foss, K.D. (1999). Injury patterns in selected high school sports: A review of the 1995-1997 seasons. *Journal of Athletic Training, 34*(3), 277. Retrieved from/www.nata.org

Queen, R. M., Charnock, B.L., Garrett, W.E., Hardaker, W.M., Sims, E.L., & Moorman, C.T. (2008). A comparison ofcleat types during two football-specific tasks on FieldTurf. *British Journal of Sports Medicine, 42*(4), 278-284. doi: 10.1136/bjsm.2007.042507

Saggini, R. & Vecchiet, L. (1994). The foot–ground reaction in the male and female soccer players. *Proceedings of the International Society of Biomechanics in Sports XII*, 213-215. Retrieved from https://isbweb.org/resources/journals

Smith, N., Dyson, R., & Janaway, L. (2004). Ground reaction force measures when running in soccer boots and soccer training shoes on a natural turf surface. *Sports Engineering, 7*(3), 159-167. doi: 10.1007/BF02844054

SportsTurf Managers Association (STMA). (2008). *A guide to synthetic and natural turfgrass for sports fields: Selection, construction and maintenance* (2nd ed.). Lawrence, KS: Author.

Sterzing, T. (2016). Soccer boots and playing surfaces. Soccer Science, 339, 179-202. doi: 10.1177/0363546507300257.

Vanrenterghem, J., Venables, E., Pataky, T., & Robinson, M.A. (2012). The effect of running speed on knee mechanical loading in females during side cutting. *Journal of Biomechanics, 45*(14), 2444-2449. doi: 10.1016/j.jbiomech.2012.06.029

Verhelst, R., Malcolm, P., Verleysen, P., Degrieck, J., De Clercq, D., & Philippaerts, R. (2008). Ground reaction force of a drop jump on different kinds of artificial turf. In T. Reilly & F. Korkusuz (Eds.), Science and football VI: The proceedings of the sixth world congress on science and football (pp. 70 - 75). New York City, NY: Routledge.

19

Instructor-led versus Video-led Exercise: A Comparison of Intensity in Obese Youth

Amanda Gier MS[1]*, Nicholas M. Edwards[2], Philip R. Khoury[3], Shelley Kirk[1], Christopher Kist[1], Robert Siegel[1]

[1]Center for Better Health and Nutrition, Cincinnati Children's 3333 Burnet Ave., MLC 5016, Cincinnati, OH, 45229, USA

[2]Orthopaedics, University of Minnesota Medical Center 2450 Riverside Ave. South, Suite R200, Minneapolis, MN, 55454, USA

[3]Heart Institute, Cincinnati Children's, 3333 Burnet Ave., MLC 7002, Cincinnati, OH 45229, USA

Corresponding Author: Amanda Gier MS, E-mail: Amanda.Gier@cchmc.org

ARTICLE INFO

Conflicts of interest: None
Funding: None

ABSTRACT

Background: Exercise is a key component in treating childhood obesity. Group exercise sessions with a trained instructor are ideal, but most treatment programs cannot offer these often enough to meet physical activity guidelines. At-home options that provide a similar-intensity workout are needed. **Objective:** To determine if exercise videos are a feasible at-home option for obese youth to meet recommended physical activity guidelines for moderate-to-vigorous exercise. **Methods:** Obese youth attended a summer camp focused on weight management. Subjects wore accelerometers to assess physical activity levels at camp. During camp, all subjects completed four exercise activities: three separate exercise sessions led by exercise physiologists (EP), as well as an exercise video (EV). Each exercise session utilized a different format: high intensity interval training (HIIT), group games (GG) and yoga. The EV, created by the same EP, included aerobic exercise and yoga. Data was analyzed to determine intensity associated with each exercise session. **Results:** Data was obtained from 16 (50%) accelerometers (9 girls, 7 boys). There was no difference in sedentary (SED) minutes per hour between activities. HIIT and GG had more moderate-vigorous physical activity (MVPA) than yoga ($p<0.0001$ and $p=0.01$) and EV ($p<0.0001$ and $p=0.01$). There was no difference in MVPA between HIIT and GG. **Conclusions:** Obese children exercised at higher intensities during instructor-led HIIT and GG exercise sessions than yoga or EV sessions.

Key words: Obesity, Pediatric Obesity, Overweight, Exercise, Instructional Films and Videos

INTRODUCTION

Over the past thirty years, prevalence of pediatric obesity has increased, placing it among the most important health care issues facing youth (Ogden et al., 2016). Though some studies suggest that pediatric obesity rates may be plateauing, a more in-depth look reveals that rates of severe obesity have increased (Ogden et al., 2016; Skinner, Perrin, & Skelton, 2016). In children and adolescents, obesity is defined as a body mass index (BMI) at the 95th percentile or above for age and gender. "Severe obesity" is classified as ≥120% of the 95th percentile for BMI (Daniels & Kelly, 2014). It is now estimated that 31.8% of youth, ages 2-19, are overweight or obese. Of those, 17% are obese, of which 5.8% can be classified as severely obese (Ogden et al, 2016; Skinner et al., 2016; Ogden, Carroll, Kit, & Flegal, 2014). Youth with overweight and obesity can develop co-morbidities such as hypertension, hyperlipidemia, fatty liver disease, Type 2 diabetes, polycystic ovarian syndrome, orthopedic concerns and obstructive sleep apnea (Kelly et al., 2013; Dietz, 1998; Maggio et al., 2014). Research by the World Obesity Federation has estimated that by 2025, if no effective treatment interventions are identified, 268 million children worldwide, ages 5-17, will be overweight or obese. Of these, an estimated 12.7 million will have impaired glucose tolerance, 4 million will have from type 2 diabetes, 27 million will have hypertension and 38 million will have hepatic steatosis (Lobstein & Jackson Leach, 2016). Pediatric obesity also often leads to adult obesity, co-morbidities and shortened lifespan (Reilly & Kelly, 2011).

Many comprehensive weight management programs for children have been established to address these issues. Physical activity and exercise are important components of these programs. Many programs offer group exercise sessions to their patients. Of 23 pediatric weight management programs surveyed, 74% offered patients the opportunity to participate in group exercise classes (Kist et al., 2016). However, these exercise classes are not always offered daily, and some patients may not be able to attend group sessions due to distance, lack of transportation or scheduling conflicts. Because of this, weight management programs also provide prescriptions for at-home exercise, often consisting of age-appropriate exercise like active play. However, children often face barriers to exercise at home. Many children don't know what type of exercise they can do indoors, especially within the confines of small space or no equipment. Lack of safe outdoor environments and equipment (Kottyan, Kottyan, Edwards, & Unaka, 2014; Lee et al., 2015) as well as extreme weather conditions (Edwards et al., 2015) can limit free play. In addition, independent free play outdoors may not be of sufficient intensity to meet activity guidelines. Previous research done by this group found that in obese youth who attended a week-long summer camp, group exercise led by an exercise physiologist was superior to self-paced exercise in achieving higher levels of moderate-to-vigorous physical activity (MVPA)(Gier et al., 2014). Ideally, exercise done by patients at home will be of sufficient intensity to meet the current guidelines set for children. Current recommendations state that children should accumulate at least 60 minutes of daily activity. Additionally, most of the 60 minutes should be aerobic in nature and of moderate or vigorous intensity. Vigorous intensity exercise should be included at least three days each week (US Department of Health and Human Services, 2008). According to the 2016 United States Report Card on Physical Activity for Children and Youth, only 22% of US children and adolescents, ages 6-19, meet the current recommendations of 60 minutes of MVPA at least 5 days per week (National Physical Activity Plan Alliance).

Exercise videos may help remove some of these barriers to achieving the recommended amount and intensity of exercise. They can be done in the safety of a patient's home with little-to-no costly equipment and overcome the barriers of distance, schedules and transportation (Killen, Barry, Cooper, & Coons, 2014). In addition, they can serve to provide patients with age-appropriate exercises of adequate intensity, recommended and demonstrated by exercise professionals (Gothe et al., 2015). Some research has been conducted using exercise videos for home workouts in various age groups and health conditions. At the conclusion of a 6-month study with older adults, those participating in a home exercise program via DVD accumulated more time in MVPA than those in the control group, when measured via accelerometers and self-report (Gothe et al., 2015). Conversely, a study of college-aged females found that subjects completed identical workouts at a higher intensity with a live personal trainer versus a pre-recorded video session (Killen et al., 2014). Regarding the use of exercise videos in children, a 2002 pilot study in a school setting found that over half of the participating first and second grade students were excited about actively following along with a 15-minute interactive video about health (Levin, Martin, McKenzie, & DeLouise). Another school-based study found that during an indoor recess, children following along to a dance video were physically active for 68% of the recess period (Erwin, Koufoudakis, & Beighle, 2013). A more recent pilot study found that pre-school children engaging in a "movement-to-music" exercise video with their mothers at home accumulated more light and MVPA than children who did not use the video (Tuominen, Husu, Raitanen, & Luoto, 2016). However, a follow-up randomized controlled trial found no significant differences in light activity, MVPA or sedentary time between children using the video and the control group (Tuominen, Husu, Raitanen, Kujala, & Luoto, 2017).

Other technology-driven interventions, such as internet-based activity or active videos games, have also been researched. A review of literature examining the use of technology in adolescent obesity interventions found that, out of eleven studies, six saw improvements in physical activity measures (Chen & Wilkosz, 2014). A review of studies looking at active video games found that they produced similar intensity levels to traditional, moderately active free play and sports (Peng, Lin, & Crouse, 2011). In addition to removing physical barriers to exercise, utilizing technology in pediatric obesity interventions may help increase motivation. Screens and technology continue to become more ever-present in the daily lives of children and adolescents. In children under the age of 8 years old, 98% have access to both televisions and mobile devices in their homes; 95% have at least one smart phone in the home, and 78% have access to tablets. In this age group, 42% have their own "personal" tablet (Common Sense, 2017). In households of "tweens," defined as children ages 8-12 years old, 94% have televisions, 79% have smart phones and 80% have tablets. In households with teenagers, ages 13-18 years old, 95% have televisions, 84% have smart phones and 73% have tablets. 24% of tweens and 67% of teens have their own smart phones, while 53% of tweens and 37% of teens have their own tablets (Common Sense, 2015).

These statistics suggest that screens are a very familiar medium for youth today. Quelly, Norris and DiPietro (2015) refer to young people as "digital natives accustomed to interacting with computers and cell phones for most of their lives." Because children have grown up with technology and seem drawn to it, it seems plausible that incorporating this technology into exercise prescriptions may serve as a way to increase motivation. A systematic review of the use of mobile apps in pediatric obesity interventions found that one study improved "positive attitudes" toward specific exercises, while three other studies demonstrated increased motivation through the use of apps (Quelly et al., 2015). A review of exergaming studies conducted in "field-based settings, such as schools, communities and homes," found three interventions demonstrating a positive outcome with regards to enjoyment and motivation to exercise through the use of active video games (Gao & Chen, 2014). For pediatric weight management programs that are unable to offer group exercise classes, or for their patients who have barriers to attending classes, it is necessary to offer motivating options for at-home exercise to help children meet guidelines for frequency, duration and intensity of daily exercise. The findings above suggest that it may be feasible to use exercise videos or other technology with obese children to increase higher intensity exercise at home. This clinical pediatric weight management program filmed its own exercise video, specifically for youth, with a goal of providing patients with a more structured, higher-intensity option for at-home exercise. The purpose of this study is to analyze the effectiveness and intensity of an exercise video when compared to similar workouts led in-person by an exercise physiologist.

METHODS

Design of Study and Participants

The Institutional Review Board at Cincinnati Children's Hospital Medical Center approved the study protocol. This is a quantitative quasi-experimental, within-subjects study of exercise intensity in overweight and obese children. Current patients of a clinical weight management program were invited to attend a 6-day summer camp. Camp consisted of a variety of daily activities of various intensity, as well as healthy meals and snacks. Participation in camp was limited to patients ages 9-13 years old. Non-English speaking patients were excluded from the study. All campers and their legal guardians were approached and offered the opportunity to participate in the study. Informed consent and assent (ages 11-13) was obtained. Thirty-two campers enrolled in the study. All subjects were assigned to the physical activity intervention. Each subject completed each of four exercise activities.

Study procedures

Accelerometers were individually programmed with gender, date of birth, height and weight of each subject. Accelerometers were labeled with each subject's study ID number. Camp counselors were provided with each subject's study ID to ensure the same accelerometer was used by each subject throughout the week. Subjects wore their accelerometers at the waist on their non-dominant side. Accelerometers were worn at all times during camp except when swimming, bathing and sleeping. Accelerometers were collected from subjects at the conclusion of camp. During the week of camp, all subjects completed four exercise activities. Three activities were led by an exercise physiologist (EP), and one activity was conducted via exercise video (EV). An EP led all subjects through exercise sessions on three separate mornings. The duration of each EP-led activity was approximately 20-30 minutes. Each EP-led exercise session utilized a different format: high intensity interval training (HIIT), yoga and active group games (GG). All EP-led sessions included a brief warm-up and cool-down. The EV activity included aerobic exercise, yoga, a warm-up and cool-down. Subjects followed along with the on-screen exercises for approximately 52 minutes. The EV was created for obese youth by the same EP guiding the instructor-led exercise activities.

Outcome Measures

The primary outcome measures of this study were sedentary minutes and moderate-to-vigorous minutes per exercise activity, objectively assessed through the use of triaxial accelerometers (RT3, Stayhealthy Research®). Activity counts per hour were assessed as a secondary outcome measure. Accelerometers were placed on subjects during their first morning at camp and continuously recorded activity throughout the week. The camp schedule of daily activities was used to establish timeframes of measurement to isolate only the EP-led and video-led exercise sessions for data analysis.

Analysis

Statistical Analysis Software (SAS®) was used to clean and process data. Mixed models repeated measures analyses were performed to account for multiple observations per subject. The covariance structure used in these analyses was compound symmetry. Exercise session and subject id were fixed effects, with id being repeated. The estimation method was restricted maximum likelihood (REML). Differences in mean levels of moderate-to-vigorous minutes, sedentary minutes and activity counts per hour between exercise activities were compared using LSMEANS. Results were considered significant at a value of $p \leq 0.05$.

RESULTS

Usable data were obtained from 16 accelerometers (50%). Data were obtained from 9 girls and 7 boys. Mean age of subjects was 11.3 ± 1.2 years. Mean BMI was 31.5 ± 5.3 kg/m² with a BMI z-score of 2.32 (Table 1). In a mixed models analysis, exercise activity had a significant effect on sedentary minutes ($F_{(4,43)}=128$, $p<0.0001$), MVPA ($F_{(4,43)}=19$, $p<0.0001$) and activity counts per hour ($F_{(4,43)}=34$, $p<0.0001$). There was no significant difference in sedentary (SED) minutes per hour between any of the activities (all $p \geq 0.19$) (Table 2). HIIT and GG produced more MVPA than yoga ($p<0.0001$ and $p=0.01$) and EV ($p<0.0001$ and $p=0.01$) (Table 3) (Figure 1). There was no significant difference in MVPA between HIIT and GG ($p=0.12$), though HIIT elicited significantly higher activity counts per hour (mean value=1002) than GG (mean value=854) ($p=0.02$) (Table 4).

DISCUSSION

While the exercise video used in this study effectively reduced sedentary time, obese children did not attain as much

Table 1. Characteristics of participants

Variables	Group (n=16)	Males (n=7)	Females (n=9)
Age (year)	11.3±1.2	11.3±1.0	11.2±1.5
Height (cm)	156.2±10.5	153.8±10.6	158.1±10.7
Weight (kg)	78.0±20.8	70.3±15.0	84.0±23.5
BMI (kg/m²)	31.5±5.3	29.5±4.0	33.1±5.9

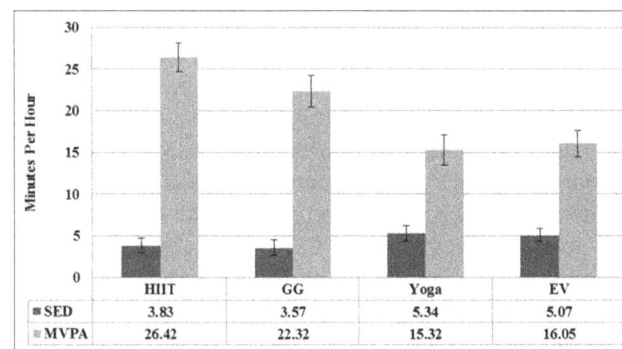

	HIIT	GG	Yoga	EV
■ SED	3.83	3.57	5.34	5.07
■ MVPA	26.42	22.32	15.32	16.05

Figure 1. Differences in sedentary and moderate-to-vigorous minutes per hour between high-intensity interval training

Table 2. Difference in sedentary minutes between per hour between exercise activities

Activity	Activity	Difference(minutes)	Standard Error	DF	t-value	p-value
GG	Yoga	−1.7692	1.3308	43	−1.33	0.1907
GG	EV	−1.5064	1.2328	43	−1.22	0.2284
GG	HIIT	−0.2592	1.3219	43	−0.20	0.8454
Yoga	EV	0.2628	1.1912	43	0.22	0.8264
Yoga	HIIT	1.5099	1.2975	43	1.16	0.2509
EV	HIIT	1.2471	1.1983	43	1.04	0.3038

High-intensity interval training (HIIT), group games (GG) and exercise video (EV)

Table 3. Difference in moderate-to-vigorous minutes per hour between exercise activities

Activity	Activity	Difference(minutes)	StandardError	DF	t-value	p-value
GG	Yoga	6.9947	2.6082	43	2.68	0.0103
GG	EV	6.2639	2.4161	43	2.59	0.0130
GG	HIIT	−4.1006	2.5907	43	−1.58	0.1208
Yoga	EV	−0.7308	2.3346	43	−0.31	0.7558
Yoga	HIIT	−11.0953	2.5428	43	−4.36	<0.0001
EV	HIIT	−10.3645	2.3486	43	−4.41	<0.0001

High-intensity interval training (HIIT), group games (GG) and exercise video (EV)

Table 4. Difference in activity counts per hour between exercise activities

Activity	Activity	Difference(counts)	Standard Error	DF	t-value	p-value
GG	Yoga	214.32	61.6352	43	3.48	0.0012
GG	EV	143.80	57.0966	43	2.52	0.0156
GG	HIIT	−147.89	61.2215	43	−2.42	0.0200
Yoga	EV	−70.52	55.1707	43	−1.28	0.2080
Yoga	HIIT	−362.21	60.0907	43	−6.03	<0.0001
EV	HIIT	−291.69	55.5005	43	−5.26	<0.0001

High-intensity interval training (HIIT), group games (GG) and exercise video (EV)

MVPA during the video as they did during EP-led group exercise, such as active games and HIIT. Children were engaged in MVPA 44% of the time spent participating in HIIT and 37% of time spent participating in GG. The difference between HIIT and GG was not significant. However, time spent in MVPA during the exercise video (27%) was significantly lower. MVPA during instructor-led yoga (25%) was comparable to the EV and lower than HIIT and GG. This suggests that obese children are more likely to meet recommendations for MVPA when completing workouts in person instead of via an exercise video. Screens and technology now occupy a large part of the everyday life of children. Common Sense Media found that children between the ages of 8 and 12 years old engage in "entertainment media" almost 6 hours per day, and teenagers average close to 9 hours daily (2015). Health interventions are increasingly capitalizing on this widespread use of technology as a new way to deliver programming. Exercise videos, in particular, are one method. The purpose of this study was to determine if the use of an EV by obese youth resulted in a similar intensity workout to a session being delivered in-person by an exercise physiologist. The results demonstrated the EV is less effective.

Children may be more willing to push themselves to work at a higher intensity with an exercise physiologist present. In the study of college-aged women completing an identical workout with a trainer and then via an exercise DVD, it was suggested that an in-person trainer provides greater levels of encouragement, leading to increased effort. The researchers arrived at this conclusion in part because the women reported no significant differences in enjoyment, comfort or confidence between the sessions (Killen et al., 2014). A study examining physical activity during indoor recess in a sample of 8- to 12-year-old students utilized custom dance videos. The students did these with no instruction or encouragement from an in-person adult. Results showed children spent approximately 22% of the indoor recess engaged in MVPA (Erwin et al., 2013), similar to the results of 27% with the exercise video in this current study. While the video was not as effective as in-person exercise sessions with an exercise physiologist, it may still yield higher exercise intensities than self-paced workouts at home. Though intended for home use, the exercise video was examined in a group summer camp setting for ease of assessment. Future research may determine if obese youth using the exercise video at home work at higher intensities than during self-chosen physical activity such as walking, biking or sports with friends in a home or community environment. Further studies could also look at effectiveness of the exercise video when obese youth do not have the option of outdoor play or exercise, due to weather or safety. Obese youth given access to an exercise video may accumulate more intense activity and less sedentary time inside versus children without a video. With this, it would be beneficial to examine delivery method of home workouts, as well. With rapidly changing technology, children may be more apt to perform exercise when they can access it through an app or streaming device versus the more outdated DVD.

One limitation of the study is that the video included both yoga and aerobic exercise, while yoga was evaluated independently when analyzing EP-led group exercise. Future research could examine only the aerobic portions of the EV to better compare intensities between EP-led and video-led exercise in obese youth, which may lead to higher percentages of time being spent in MVPA during an EV (Gier et al., 2015). This study had other limitations. Sample size was small, limited by total number of accelerometers available and reliability of devices – only 16 accelerometers (50%) had usable data. This study does not examine long-term adherence to exercise videos in a pediatric population. Future research could examine this, as well as age or gender differences associated with enjoyment, effort and intensity levels when using exercise videos for home workouts.

CONCLUSION

A variety of exercise formats can be used in exercise prescriptions to improve health and BMI in obese youth by reducing sedentary time and meeting the guidelines of 60 minutes of daily MVPA. Thus, while exercise videos were not as effective as instructor-led workouts to elicit MVPA, they can be offered to obese youth as a safe, low-cost, potentially motivating option for at-home exercise.

REFERENCES

Chen, J.L., & Wilkosz, M.E. (2014). Efficacy of technology-based interventions for obesity prevention in adolescents: a systematic review. *Adolescent Health, Medicine and Therapeutics, 5,* 159-170.

Common Sense Media. (2015). *The Common Sense census: media use by tweens and teens.* Retrieved from http://cdn.cnn.com/cnn/2017/images/11/07/commonsense-census.mediausebytweensandteens.2015.final.pdf.

Daniels, S.R., & Kelly, A.S. (2014). Pediatric severe obesity: time to establish serious treatments for a serious disease. *Childhood Obesity, 10*(4), 283-284.

Dietz, W.H. (1998). Health consequences of obesity in youth: childhood predictors of adult disease. *Pediatrics, 101*(3 pt 2), 518-525.

Edwards, N.M., Myer,G.D., Kalkwarf, H.J., Woo, J.G., Khoury, P.R., Hewett, T.E., & Daniels, S.R. (2015). Outdoor temperature, precipitation, and wind speed affect physical activity levels in children: a longitudinal cohort study. *Journal of Physical Activity and Health, 12*(8):1074-81.

Erwin, H., Koufoudakis, R., & Beighle, A. (2013). Children's physical activity levels during indoor recess dance videos. *Journal of School Health, 83*(5), 322-327.

Gao, Z., & Chen, S. (2014). Are field-based exergames useful in preventing childhood obesity? A systematic review. *Obesity Reviews, 15*(8), 676-691.

Gier, A., Edwards, N.M., Jimenez-Vega, J., Kist, C., Khoury, P.R., Siegel, R., & Kirk, S. (2014). Physical activity: intensity and associated energy expenditure during a youth weight management camp. *Medicine and Science in Sports and Exercise, 46*(5S), 227.

Gier, A., Edwards, N.M., Khoury, P.R., Kirk, S., Kist, C., & Siegel, R. (2015). Instructor-led vs. video-led group exercise: comparison of intensity in obese youth. *Medicine and Science in Sports and Exercise, 47*(5S), 385.

Gothe, N.P., Wójcicki, T.R., Olson, E.A., Fanning, J., Awick, E., Chung, H.D.,…McAuley, E. (2015). Physical activity levels and patterns in older adults: the influence of a DVD-based exercise program. *Journal of Behavioral Medicine, 38,* 91-97.

Kelly, A.S., Barlow, S.E., Rao, G., Inge, T.H., Hayman, L.L., Steinberger, J.,…Daniels, S.R. (2013). Severe obesity in children and adolescents: identification, associated health risks, and treatment approaches. A scientific statement from the American Heart Association. *Circulation, 128*(15), 1689-1712.

Killen, L.G., Barry, V.W., Cooper, C., & Coons, J.M. (2014). Live vs. digital video disk exercise in college-aged females. *Journal of Strength and Conditioning Research, 28*(12), 3393-3398.

Kist, C., Gier, A., Tucker, J., Barbieri, T.F., Johnson-Branch, S., Moore, L.,…Coleman, N. (2016). Physical activity in clinical pediatric weight management programs: current practices and recommendations. *Clinical Pediatrics, 55*(13), 1219-1229.

Kottyan, G., Kottyan, L., Edwards, N.M., & Unaka, N.I. (2014 Jun). Assessment of active play, inactivity and perceived barriers in an inner city neighborhood. *Journal of Community Health, 39*(3):538-44.

Lee, H., Tamminen, K.A., Clark, A.M., Slater, L., Spence, J.C., & Holt, N.L. (2015). A meta-study of qualitative research examining determinants of children's independent active free play. *International Journal of Behavioral Nutrition and Physical Activity, 12*(5).

Levin, S., Martin, M.W., McKenzie, T.L., & DeLouise, A.C. (2002). Assessment of a pilot video's effect on physical activity and heart health for young children. *Family and Community Health, 25*(3), 10-17.

Lobstein, T., & Jackson-Leach, R. (2016). Planning for the worst: estimates of obesity and comorbidities in school-age children in 2025. *Pediatric Obesity, 11*(5), 321-325.

Maggio, A.B.R., Martin, X.E., Gasser, C.S., Gal-Duding, C., Beghetti, M., Farpour-Lambert, N.J., & Chamay-Weber, C. (2014). Medical and non-medical complications among children and adolescents with excessive body weight. *BMC Pediatrics, 14,* 232.

National Physical Activity Plan Alliance. (2016). *2016 US report card on physical activity for children and youth.* Retrieved from http://www.physicalactivityplan.org/

projects/reportcard.html.

Ogden, C.L., Carroll, M.D., Lawman, H.G., Fryar, C.D., Kruszon-Moran, D., Kit, B.K., & Flegal, K.M. (2016). Trends in obesity prevalence among children and adolescents in the United States, 1988-1994 through 2013-2014. *Journal of the American Medical Association, 315*(21), 2292-2299.

Ogden, C.L., Carroll, M.D., Kit, B.K., & Flegal, K.M. (2014). Prevalence of childhood and adult obesity in the United States, 2011-2012. *Journal of the American Medical Association, 311*(8), 806-814.

Peng, W., Lin, J.H., & Crouse, J. (2011). Is playing exergames really exercising? A meta-analysis of energy expenditure in active video games. *Cyberpsychology, Behavior, and Social Networking, 14*(11), 681-688.

Quelly, S.B., Norris, A.E., & DiPietro, J.L. (2015). Impact of mobile apps to combat obesity in children and adolescents: a systematic review. *Journal for Specialists in Pediatric Nursing, 21*(1), 5-17.

Reilly, J.J., & Kelly, J. (2011). Long-term impact of overweight and obesity in childhood and adolescence on morbidity and premature mortality in adulthood: systematic review. *International Journal of Obesity, 35*(7), 891-898.

Skinner, A.C., Perrin, E.M., & Skelton, J.A. (2016). Prevalence of obesity and severe obesity in US children, 1999-2014. *Obesity, 24*(5), 1116-1123.

Tuominen, P.P.A., Husu, P., Raitanen, J., Kujala, U.M., & Luoto, R.M. (2017). The effect of a movement-to-music video program on the objectively measured sedentary time and physical activity of preschool-aged children and their mothers: a randomized controlled trial. *PLOS One, 12*(8), e0183317. https://doi.org/10.1371/journal.pone.0183317.

Tuominen, P.P.A., Husu, P., Raitanen, J., & Luoto, R.M. (2016). Differences in sedentary time and physical activity among mothers and children using a movement-to-music video program in the home environment: a pilot study.

SpringerPlus, 5(93). doi: 10.1186/s40064-016-1701-z. US Department of Health and Human Services. (2008). Active Children and Adolescents. In *2008 Physical activity guidelines for Americans; ODPHP Publication No. U0036* (Chapter 3). Retrieved from https://health.gov/paguidelines/pdf/paguide.pdf.

20

Four Weeks of Muscular Endurance Resistance Training Does Not Alter Fatigue Index

John W. Farrell , Daniel J. Blackwood, Rebecca D. Larson,

Department of Health and Exercise Science, University of Oklahoma 1401 Asp Ave, Norman, OK 73019, USA

Corresponding Author: John Farrell, E-mail: John.W.Farrell-1@ou.edu

ARTICLE INFO

Conflicts of interest: None
Funding: None

ABSTRACT

Background of Study: The implementation of a muscular endurance resistance training (MERT) program has been shown to be beneficial in augmenting the onset of blood lactate accumulation (OBLA). However, the effects of MERT on local muscular endurance has not been investigated. **Objectives:** The purposes of the current study were to investigate the effects of 4 weeks of MERT on local muscular endurance, and the relationship between OBLA and fatigue index (FI). **Methods:** Endurance trained males were randomly designated to either the experimental (EX) or control (CON) group: 9 EX and 8 CON. All participants continued current aerobic training. Baseline measures included OBLA, 1 repetition maximum (1RM) for: leg press (LP), leg curl (LC), and leg extension (LE). FI of the quadriceps was assessed via a dynamometer and the Thorstesson protocol. In addition, the EX group performed supervised MERT training for four weeks. A two way ANOVA was used to assess group and time differences in performance measures. The relationship between OBLA and FI was assessed using Pearson's Correlation. **Results**: No significant group differences were observed in all baseline measurements ($p > 0.05$). There were no significant group or time differences for OBLA and FI ($p > 0.05$). Pearson's correlation revealed no significant relationship ($p > 0.05$, $r = <0.01$) existed between FI and OBLA. **Conclusions:** It was observed that four weeks of MERT provided an insufficient stimulus to improve OBLA and FI, and no significant relationship existed between OBLA and FI. Athletes using MERT should include additional mesocycles for favorable adaptations to local muscular endurance and OBLA.

Key words: Lactate, Physical Endurance, Strength Training, Fatigue

INTRODUCTION

Endurance sports and events consist of performing muscular contractions at submaximal intensities for either a prolonged period of time or for numerous repetitions. The nature and physiological demands of endurance sports enhance the susceptibility of participants to the development of fatigue. Due to the complex nature of fatigue several different definitions are used to describe it in the field of exercise physiology. One that seems to encompass its many facets defines fatigue as "the sensation of tiredness and associated decrements in muscular performance and function (Abbiss & Laursen, 2005; Green, 1997; Kay et al., 2001)." Performance in most endurance sports or events is mainly determined by the maximal sustainable power or speed/pace for a given competition distance (Rønnestad & Mujika, 2014). As fatigue develops, the ability to maintain greater power production or speed/pace is inhibited (Abbiss & Laursen, 2005; Rønnestad & Mujika, 2014). Due to this inhibition, endurance athletes and coaches focus on utilizing training methodologies that enhance performance through improved fatigue resistance. Previous research suggests metabolite, e.g. lactate, accumulation during exercise exacerbates the development of fa-

tigue. A strong correlation has been shown to exist between increases in lactate concentration and decreases in cycling performance (Abbiss & Laursen, 2005; Ainsworth, Serfass, & Leon, 1993; Liedl, Swain, & Branch, 1999). An important threshold used by researchers and practitioners to mark shifts and improvements in lactate kinetics is the onset of blood lactate accumulation (OBLA) (Santos-Concejero et al., 2013; TANAKA, 1990). OBLA is the exercise intensity that corresponds to 4mmol/L of blood lactate concentration, and also marks the transition from a tolerable exercise intensity or workload to one that is considered severe (Chmura & Nazar, 2010; Figueira, Caputo, Pelarigo, & Denadai, 2008). A rightward shift in OBLA to a higher workload or percentage of VO_2max will theoretically result in reduced levels of fatigue and improved endurance performance (Faude, Kindermann, & Meyer, 2009; Hostrup & Bangsbo, 2017).

Evidence shows that endurance training supplemented with resistance training has an additive effect on endurance performance through enhanced improvements in exercise economy, anaerobic capacity, maximal power and speed/pace (Farrell III, Lantis, Ade, Bemben, & Larson, 2017; Farrell III, Lantis, Ade,

Cantrell, & Larson, 2018; Lantis, Farrell, Cantrell, & Larson, 2017; Losnegard et al., 2011; Rønnestad & Mujika, 2014). Resistance training utilizing higher repetitions with lower resistance and short recovery periods between sets has been used as a potential stimulus for enhancing muscular endurance and fatigue resistance (Farrell III et al., 2017; Farrell III et al., 2018; Lantis et al., 2017). Muscular endurance resistance training (MERT) consists of performing multiple sets of 12 to 15 repetitions at 50% of 1RM with ≤ 1 minute of rest between sets of exercise (Farrell III et al., 2017; Farrell III et al., 2018; Lantis et al., 2017). A bout of MERT has been shown to induce an accumulation of blood lactate to values similar to that reported by HIT, and induce improvements in OBLA and 1RM strength when combined with aerobic training in aerobically active individuals (Edge, Hill-Haas, Goodman, & Bishop, 2006; Farrell III et al., 2017; Farrell III et al., 2018; Lantis et al., 2017; Rogatzki, Wright, Mikat, & Brice, 2014). However, there has been little research into the effects a concurrent training program, consisting of both endurance and MERT, has on local muscular endurance and how muscular endurance relates to endurance performance variables. It can be speculated that a positive relationship between muscular endurance and OBLA exists. Individuals that are capable of maintaining high levels of strength over several repetitions theoretically should possess enhanced lactate kinetics. Also, it can be speculated that performing MERT, which has been shown to improve OBLA, should increase fatigue resistance as indicated by sustained strength while performing several repetitions. Therefore, the purpose of the current study is to examine the relationship between OBLA and local muscular endurance. Additionally, the current study aims to investigate the adaptations of both local muscular endurance and OBLA to a mesocycle (4 weeks) of MERT. The current researchers hypothesize that local muscular endurance and OBLA will exhibit a significant relationship. Also, it is hypothesized that both local muscular endurance and OBLA will exhibit significant improvements following one mesocycle of MERT.

METHODS

Subjects and Design of Study

Nineteen participants (18-37 years old) were recruited for this randomized controlled trial. 17 participants completed the study with 2 participants dropping out due to time commitment issues. Subjects were randomly divided into an experimental (EX) group, whose regular aerobic training was supplemented with a MERT program, or a control (CON) group, who continued their regular aerobic exercise training without the addition of MERT. All subjects were considered to be aerobically active and had not participated in any resistance training for 6 months prior to start of the study, determined by a self-reported physical activity questionnaire. Aerobically active was defined as having participated in aerobic exercise at least one hour per day for 3 days per week for the past 6 months. The current cohort consisted of 8 runners, 8 cyclist, and 1 triathlete. All subjects were required to reach a VO_2max of at least 40 ml/kg/min to participate in the study. This threshold has been used previously in similar studies and indicates an aerobic capacity of good/excellent (Farrell III et al., 2017; Farrell III et al., 2018;

Heyward, 1992; Lantis et al., 2017). This study was approved by the Institutional Review Board at the University of Oklahoma; each subject gave a verbal and written informed consent before participation. All testing and training was completed in an air-conditioned laboratory at a temperature 20-25˚C.

Experimental Protocol

Prior to and following the 4 week training period both groups performed a staged graded exercise test to determine OBLA and VO_2max. The Thorstennson protocol was used to assess the fatigue rate of the knee extensor muscle group of the dominant leg (Thorstensson & Karlsson, 1976). All subjects were instructed to continue their low-intensity aerobic training without making alterations to volume or intensity. In addition to their current low-intensity aerobic training the EX group returned to the laboratory two times per week for four weeks to perform MERT under the supervision of the researchers.

Incremental exercise test

The incremental exercise test protocol utilized has been described elsewhere (Farrell III et al., 2017; Farrell III et al., 2018; Lantis et al., 2017). In short, a resting fingertip capillary blood sample was collected to determine whole blood lactate concentration prior to testing using a commercial lactate meter (Lactate Plus, Nova Biomedical, Waltham, MA). The staged exercise test was initiated at a work rate of 125 watts (W) and increased by 25 W every three minutes until the participant reached task failure indicated by a pedal rate dropping below 50 revolutions per minute. At the end of each of the three-minute stages blood lactate and rating of perceived exertion (RPE), based on the Borg Scale, were measured (Borg, 1971). The W corresponding to 4.0 mmol/L (OBLA) was calculated by plotting W against blood lactate concentration and using linear interpolation (Faude et al., 2009). Metabolic and ventilatory data were continuously measured and averaged over 30 second intervals.

Fatigue index

The fatigability of the knee extensors were assessed following the Thorstensson protocol using a Kin Com dynamometer (KinCom model: KC125AP, Isokinetic International, East Ridge, TN 37412) (Thorstensson & Karlsson, 1976). Subjects performed 50 knee extensions with the dominant leg from the knee joint angle of 90° to 0° (knee fully extended). Constant angular velocity was set at 180°/s. Subjects were instructed to perform extensions with maximal effort and to return to the starting position passively between contractions. Peak force from the load range portion of each contraction was recorded at 1000 Hz. Fatigue Index (FI) was calculated using the following equation:

$$\text{Fatigue Index} = \left[\frac{\left(\text{Average of initial three extensions}\right) - \left(\text{Average of final three extensions}\right)}{\left(\text{Average of initial three extensions}\right)} \right] \times 100$$

Aerobic exercise

Based on previous studies, subjects were instructed to maintain current aerobic training volume and intensity throughout the study (Farrell III et al., 2017; Farrell III et al., 2018; Karsten, Stevens, Colpus, Larumbe-Zabala, & Naclerio, 2016; Lantis et al., 2017). If subjects indicated a decrease of > 1/3 or an increase of > 5% in training volume they were excluded from the study to prevent detraining or additional aerobic adaptations (Fleck, 1994; Haff & Triplett, 2015; Zupan & Petosa, 1995). Also, any indications of an increase in aerobic training intensity resulted in exclusion from the study.

Muscular endurance resistance training

The current training program has been described elsewhere (Farrell III et al., 2017). In short, the training program consisted of supervised sessions on 2 days*wk^{-1} over a four week period to supplement participants' aerobic training program. Participants were instructed to not perform any resistance training outside of the study. Each resistance training session included a warmup consisting of several repetitions at 30 to 40 percent of their 1RM followed by four sets of 12 to 15 repetitions at 50% of the subject's established 1-RM for LP, LC, and LE (Cybex Strength Systems) with 30 seconds of rest between sets and 3 minutes of rest between exercises. If an individual was able to complete four sets of 15 repetitions after 2 weeks (4 training sessions) the training weight was increased by 4.54 kilograms (a 2 to 4% increase) to compensate for any strength gains (Haff & Triplett, 2015; Kraemer & Ratamess, 2004). If participants were unable to complete four sets of 15 repetitions after two weeks the training weight was kept the same.

Statistical analysis

Data are presented as means ± SD. Independent t-tests were utilized to determine if significant between group differences existed for subject characteristics. Data was found to be normally distributed. To determine differences in physiological variables between groups at pre- and post-training a two-way repeated measures analysis of variance (ANOVA) (time and group as factors) was utilized. If the ANOVA reached significance, a Bonferroni-post hoc analysis was performed. Pearson's r correlations were performed to determine the relationship between FI and performance measurements assessed during the GXTs. All statistical analyses were performed using SigmaPlot (Version 12.5, Systat Software Inc., San Jose, CA). Cohen's d effect sizes (ES) were reported for all significant measures. A value of ≤ 0.20 was considered a weak effect, a value of ≤ 0.50 was considered a moderate effect, and a value of ≥ 0.80 was considered a strong effect (Cohen, 1988). An alpha level of $p \leq 0.05$ was set for the level of significance.

RESULTS

Subject Characteristics and Training Compliance

Descriptive characteristics are summarized in Table 1. No statistical differences (p>0.05) existed between groups for age, height, and body mass. Of the 9 subjects included in the EX group all participants completed at least 12 repetitions per set for all training sessions. All subjects met the requirements for increasing training load after the 4th training session.

Performance Measurements

Performance measures collected and assessed are presented in Table 2. No statistically significant differences (p>0.05) were present between groups for VO$_2$max, OBLA, and FI prior to the training intervention. Post-training statistical analysis indicated no significant group X time interaction for all performance variables with no main effects for group or time.

Correlations

Pearson's r correlations were performed to examine the relationship between FI and OBLA. Since no significant differences were observed between groups and between pre- and post-training, both groups and time points were pooled for analysis. It was revealed that no statistically significant relationship between FI and OBLA (r = -0.01 and p = 0.44) exists. This relationship is illustrated in Figure 1.

DISCUSSION

The purposes of the current study were: (1) to examine the effects of aerobic exercise supplemented with 4 weeks of MERT on local muscular endurance, assessed via the FI of the quadriceps, and (2) to examine the relationship between local muscular endurance and variables related to endurance performance, OBLA and VO$_2$max. Analysis from the current study revealed no significant improvements in FI in following the prescribed training intervention. Additionally, no significant relationships were detected between FI and the aerobic performance variables: OBLA and VO$_2$max. The current study did not observe any significant improvements in the FI of the quadriceps following 4 weeks of MERT. This is an interesting finding as previous research pertaining to resistance training using lower loads and higher repetitions have seen improvements in local muscular endurance as well as hypertrophy of Type I muscle fibers (Campos et al., 2002; Mitchell et al., 2012; Brad J. Schoenfeld, Grgic, Ogborn, & Krieger, 2017; Brad J Schoenfeld, Peterson, Ogborn, Contreras, & Sonmez, 2015; Vinogradova et al., 2013). Schoenfeld et al. 2015 prescribed participants to perform 3 sets of 25-35 repetitions at 30 to 50% of 1RM 3 time per week for 8 weeks (Brad J Schoenfeld et al., 2015). It was observed that after completing the training intervention participants saw a significant improvement (16.6%) in the number of repetitions performed to failure for bench press at 50% of 1RM. Additionally, significant increases in the muscle thickness of the elbow flexors and extensors and quadriceps were observed (8.6%, 5.2%, and 9.3% respectively). Differentiation between the Type II (fast twitch) and Type I (slow twitch) fibers was not described in the study by Schoenfeld et al. 2015 (Brad J. Schoenfeld et al., 2017). Previous research has

Table 1. Subject characteristics (Mean ± SD)

| Variables | Groups | | | |
| | Experimental (n = 9) | | Control (n = 8) | |
	Pre	Post	Pre	Post
Age (years)	21.4 ± 2.1	21.6 ± 2.1	25.5 ± 6.4	25.6 ± 6.3
Height (cm)	180.2 ± 5.3	180.2 ± 5.3	179.5 ± 3.9	179.5 ± 3.8
Body mass (kg)	75.2 ± 10.0	75.2 ± 8.6	77.2 ± 11.8	76.6 ± 11.4

Differences if present were denoted using *(p<0.05). Standard deviations represent variability

Table 2. Physiological variables (Mean±SD)

| Variables | Groups | | | | | |
| | Experimental (n = 9) | | | Control (n = 8) | | |
	Pre	Post	Δ%	Pre	Post	Δ%
VO$_2$ max (ml/kg/min)	50.2 ± 7.03	50.9 ± 7.81	1.22 ± 5.81	46.2 ± 3.95	47.3 ± 4.43	2.34 ± 5.16
OBLA (W)	198.3 ± 46.2	191.1 ± 46.5	−3.6 9 ± 6.08	179.5 ± 34.2	183.1 ± 37.3	1.92 ± 5.37
Fatigue index (%)	54.0 ± 18.3	53.9±10.7	−0.01 ± 17.6	57.3 ± 13.1	58.7 ± 14.6	1.40 ± 10.8

Differences if present were denoted using *(p<0.05). Standard deviations represent variability

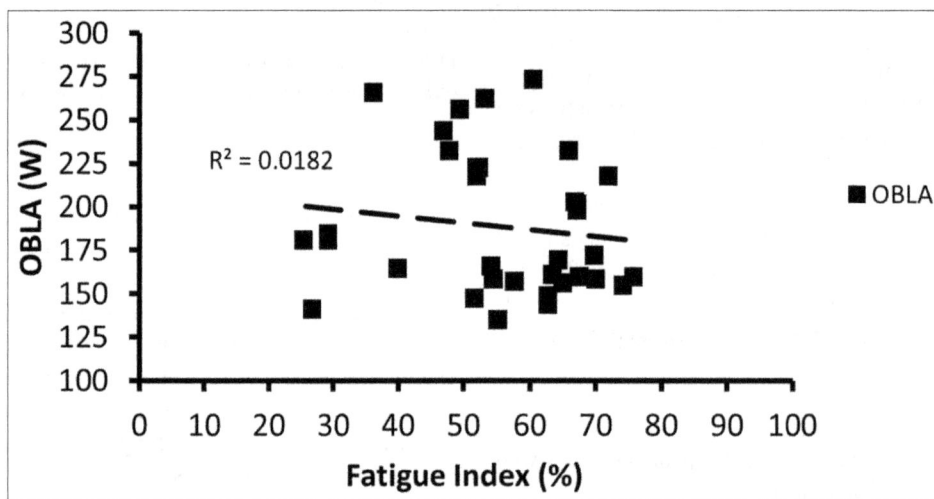

Figure 1. Relationship between FI and OBLA

demonstrated a direct relationship between the growth of muscle fiber types and training load utilized (Brad J. Schoenfeld et al., 2017; Vinogradova et al., 2013). The beneficial effects observed on muscular endurance that training with lower loads has induced in previous studies can been speculated to be partly due to favorable phenotypic adaptions, such as increases in size and proportion, to Type I muscle fibers (Brad J. Schoenfeld et al., 2017; Brad J Schoenfeld et al., 2015).

When utilizing lower loads with higher repetitions longer time-under-load occurs, resulting in a greater increase in metabolic stress compared to traditional resistance training (Burd et al., 2010; Brad J. Schoenfeld et al., 2017; Brad J Schoenfeld et al., 2015; Vinogradova et al., 2013). Metabolic stress is indicated by an increase in calcium flux as well as an accumulation in lactate and hydrogen ions. This stress has been hypothesized to mediate muscle hypertrophy. It has also been shown to favorably affect mitochondrial protein synthesis that may enhance cellular energetics in a manner

that favors fatigue resistance. MERT has been shown to induce a significant increase in metabolic stress indicated by large accumulations of lactate (Farrell III et al., 2017). Theoretically, this accumulation should have provided a stimulation of the proper magnitude to induce adaptations associated with fatigue resistance. However, differences in the volume of stimulus provided through resistance training differs between the current study and previous research, and could provide an explanation for the lack of favorable adaptations (Farrell III et al., 2018; Lantis et al., 2017; Brad J Schoenfeld et al., 2015; Vinogradova et al., 2013). The current researchers speculate that the reason for the lack of improvements in muscular endurance, as seen in previous literature, may be due to differences in length of the current training intervention, total training volume, and training status of participants compared to previous research (Farrell III et al., 2018; Lantis et al., 2017; Brad J. Schoenfeld et al., 2017; Brad J Schoenfeld et al., 2015). Previous research pertaining to MERT and resistance training utilizing low loads and high repetitions, which have observed significant improvements in variables related to fatigue resistance, have been at least 8 weeks in length with 2-3 training sessions per week (Farrell III et al., 2018; Lantis et al., 2017; Brad J Schoenfeld et al., 2015). The current study consisted of 2 training sessions per week for 4 weeks. The length of the current study was chosen to mimic that of the typical length of a training mesocycle. It can be concluded that 4 weeks of MERT with 2 sessions per week is not a sufficient physiological stimulus to induce fatigue resistant adaptions. The current training intervention was concurrent in nature, consisting of both MERT and aerobic training. Although several previous studies have shown that concurrent training has additive effects on endurance performance, it has been shown that concurrent training attenuates adaptations associated with resistance training. It can be speculated that the aerobic training performed in the current study may have attenuated some adaptations compared to if the resistance training had been performed independently (Farrell III et al., 2018; Lantis et al., 2017; Rønnestad & Mujika, 2014). Previous research has speculated that the utilization of low loads during resistance training induces adaptations preferentially to the Type I muscle fibers (Brad J. Schoenfeld et al., 2017; Brad J Schoenfeld et al., 2015; Vinogradova et al., 2013). These previous studies have used both untrained and resistance trained individuals who perhaps possessed underdeveloped Type I muscle fibers, resulting in large adaptations (Brad J Schoenfeld et al., 2015). However, the current study utilized individuals who were aerobically trained, and it can be speculated that these individuals had a much greater degree of development of Type I muscle fibers or Type IIa fibers that were shifted more towards the aerobic end of the spectrum. The greater degree of aerobic adaptions in the current cohort may have blunted the response, and may indicate the need for a greater stimulus to induce a favorable response.

The current study did not observe any improvements in OBLA in the EXP group following the training intervention. Previous research using MERT in aerobically trained individuals has shown improvements in lactate kinetics via an increase in the power output and percentage of VO_2max at which OBLA occurred during a GXT (Farrell III et al., 2018; Lantis et al., 2017). However, as previously mentioned the current training intervention was 4 weeks in length compared to 8 weeks used by previous research (Farrell et al., 2018; Lantis et al., 2017). This finding may provide additional insight into the proper length of training needed to induce favorable adaptions for both OBLA and local muscular endurance in aerobically trained individuals. Additionally, it can be speculated that the due to the current cohort participating in aerobic training they may have possessed a large percentage of Type I muscle fibers and thus an enhanced ability to remove and oxidize lactate from the blood stream. A greater training stimulus maybe required to induce any desired adaptions associated with enhancing lactate kinetics in the current cohort due to their physiological profile and previous training prior to the start of the current training intervention. The same reasoning for the lack of improvements in OBLA may also explain the lack of improvement in the FI of the quadriceps. As previously mentioned the current cohort may

have possessed a large percentage of Type I muscle fibers and previous training was designed to further develop these fibers. This may have reduced the physiological impact that the current training intervention had on the cohort. When examining the relationship between FI and OBLA in the current data set, it appears that no significant relationship exists. The reasoning for the absence of a significant relationship could pertain to the nature of the Thorstensson test and lack of specificity in regards to the aerobic activities performed by the current cohort (Thorstensson & Karlsson, 1976).

The current study is not without its limitations. The assessment of the fatigue index via the Thorstensson protocol may have lacked specificity to not only the aerobic activities that the current cohort participated in, but also the current training intervention. Future studies examining local muscular endurance following a training intervention of MERT may chose to use testing that better reflects the movements and number of repetitions used during the training intervention. Future studies examining the effects of MERT on local muscular endurance should also utilize an intervention closer in length to that used by previous studies (Farrell et al., 2018, Lantis et al., 2017).

CONCLUSION

The current study observed: 1) that 4 weeks (8 training sessions) of MERT did not induce favorable adaptions associated with improved muscular endurance and fatigue resistance and 2) that FI, assessed via the Thorstennson protocol, did not exhibit a significant relationship with OBLA and VO_2max. The current study provides insight into the proper programming of MERT for adaptions associated with fatigue resistance in aerobically active individuals. It appears that 4 weeks, or one mesocycle, is indeed not a sufficient stimulus to induce adaptations. Trainers and coaches should aim to integrate more than one mesocycle of MERT into an endurance athlete's program to allow for an appropriate length of time for adaptations.

ACKNOWLEDGMENTS

No external funding was used to support the current study. The authors have no relationships with any companies who will benefit from the results of the present study.

REFERENCES

Abbiss, C. R., & Laursen, P. B. (2005). Models to explain fatigue during prolonged endurance cycling. *Sports Medicine, 35*(10), 865-898.

Ainsworth, B. E., Serfass, R. C., & Leon, A. S. (1993). Effects of recovery duration and blood lactate level on power output during cycling. *Canadian Journal of Applied Physiology, 18*(1), 19-30.

Borg, G. (1971). The perception of physical performance. *Frontiers of fitness*, 280-294.

Burd, N. A., West, D. W., Staples, A. W., Atherton, P. J., Baker, J. M., Moore, D. R., Baker, S. K. (2010). Low-load high volume resistance exercise stimulates muscle protein synthesis more than high-load low volume resistance exercise in young men. *PLoS One, 5*(8), e12033.

Campos, G. E., Luecke, T. J., Wendeln, H. K., Toma, K., Hagerman, F. C., Murray, T. F., Staron, R. S. (2002). Muscular adaptations in response to three different resistance-training regimens: specificity of repetition maximum training zones. *European journal of applied physiology, 88*(1-2), 50-60.

Chmura, J., & Nazar, K. (2010). Parallel changes in the onset of blood lactate accumulation (OBLA) and threshold of psychomotor performance deterioration during incremental exercise after training in athletes. *International Journal of Psychophysiology, 75*(3), 287-290.

Cohen, J. (1988). *Statistical power analysis for the behavioral sciences (2nd ed.)*. Hillsdale, NJ: Erlbaum.

Edge, J., Hill-Haas, S., Goodman, C., & Bishop, D. (2006). Effects of Resistance Training on H$^+$ Regulation, Buffer Capacity, and Repeated Sprints. *Medicine and Science in Sports and Exercise, 38*(11), 2004.

Farrell III, J. W., Lantis, D. J., Ade, C. J., Bemben, D. A., & Larson, R. D. (2017). Metabolic Response to Four Weeks of Muscular Endurance Resistance Training. *International Journal of Kinesiology & Sports Science, 5*(4), 10.

Farrell III, J. W., Lantis, D. J., Ade, C. J., Cantrell, G. S., & Larson, R. D. (2018). Aerobic exercise supplemented with muscular endurance training improves onset of blood lactate accumulation. *The Journal of Strength & Conditioning Research, 32*(5), 1376-1382.

Faude, O., Kindermann, W., & Meyer, T. (2009). Lactate threshold concepts. *Sports Medicine, 39*(6), 469-490.

Figueira, T. R., Caputo, F., Pelarigo, J. G., & Denadai, B. S. (2008). Influence of exercise mode and maximal lactate-steady-state concentration on the validity of OBLA to predict maximal lactate-steady-state in active individuals. *Journal of Science and Medicine in Sport, 11*(3), 280-286.

Fleck, S. J. (1994). Detraining: Its Effects on Endurance and Strength. *Strength & Conditioning Journal, 16*(1), 22-28.

Green, H. (1997). Mechanisms of muscle fatigue in intense exercise. *Journal of Sports Sciences, 15*(3), 247-256.

Haff, G. G., & Triplett, N. T. (2015). *Essentials of Strength Training and Conditioning 4th Edition*: Human kinetics.

Heyward, V. H. (1992). Advanced Fitness Assessment and Exercise Prescription. *Medicine & Science in Sports & Exercise, 24*(2), 278.

Hostrup, M., & Bangsbo, J. (2017). Limitations in intense exercise performance of athletes–effect of speed endurance training on ion handling and fatigue development. *The Journal of Physiology, 595*(9), 2897-2913.

Karsten, B., Stevens, L., Colpus, M., Larumbe-Zabala, E., & Naclerio, F. (2016). The effects of a sports specific maximal strength and conditioning training on critical velocity, anaerobic running distance and 5-km race performance. *International journal of sports physiology and performance, 11*(1), 80-85.

Kay, D., Marino, F. E., Cannon, J., St Clair Gibson, A., Lambert, M. I., & Noakes, T. D. (2001). Evidence for neuromuscular fatigue during high-intensity cycling in warm, humid conditions. *European journal of applied physiology, 84*(1), 115-121.

Kraemer, W.J., & Ratamess, N.A. (2004) Fundamentals of resistance training: progression and exercise prescription. *Medicine and science in sports and exercise, 36 (4), 674-688.*

Lantis, D. J., Farrell, J. W., Cantrell, G. S., & Larson, R. D. (2017). Eight Weeks of High Volume Resistance Training Improves Onset of Blood Lactate in Trained Individuals. *The Journal of Strength & Conditioning Research.*

Liedl, M. A., Swain, D. P., & Branch, J. D. (1999). Physiological effects of constant versus variable power during endurance cycling. *Medicine and Science in Sports and Exercise, 31*(10), 1472-1477.

Losnegard, T., Mikkelsen, K., Rønnestad, B., Hallén, J., Rud, B., & Raastad, T. (2011). The effect of heavy strength training on muscle mass and physical performance in elite cross country skiers. *Scandinavian journal of medicine & science in sports, 21*(3), 389-401.

Mitchell, C. J., Churchward-Venne, T. A., West, D. W., Burd, N. A., Breen, L., Baker, S. K., & Phillips, S. M. (2012). Resistance exercise load does not determine training-mediated hypertrophic gains in young men. *Journal of applied physiology, 113*(1), 71-77.

Rogatzki, M. J., Wright, G. A., Mikat, R. P., & Brice, A. G. (2014). Blood ammonium and lactate accumulation response to different training protocols using the parallel squat exercise. *The Journal of Strength & Conditioning Research, 28*(4), 1113-1118.

Rønnestad, B. R., & Mujika, I. (2014). Optimizing strength training for running and cycling endurance performance: A review. *Scandinavian journal of medicine & science in sports, 24*(4), 603-612.

Santos-Concejero, J., Granados, C., Bidaurrazaga-Letona, I., Zabala-Lili, J., Irazusta, J., & Gil, S. M. (2013). Onset of blood lactate accumulation as a predictor of performance in top athletes. *Retos. Nuevas tendencias en Educación Física, Deporte y Recreación, 23*, 67-69.

Schoenfeld, B. J., Grgic, J., Ogborn, D., & Krieger, J. W. (2017). Strength and Hypertrophy Adaptations Between Low- vs. High-Load Resistance Training: A Systematic Review and Meta-analysis. *The Journal of Strength & Conditioning Research, 31*(12), 3508-3523. doi: 10.1519/jsc.0000000000002200

Schoenfeld, B. J., Peterson, M. D., Ogborn, D., Contreras, B., & Sonmez, G. T. (2015). Effects of low-vs. high-load resistance training on muscle strength and hypertrophy in well-trained men. *The Journal of Strength & Conditioning Research, 29*(10), 2954-2963.

Tanaka, K. (1990). Lactate-related factors as a critical determinant of endurance. *The Annals of physiological anthropology, 9*(2), 191-202.

Thorstensson, A., & Karlsson, J. (1976). Fatiguability and fibre composition of human skeletal muscle. *Acta Physiologica, 98*(3), 318-322.

Vinogradova, O. L., Popov, D. V., Netreba, A. I., Tsvirkun, D. V., Kurochkina, N. S., Bachinin, A. V., Orlov, O. I. (2013). Optimization of training: New developments in safe strength training. *Human Physiology, 39*(5), 511-523. doi: 10.1134/s0362119713050162

Zupan, M. F., & Petosa, P. S. (1995). Aerobic and Resistance Cross-Training for Peak Triathlon Performance. *Strength & Conditioning Journal, 17*(5), 7-12.

21

Effect of Nasal Versus Oral Breathing on Vo$_2$max and Physiological Economy in Recreational Runners Following an Extended Period Spent Using Nasally Restricted Breathing

George M. Dallam[1]*, Steve R. McClaran[1], Daniel G. Cox[2], Carol P. Foust[1]

[1]Department of Exercise Science, Health Promotion, and Recreation, Colorado State University – Pueblo; Pueblo.2200 Bonforte Boulevard, Pueblo, CO, USA 81001-4901

[2]Staff TherapistArizona Orthopedic Physical Therapy 9980 W. Glendale Rd ste 110 Glendale, AZ 85307

Corresponding Author: George M. Dallam, E-mail: George.Dallam@CSUPueblo.edu

This research was funded by a faculty seed grant from Colorado State University –Pueblo.

ARTICLE INFO

Conflicts of interest: None
Funding: None

ABSTRACT

Background: In subjects who do not practice nasally restricted breathing, peak oxygen uptake (VO$_2$max) and time to exhaustion in a graded exercise protocol (GXT TE) are impaired while breathing nasally versus orally. **Objective:** This study investigated the effect of oral versus nasal breathing on VO$_2$max, GXT TE and physiological economy (PE) in subjects who had previously self-selected a nasal only breathing approach during training and racing. **Methods**: A mixed gender sample (N=10, 5 male and 5 female) of nasal breathing recreational runner's completed a maximal GXT and high level steady state trial at 85% of their maximal GXT running velocity (SS85) in both nasally and orally restricted breathing conditions. **Results:** In the GXT trials the subjects exhibited no significant mean difference in GXT TE, VO$_2$max or peak lactate. However, in the nasally restricted breathing condition they demonstrated a significantly lower mean ventilatory equivalent for both oxygen (VE/VO$_2$) (p = 0.002), and carbon dioxide (VE/VCO$_2$) (p = 0.043) at VO$_{2max}$ with large effect sizes. During the SS85 trials the subjects exhibited a significantly better PE (P = 0.05) and no significant difference in lactate production, as well as a significantly lower mean VE/VO$_2$ (p = 0.002) and VE/VCO$_2$ (p = 0.002) with large effect sizes. **Conclusion:** This study supports the ability of recreational runners to utilize a nasally restricted breathing pattern at all levels of running intensity without loss in VO$_2$max or GXT TE, and with superior PE and VE/VO$_2$, following an extended training period using this practice.

Key words: Lactate, Bronchoconstriction, Ventilatory, Efficiency, Oropharynx, Nasopharynx

INTRODUCTION

Within the last decade, a variety of health professionals and others have posted articles/blogs on the internet describing the value of breathing restricted to the nasopharynx during exercise (Cap, 2016; Mercola, 2013; Rakimov, 2004; Raman, 2006; Ruth, 2015). In general, the largely unexamined theoretical rationale they provide for doing so can be summarized as follows: 1) nasally restricted breathing during exercise allows for the filtration, humidification and temperature regulation of inhaled air in the nasopharynx thereby avoiding the health problems associated with breathing large volumes of unfiltered, non-humidified and non-temperature regulated air while breathing predominately through the oropharynx during exercise, 2) nasally restricted breathing improves oxygenation locally through the release of nitric oxide (NO), a potent vasodilator, and through increased serum carbon dioxide (CO$_2$); a competitive binder of hemoglobin with oxygen (O$_2$), thereby resulting in increased O$_2$ release from hemoglobin at the active tissues. However, many commenters to these same posts describe the sensation of air hunger while attempting to breathe in a nasally restricted manner during exercise, thereby rejecting the notion that such breathing is effective to support high intensity exercise (Cap, 201; Mercola, 2013; Rakimov, 2004; Ramon, 2006). The published research on the use of nasally restricted breathing during exercise is limited, however the following observations have been made. The vast majority of individuals appear to breathe through the mouth during intensive exercise (Veli, 1983). Most individuals will spontaneously switch from predominately nasal breathing to predominately oral breathing or oronasal breathing at some point during a graded exercise test, with a ventilation rate of approximately 40 liters per minute as the upper threshold for nasally restricted breathing (Saibene, et al., 1978). This switching point has been theorized to be related to the increased work of breathing (Fregosi & Lansing, 1995) or alternatively as an indirect effect of hypoventilation (Saibene, et al., 1978). A theoretical case can also be made that oral breathing during heavy exercise may precipitate the development of exercise induced bronchospasm (EIB) in athletes (Carlsen, 2012; Fitch, 2012; Price et al., 2013), and that the incidence of EIB is increased by those participating in competitive endurance sports (Rundell & Jenkinson, 2002). However, two studies strongly suggest that breathing in a nasally restricted manner will eliminate the EIB response in asthmatic patients at lower levels of exercise (Mangla & Menon, 1981; Shturmman-Ellstein et al., 1978), and nasal breathing has also been suggested as a possible strategy to reduce the occurrence of EIB in otherwise healthy athletes (Anderson & Kippelen, 2012).

In support of the possibility of using a nasally restricted breathing approach as a practical intervention, a recent study examining nasally restricted versus orally restricted and oronasal breathing in normal subjects (LaComb et al., 2017) suggests that healthy individuals can breathe entirely nasally at the lower levels of work necessary to improve aerobic fitness in healthy normal populations without any specific adaptation to the process. A second study from the same laboratory (Recinto et al., 2017) examined the effect of nasal breathing on maximal anaerobic work in active healthy students using a Wingate protocol and found no reduction in the peak work achieved. However, the only currently published study examining the ability of healthy normal subjects to complete maximal aerobic work while breathing in a nasally restricted manner demonstrated a significant reduction in both $VO2_{max}$ and the peak work accomplished in the nasal breathing condition in comparison to the oral and oronasal conditions (Morton et al., 1995). The last finding is strongly discouraging to most sport scientists, coaches and athletes who might consider adopting a nasally restricted breathing strategy, as it suggests that peak work capacity will be reduced and training intensity impaired. A recent article addressing various methods for preventing the development of EIB in elite athletes strongly suggests that a nasal breathing approach is untenable due to the previously described upper limits of ventilation at which previous research subjects switched to oral breathing (Fitch et al., 2012). Recently however, we published a case study design (Hostetter et all., 2016) supporting the claim of a highly trained triathlete that, following a 6 month training period spent using nasally restricted breathing, he was able race and train at all levels of running intensity while breathing only nasally without loss in performance ability or undue air hunger, as a means of eliminating his own EIB problems. Consequently, the purpose of this study was to extend those findings to determine if recreational runners, following an extended period of self-selected adaptation to nasally restricted breathing, can complete a maximal GXT and high level (85% of maximal velocity) steady state protocol without loss in VO_2max, peak running velocity or physiological economy.

METHODS

Subjects

The subjects were 10 mixed gender (5 males, 5 females) recreational runners who met inclusion criteria which required them to have utilized a nasally restricted breathing pattern during all training and racing for a minimum of 6 months. They were required to be in a good state of health and willing to maintain constant training conditions during the course of the study. The subjects were recruited from the Pueblo, Colorado community via flyer, internet postings and word of mouth. The subjects then signed an informed consent approved by the CSU-Pueblo Institutional Review Board, completed the American College of Sports Medicine screening procedure prior to participation (23), and were all assigned a low risk. Subject demographics by gender appear in Table 1, 3.1 in Results.

Study Design

The study design consisted of a repeated measures comparison of 10 participants across two conditions (nasally restricted versus orally restricted breathing) in randomized testing order, following a familiarization trial. The study was approved by the Institutional Review Board at Colorado State University – Pueblo and conducted there at an elevation of 1450 meters above sea level over a 2.5 year period.

Procedures

Upon arrival to the laboratory for the first test session, participants were weighed using a balance beam scale and had their height measured using a stadiometer (Detecto 439 Eye Level Beam Physician Scale, Detecto Scale Company, Webb City, MO). Upon returning for subsequent trials they were re-weighed in the same manner. In each trial, the participants first completed the same individualized graded exercise test (GXT) protocol designed to elicit a maximum workload and oxygen uptake within six to ten minutes on a motorized treadmill (TRUE Commercial Series 8.0 Treadmill, True Fitness, St. Louis, Missouri, USA.). The starting velocity was determined from the most recent performance data each participant was able to report. The protocol increased workload by 0.3 mph every 30 seconds until the subject reached voluntary termination. The time from the beginning of the protocol until volitional termination was recorded and is reported in seconds as GXT Time to Exhaustion (GXT TE). The ramping approach allowed for greater resolution at the end point in determining differences in run performance across conditions. Ten minutes after the maximal protocol the subject completed a six minute steady state protocol (SS85) at 85% of the maximal velocity achieved in their familiarization protocol and then used in both subsequent experimental trials. This protocol was designed to allow the subject to work at an achievable high level pace over a full six minutes whereby they would reach steady state values for the

Table 1. Participant descriptive by gender

Variable (M±s)	Males (n=5)	Females (n=5)
Age (yr)	34.8±15.64	23.2±3.27
Running (yr)	18.4±12.30	6.1±5.38
Nasal breathing (yr)	5.75±3.36	3.25±3.5
Mass (kg)	71.09±5.32	58.09±3.98
Height (m)	1.81±0.07	1.66±0.08
Body mass index (kg/m²)	21.60±1.95	21.04±2.04
VO_2 max (ml/kg/min)	48.14±5.19	37.58±4.41

various cardiorespiratory measures by the final two minutes. The oral condition was created by having the subject wear a swimming nose clip (Speedo Profile Nose Clip, Speedo, New York, NY, USA) underneath a full face style mask (VacuMed Full Face Ventilation Mask,-R113485- R113489, VacuMed, Ventura, CA, USA). The nasal condition was created by using the same mask with the mouth taped shut and a nasal splint placed on the nose to offset the slight pressure effect created by the mask on the nasal flares. Metabolic functions were measured using a metabolic cart (Medgraphics Ultima PFX, MGC Diagnostics Corporation, Saint Paul, MN, USA). Peak heart rate (HR_{peak}) was measured at volitional termination of the GXT protocol and steady state heart rate (HR_{ss}) was measured as an average during the final two minutes of the SS85 using a heart rate monitor (Polar FT1, Polar Electro Inc., Lake Success, NY, USA). Blood lactate concentrations were measured immediately post GXT (LA_{peak}) and again post SS85 (LA_{ss}) using a validated (Pyne et al., 2000) lactate meter (Lactate Pro LT-1710, ARKRAY USA, Minneapolis, MN, USA). The complete testing procedure was performed on successive weeks for familiarization first and then randomly following for both nasal and oral breathing conditions. The trials were conducted at the same time of day one week apart over three successive weeks. The subjects were blinded as to work output and physiological responses throughout the trials. The subjects verbally reported completing similar training volume, intensity and microcycle periodization in the weeks prior to each testing session and the testing was scheduled at the same time and day on subsequent weeks. Subjects were requested to maintain normal hydration and dietary intake during the course of the study, as well as to refrain from entering races.

During the GXT protocols, individual subject values for maximal oxygen consumption (VO_2max) and carbon dioxide production (VCO_2max), ventilation (VE), ventilatory equivalents for VO_2 (VE/VO_2) and CO_2 (VE/VCO_2), respiratory rate (RR), tidal volume (V_T), end tidal pulmonary partial pressure for oxygen (PET_{O2}) and carbon dioxide (PET_{CO2}), the fraction of expired oxygen (FE_{O2}) and carbon dioxide (FE_{CO2}) and the respiratory exchange ratio (RER), were obtained from 30 second averages of breath by breath data derived from the metabolic cart at VO_2max. The subject's maximal level of exertion reached in each GXT protocol was examined by recording the original Borg scale (6-20) rating of perceived exertion (RPE) reached after each subject self-terminated the protocol; by measuring the maximal 30 second average RER reached in the protocol; and by evaluating the final several 30 second average measurements of VO_2 for leveling or dropping prior to each subject's volitional termination of the maximal protocol. During the SS85 protocols the last two minutes of data were averaged for the same metabolic variables to produce each subject value with the VO_2 measures interpreted as measure of physiological economy at steady state (VO_{2ss}).

Statistical Analysis

Data analysis was completed using a spreadsheet (Microsoft EXCEL - Version 2013, Microsoft Corporation, Redmond, Washington). The mean and standard deviation were calculated and reported for the participant's demographic variables by gender. Means and standard errors were calculated and reported for the experimental measures. Student's paired samples t tests were used to analyze differences in the mean scores of the dependent variables between experimental trials. Statistical significance was established at $p < 0.05$. Effect sizes were calculated using the formula ($t/\sqrt{n}$) and reported as Cohen's d values. Moderate effects were interpreted as d = 0.50 – 0.80 and large effects were interpreted when d > 0.80. The small sample size (n=10) resulted from the difficulty in identifying participants who met the highly selective entry criteria described previously.

RESULTS

Subject Descriptives

The subjects (N=10) consisted of 5 female and 5 male recreational runners with diverse abilities and physical characteristics as seen in Table 1.

Maximal GXT Results

In the maximal GXT trials the subjects exhibited no significant mean difference in GXT TVE, VO_2max or LA_{peak} All subjects reported an RPE of 20 following each GXT. In addition, there were no significant differences in RER, or HR_{peak} between trials. However, in the nasally restricted breathing condition the subjects demonstrated a significantly lower VE/VO_2 and VE/VCO_2 at VO_2max, with large and moderate effect sizes respectively. In addition, the nasal breathing condition produced a significantly lower maximal RR, VE, FE_{O2} and PET_{O2}, with large effect sizes, along with a significantly higher FE_{CO2} and PET_{CO2} with large and moderate effect sizes respectively, and no significant difference in V_T, The subjects also demonstrated a significantly lower VCO_2max with a moderate effect size during nasal breathing as well. Complete data may be observed in Table 2.

Steady State Results

During the SS85 trials the subjects exhibited no significant difference in LA, RER, RPE or HR between trials. However, in the nasally restricted breathing condition they again demonstrated a significantly lower mean VE/VO_2 and VE/VCO_2, with large effect sizes, as well as a significantly lower $VO2_{ss}$.

In addition, the nasal breathing condition during steady state work produced a significantly lower RR, VE, FE_{O2} and PET_{O2}, with large effect sizes, along with a significantly higher PET_{CO2}, with a large effect size, and no significant difference in V_T, FE_{CO2} or VCO_2. Complete data may be observed in Table 3.

DISCUSSION

This study is the first to examine the effect of prior training using a nasally restricted breathing approach on running economy, the ability to produce peak work, and the ability

Table 2. Effect of breathing route on performance and cardiorespiratory variables at VO_{2max} in the GXT (n=10)

Variable	Mean±standard error		p-value *significant at 0.05	Effect size (d) *moderate ** large
	Nasal condition	Oral condition		
GXT TE (s)	428±24	421±18	0.74	0.11
VO_2 max (L/min)	2.55±0.25	2.75±0.25	0.09	0.60*
VCO_2 max (L/min)	3.19±0.36	3.55±0.33	0.02*	0.93**
LA_{peak} (mg/dl)	7.20±0.76	7.03±0.76	0.74	0.11
RER	1.31±0.06	1.28±0.03	0.53	0.21
RR (bpm)	39.20±2.13	49.40±2.53	0.008*	1.06**
HR_{peak} (bpm)	180.50±3.92	185.40±3.57	0.16	0.48
RPE (Borg 6-20)	20.00	20.00	n/a	n/a
VE (L/min)	90.50±9.92	117.76±12.73	0.001*	1.42**
V_T (L/min)	2.33±0.21	2.35±0.19	0.812	0.08
FE_{O2} (%)	16.28±0.15	16.89±0.16	0.002*	1.35**
PET_{O2} (mm/hg)	85.60±1.11	89.70±1.21	0.007*	1.07**
VE/VO_2	35.20±1.34	41.30±1.59	0.002*	1.35**
FE_{CO2} (%)	7.67±0.24	6.92±0.28	0.028*	0.82**
PET_{CO2} (mm/hg)	44.70±1.55	40.20±1.46	0.035*	0.78*
VE/VCO_2	29.40±1.33	32.80±1.13	0.043*	0.74*

Table 3. Effect of breathing route on cardiorespiratory variables at 85% of maximal GXT velocity for six minutes at steady state (n=10)

Variable	Mean±standard error		p-value *significant at 0.05	Effect size (d) *moderate ** large
	Nasal condition	Oral condition		
VO_{2ss} (L/min)	2.64±0.27	2.76±0.25	0.05*	0.71*
VCO_{2ss} (L/min)	2.98±0.31	3.10±0.24	0.40	0.28
LA_{ss} (mg/dl)	9.05±0.88	7.92±0.98	0.11	0.57*
RER	1.19±0.04	1.11±0.03	0.13	0.53*
RR (bpm)	36.45±1.78	43.28±2.27	0.01*	0.99**
HR (bpm)	182.70±4.39	181.20±5.27	0.27	0.37
RPE (Borg 6-20)	14.40±0.65	15.10±0.38	0.24	0.40
VE (L/min)	84.41±8.48	102.14±8.22	0.0001*	1.94**
V_T (L/min)	2.32±0.19	2.39±0.18	0.53	0.20
FE_{O2} (%)	16.07±0.12	16.55±0.12	0.004*	1.19**
PET_{O2} (mm/hg)	85.05±0.80	88.25±1.06	0.03*	0.84**
VE/VO_2	32.43±0.77	36.70±1.03	0.002*	1.40**
FE_{CO2} (%)	7.52±0.29	6.96±0.94	0.13	0.52*
PET_{CO2} (mm/hg)	44.63±1.17	40.20±1.46	0.01*	0.94**
VE/VCO_2	28.47±0.68	32.92±0.92	0.002*	1.37**

maintain a high aerobic capacity while breathing nasally versus orally. In the only previously published study addressing the effect of nasally restricted versus orally restricted breathing on VO_2max and peak work, both were substantially reduced in the nasally restricted breathing condition (Morton et al., 1995). However, the participants in that study were normal healthy volunteers who had made no specific attempt to utilize a nasally restricted breathing approach prior to the study. In our study of self-selected nasal breathers, the participants had specifically chosen to utilize a nasally restricted breathing pattern over a minimum of 6 months prior

to their inclusion in the study. Subsequently, these participants were able to achieve the same peak work and maximal oxygen consumption in a GXT while breathing nasally that they achieved while breathing orally. As in the previously mentioned Morton et al. study (Morton et al., 1995), our participants exhibited a significantly reduced RR and VE at VO_{2max} in the nasal breathing condition. On average, VE was reduced by 22%. However, unlike the previous study, they were still able achieve adequate oxygenation in this condition and continue to increase work to levels as high as in the oral breathing condition with no significant difference in anaerobic energy contribution. By contrast, Morton's participants experienced a 35% reduction in maximal VE, a 10.2% reduction in VO_2max, and an 8.4% reduction in their GXT TE (Morton et al., 1995). These differences in results between studies strongly suggest that our study's subjects achieved an adaptation as a result of their extended time spent using nasally restricted breathing. This study's subjects achieved adequate oxygenation in spite of a reduced ventilation while breathing nasally by increasing their total oxygen diffusion breath to breath. This is evidenced by the decreased PET_{O2} and FE_{O2} in their expired air at VO_{2max} at the same V_T. Assuming the concentration of oxygen in the ambient air is constant, by inhaling and exhaling the same volume of air (V_T) with each breath and achieving a lower fraction of oxygen at the end of each exhalation (FE_{O2}), the partial pressure of oxygen was reduced at the end of each exhalation (PET_{O2}) indicating that a larger volume of oxygen was removed during nasal breathing. This phenomenon is very likely the direct result of the lower RR necessitated by breathing exclusively through the nasal passage, thereby allowing greater time for diffusion with each breath, and has been observed in other studies examining nasal breathing during exercise (LaComb et al 2017; Morton et al., 1995). In support of this hypothesis, Nalbandian, et al. (Nalbandian, et al., 2017) demonstrated a similar outcome by reducing RR without changing the breathing route during cycling. In their study, peak work and VO_2max were similarly maintained across three RRs of 30, 45 and 60 breaths per minute.

However, the participants in this study also demonstrated an increased flux of CO_2 breath to breath during nasal breathing as established by their increased PET_{CO2} and FE_{CO2} at the same V_T at both VO_2max and during steady state running. This is significant because the available resting state evidence suggests that an increase in PET_{CO2} is associated with increased air hunger (Banzett et al., 1996). In addition, nasal breathing at rest also increases PET_{CO2} (Tanaka et al., 1988) so this effect during exercise is not surprising. This may be the mechanism by which those not adapted to nasally restricted breathing during exercise experience an unacceptable sensation of air hunger at some level of intensity, causing them to switch over to an oral breathing pattern at a relatively low ventilation rate, thereby reducing PET_{CO2} and air hunger for a given level of exertion. In addition, experimental resting data suggests that sustained exposure to breathing conditions that increase PET_{CO2} and air hunger over normal also results in a loss of air hunger over time (Bloch-Salisbury et all., 1996), very likely as a result of down regulation of the receptor response to the increased flux of CO_2 breath to breath. Although previous work suggests that the mechanism driving the spontaneous switch to oral breathing patterns during increasing exercise intensities is related to a disproportionate increase in nasal resistance associated with increased turbulence (Fregosi & Lansing, 1995), our study suggests that this may manifest itself via the volume of breath to breath CO_2 flux and its effect on the sensation of airlessness. In support of this possible mechanism are numerous anecdotal accounts of experiencing a sense of air hunger upon initially attempting to exercise while breathing in a nasally restricted manner and the gradual loss of

that sensation in those who persist (Davidson, 2012; Fields, 2004; Hostetter et al., 2016; Smith, 2013). This phenomenon may also represent the primary mechanism by which athletes are able to gradually adapt to a nasally restricted breathing pattern during exercise and avoid switching to oral breathing as work intensity is increased. In light of this interpretation, it is also not surprising that few individuals choose spontaneously to breathe in a nasally restricted manner during heavy exercise (Saibene et al., 1978). In addition, the data from our study, along with the Nalbandian study data (Nalbandian et al., 2017) suggests that total ventilation is not a primary limiter to oxygenation and peak work regardless of breathing route.

During the SS85 the participants exhibited the same results as in the GXT, suggesting that they were not limited in the sustained work they could achieve while breathing nasally. Interestingly, this protocol produced even higher VE and VO_2 values than the preceding GXT, possibly as a result of the increase in total body cooling necessary to sustain high level work on a treadmill. However, the HR, RPE and LA were not significantly different in the two breathing conditions. In addition, VE, VO2, VE/VO_2, and VE/VCO_2 were all significantly lower in the nasally restricted breathing condition, further supporting the case that nasal breathing produces superior ventilatory efficiency and a reduced oxygen cost in comparison to oral breathing during exercise as also observed in other published studies examining a comparison between nasal and oral breathing routes (Hostetter et al., 2016; LaComb et al., 2017; Morton et al., 1995; Recinto et al., 2017).

This study produced a significantly lower VO_2 at steady state while breathing nasally which is similar to the findings of LaComb (LaComb et al., 2017) and Morton (Morton et al., 1995). However, in contrast with the LaComb et al. interpretation that the lower VO_2 they measured during nasal only breathing represented an inefficiency (LaComb et al., 2017), an alternative explanation is that the nasal breathing condition requires less metabolic energy production to produce the same external work (lower VO_2, VCO_2 and the same RER, RPE and LA while breathing nasally) and is more physiologically economic as a result. This seems reasonable in light of the consistent observation across our participants and across studies (Hostetter et al., 2016; LaComb et al., 2017; Morton et al., 1995; Recinto et al., 2017) that nasal breathing reduces total VE at a given level of work by approximately 22%. As VE is produced by muscular work, a reduced VE logically reflects a reduced work of breathing which might result in a reduced gross metabolic cost during exercise, further resulting in a small improvement in gross economy. This concept has been demonstrated theoretically by measuring the independent cost of high ventilation rate breathing as a percentage of overall metabolic cost of exercise (Aaron et al., 1992) and by demonstrating that increases and decreases in overall oxygen costs during cycling can be produced by artificially increasing and decreasing the work of breathing respectively, while keeping exercise work constant (Harms, et al., 2000). In addition, other studies have demonstrated that potential improvements in performance occur through the application of specific respiratory muscle training which results in improved ventilatory efficiency (HanjGhanbari et al., 2013; Sheel, 2002).

In this study, the mean reduction in oxygen consumption during nasal breathing while running at 85% of the velocity at VO_2max was approximately 4%, which contrasts with the findings of LaComb who reported greater reductions of 8-10% at lower relative exercise intensities while breathing nasally during cycling (LaComb et al., 2017). However, our findings align with the Morton study, which found a 5% reduction in oxygen consumption in their participants while running in a steady state trial at 12 kilometers per hour (Morton et al., 1995). Further, these improvements in economy can be considered comparable to those achieved by an intervention using explosive weight training in highly competitive collegiate runners which resulted in an approximately 5-6% reduction in oxygen cost and a parallel improvement in running performance of approximately 3% (Paavolainen et al., 1999). Should this improvement in physiological economy prove to be the case in future studies, nasally restricted breathing during exercise might be viewed as not only a means of preventing/treating EIB, but also as a potential way to improve performance in endurance events whereby economy is a critical performance factor (Joyner & Coyle, 2008).

The primary limitation in performing this study was the difficulty in finding subjects who met the inclusion criteria of running and racing using a nasally restricted breathing approach over an extended period as this practice is very rare (Veli, 1983). Consequently, our low subject number was achieved only after 2.5 years spent recruiting and testing subjects. Another reasonable concern in regards to our methodology was that our participants might, by self-selecting a nasally restricted breathing pattern prior to the study, logically hold a bias predisposing them to limit their peak work in the oral breathing condition to validate their own beliefs. We attempted to reduce the possible influence of such bias by blinding the participants as to output during the testing, by controlling the use of nasal versus oral breathing through the test apparatus and by using short 30 second stages in the GXT protocol making the tracking of stages difficult. Further, the participants reached a similarly high RER in each condition, as well as having no significant differences in maximal HR, RPE or LA. This strongly suggests that the subjects made a maximal effort in both breathing conditions. It should be noted that our decision to use a nasal strip in the nasal breathing condition may have altered our results somewhat, as such devices have been shown to increase maximal inspiratory flow while breathing nasally (Di Somma, 1999), increase the volitional switching point from nasal to oronasal breathing during incremental exercise (Seto-Poon et al., 1999), and increase time to exhaustion at submaximal work rates while breathing in a nasally restricted state (Tong et al., 2001). Our choice to use the nasal strips was made following pilot testing, as we found that any pressure created by the face mask on the nasal flares drastically reduced some of our participant's ability to breathe nasally during testing. In addition, because we were not able to collect data on VO_2max prior to the participant's self-selected nasally restricted breathing process, we cannot determine what effect, if any, their choice may have had on their prior aerobic capacities. Further, our study did not include a measure of the work outcomes while breathing in an oronasal condition. However, Morton et al. did include an oronasal condition in their study and found no significant difference in VO_2max or VEmax in comparison to the oral only condition (Morton et al., 1995), strongly suggesting that there is no meaningful contribution of nasal breathing while breathing oronasally at high exercise intensities. Finally, our mixed gender sample (5 males, 5 females) suggested the use of a factorial analysis to examine the possible effect of gender. However, we employed the use of t-tests due to prior evidence that gender has no effect on the response of cardiorespiratory variables to the nasal versus oral breathing intervention (LaComb et al., 2017). In addition, our low participant number was insufficient to produce adequate power in a factorial analysis. While our study confirms the assumption that nasally restricted breathing results in a lower peak VE, it further demonstrates that VO_2max and peak work output can be maintained following a period of training using nasally restricted breathing. One possible explanation for this phenomenon is that individuals who choose to do so adapt to nasally restricted breathing by increasing their tolerance to CO_2 flux breath to breath before experiencing air hunger. These findings suggest that it may be beneficial to advocate that exercisers, and particularly endurance athletes, attempt to adapt to a nasally restricted breathing pattern as a means of maintaining respiratory health and improving performance. Beyond this most basic implication, it will be important for future research to further establish that such an adaptation occurs, as well as to investigate the validity of other suggested benefits of using a nasally restricted breathing pattern during exercise. Possible additional benefits of breathing in a nasally restricted manner during exercise that should be explored include increased parasympathetic influence and relaxation, increased pulmonary and cardiac blood flow, and a reduced exposure to airborne particulate matter and pathogens.

CONCLUSION

This study supports the ability of recreational runners to utilize a nasally restricted breathing pattern at all levels of running intensity without loss in VO_2max or GXT TE and with superior PE and ventilatory efficiency, following an extended training period using this practice. These findings suggest that a nasally restricted breathing pattern may be successfully utilized by recreational runners as means of improving health, without sacrificing performance ability, following an extended period of time spent adapting to this practice.

REFERENCES

Aaron EA, Seow KC Johnson BD, and Dempsey JA. (1992). Oxygen cost of exercise hyperpnea: implications for performance. *Journal of Applied Physiology*, 72(5): 1818-1825. DOI: 10.1152/jappl.1992.72.5.1818

Anderson SD and Kippelen P. (2012). Assessment and prevention of exercise-induced bronchoconstriction. *British Journal of Sports Medicine.* 46(6): 391-6. DOI: 10.1136/bjsports-2011-090810

Banzett RB, Lansing RW, Evans KC and Shea SA. (1996). Stimulus-response characteristics of CO2-induced air hunger in normal subjects. *Respiratory Physiology,* 103(1):19-31. https://doi.org/10.1016/00345687(95)00050-X

Bloch-Salisbury E, Shea SA, Brown R, Evans K, and Banzett RB. (1996). Air hunger induced by acute increase in PCO2 adapts to chronic elevation of PCO2 in ventilated humans. *Journal of Applied Physiology,* 81(2):949 56. DOI: 10.1152/jappl.1996.81.2.949

Cap, Adam. (2016). The Nose Knows: A Case for Nasal Breathing During High Intensity Exercise [internet] *Adam Cap,* November 4. [accessed 2017, January 19]. Available from: https://adamcap.com/2013/11/29/nose-knows-case nasal-breathing-high-intensity-exercise

Carlsen, K. (2012). Mechanisms of asthma development in elite athletes. *Breathe,* 8:278-284. DOI: 10.1183/20734735.009512

Davidson, S. (2012). *Blow it out your (nose) hole* [internet]. Cycling in the South Bay. [accessed 2017 January 20] Available from: https://pvcycling.wordpress.com/2012/09/15/blow-it-out-your-nose-hole

Di Somma EM, West SN, Wheatley JR and Amis TC. (1999). Nasal dilator strips increase maximum inspiratory flow via nasal wall stabilization. *Laryngoscope,* 109(5):780-4. https://doi.org/10.1097/00005537-199905000-00018

Fields, P. (2004). *Breathing for Athletes - Proper Breathing is Essential for Athletes and Non-Athletes Alike* [internet]. Dennis Lewis. [accessed 2017 January 20] Available at: https://www.dennislewis.org/articles-other-writings/articles-essays/breathing-athletes

Fitch KD, Anderson SD, Bougault BV, Rundell KW, Malcolm S, McKenzie CD and Kippelen P. (2012). Respiratory health of elite athletes – preventing airway injury: a critical review. *British Journal of Sports Medicine.* 46:471-476. http://dx.doi.org/10.1136/bjsports-2012-091056

Fitch, KD. (2012). An overview of asthma and airway hyper-responsiveness in Olympic athletes. *British Journal of Sports Medicine.* 46:413-416. DOI: 10.1136/bjsports-2011-090814

Fregosi RF and Lansing RW. (1995). Neural drive to nasal dilator muscles: influence of exercise intensity and oronasal flow partitioning. *Journal of Applied Physiology,* 79 (4): 1330-1337. DOI: 10.1152/jappl.1995.79.4.1330

HajGhanbari B, et al. (2013). Effects of respiratory muscle training on performance in athletes: a systematic review with meta-analyses. *The Journal of Strength & Conditioning Research,* 27(6): 1643-1663. DOI: 10.1519/JSC.0b013e318269f73f

Paavolainen, L, Hakkinen, K, Hamalainen, I, Nummela and Rusko, H. (1999). Explosive strength training improves 5 km running time by improving running economy and muscle power. *Journal of Applied Physiology,* 86(5):1527-1533. DOI: 10.1152/jappl.1999.86.5.1527

Harms CA, Wetter TJ, St. Croix CM, Pegelow DF and Dempsey JA. (2000). Effects of respiratory muscle work on exercise performance. *Journal of Applied Physiology,* 89(1): 131-138. DOI: 10.1152/jappl.2000.89.1.131

Hostetter K, McClaran SR, Cox DG and Dallam GM. (2016). Triathlete Adapts to Breathing Restricted to the Nasal Passage Without loss in VO2max or vVO2max. *Journal of Sport and Human Performance,* 4(1), 1-7. DOI: https://doi.org/10.12922/jshp.v4i1.70

Joyner MI and Coyle, EF. (2008). Endurance exercise performance: the physiology of champions. *The Journal of Physiology,* 586, (1): 35–44. DOI: 10.1113/jphysiol.2007.143834

LaComb, CO, Tandy, RD, Lee, SP, Young, JC and Navalta, JW. (2017). Oral versus Nasal Breathing during Moderate to High Intensity Submaximal Aerobic Exercise. *International Journal of Kinesiology and Sports Science,* 5(1), 8-16. DOI: http://dx.doi.org/10.7575//aiac.ijkss.v.5n.1p.8

Mangla PK and Menon MP. (1981). Effect of nasal and oral breathing on exercise-induced asthma. *Clinical Allergy,* 11(5): 433-9. https://doi.org/10.1111/j.1365-2222.1981.tb01616.x

Mercola, Joseph. (2013). *Mouth Breathing During Exercise May Increase Your Risk for Asthma and Cardiac Problems* [blog]. Mercola.com. [accessed 2017, January 19]. Available at: http://fitness.mercola.com/sites/fitness/archive/2099/12/31/proper-exercise-breathing.aspx

Morton AR, King K, Papalia S, Goodman C, Turley KR, et al. (1995). Comparison of maximal oxygen consumption with oral and nasal breathing. *Australian Journal of Science and Medicine in Sport.* 27(3): 51-5. https://www.ncbi.nlm.nih.gov/pubmed/8599744

Nalbandian M, Radak Z, Taniguchi, J, and Masaki T. (2017). How different respiratory rate patterns affect cardiorespiratory variables and performance. *International Journal of Exercise Science,* 10(3): 322 329. PMCID: PMC5421979

Pescatello, LS, Arean, R., Riebe, D, and Thompson, PD. (2014). *ACSM's Guidelines for Exercise Testing and Prescription.* 9th Ed. Wolters Kluwer/Lippincott Williams & Wilkins, Philadelphia, PA.

Price OJ, Ansley L, Menzies-Gow A, Cullinan P, Hull JH. (2013). Airway dysfunction in elite athletes – an occupational lung disease? *Allergy,* 68: 1343–1352. DOI: 10.1111/all.12265

Pyne DB, Boston T, Martin DT, and Logan, A. (2000). Evaluation of the Lactate Pro blood lactate analyser. *European Journal of Applied Physiology,* 82(1): 112–116. DOI: 10.1007/s004210050659

Rakhimov, A. (2004). *NormalBreathing.com* [Internet]. Dr. Artour Rakhimov. [accessed 2017, January 19] Available at: http://www.normalbreathing.com

Raman, R. (2006). *Lower Stress and Increase Endurance by Breathing Better* [internet]. Ravi Raman. [accessed 2017 January 19]. Available at: http://raviraman.com/lower-stress-and-increase-endurance-by-breathing-better

Recinto, C, Efthemeou, T., Bofelli, PT, and Navalta, JW. (2017). Effects of Nasal or Oral Breathing on Anaerobic Power Output and Metabolic Responses. *International Journal of Exercise Science,* 10(4): 506-514. PMCID: PMC5466403

Rundell KW, Jenkinson DM. (2002). Exercise-Induced Bronchospasm in the Elite Athlete. *Sports Medicine,* 32(9): 583-600. https://doi.org/10.2165/00007256-200232090-00004

Ruth, A. (2015). *Health Benefits of Nose Breathing* [online journal]. Nursing in General Practice. [accessed 2017 January 19] (1): 40-42, 2015. http://www.lenus.ie/hse/bitstream/10147/559021/1/JAN15Art7.pdf

Saibene F, Mognoni P, Lafortuna CL and Mostardi R. (1978). Oronasal breathing during exercise. *Pflügers Archives,* 378(1): 65-69. https://doi.org/10.1007/BF00581959

Seto-Poon M, Amis TC, Kirkness JP, Wheatley JR. (1999). Nasal dilator strips delay the onset of oral route breathing during exercise. *Canadian Journal of Applied Physiology.* 24(6): 538-47. https://doi.org/10.1139/h99-035

Sheel, A.W. (2002). Respiratory muscle training in healthy individuals: physiological rationale and implications for exercise performance. *Sports Medicine.* 32(9): 567-581. https://doi.org/10.2165/00007256-200232090-00003

Shturman-Ellstein, R., Zeballos, R J, Buckley JM, Souhrada, JF. (1978). The Beneficial Effect of Nasal Breathing on Exercise-Induced Bronchoconstriction. *American Review of Respiratory Disease,* 118(1): 65-73. DOI: 10.1164/arrd.1978.118.1.65

Smith, G. (2013). *Breathe Through Your Nose* [internet] 180 Degree Health. [accessed 2017 January 20] Available at: http://180degreehealth.com/breathe-nose

Tanaka Y, Morikawa T and Honda Y. (1988). An assessment of nasal functions in control of breathing. *Journal of Applied Physiology,* 65(4):1520-4. DOI: 10.1152/jappl.1988.65.4.1520

Tong TK, Fu FH and Chow BC. (2001). Nostril dilatation increases capacity to sustain moderate exercise under nasal breathing condition. *Journal of Sports Medicine and Physical Fitness,* 41(4): 470-8. PMID: 11687766

Veli, N. (1983). Oronasal airway choice during running. *Respiration Physiology,* 53(1): 129–133. PMID: 6622862

22

Test-Retest Reliability and the Learning Effect on Isokinetic Fatigue in Female Master's Cyclists

Jordan M. Glenn[1], Michelle Gray[2], Nicole E. Moyen[3], Jennifer L. Vincenzo[4], Kylie K. Harmon5, Lee E. Brown[6]*

[1]Neurotrack Technologies Inc.399 Bradford St #101, Redwood City, CA 94063

[2]Exercise Science Research Center, University of Arkansas HPER 321-E, University of Arkansas, Fayetteville, AR 72701

[3]Hopkins Marine Station of Stanford University Pacific Grove, CA 93950

[4]Department of Physical Therapy, University of Arkansas for Medical Sciences Fayetteville, Arkansas 72703

[5]Neuromuscular Physiology Lab, University of Central Florida 12354 Research Pkwy, St #221, Orlando, FL 32826

[6]University of West Florida 7178 Loysburg St., Navarre, FL 32566

Corresponding Author: Lee E. Brown, E-mail: leebrown1220@gmail.com

ARTICLE INFO

Conflicts of interest: None
Funding: None

ABSTRACT

Background: Isokinetic exercise is commonly used as a benchmark for strength and performance. **Objective:** The purpose of this investigation was to establish isokinetic fatigue test-retest reliability and examine the learning effect when testing without familiarization. **Methods:** 22 masters-aged [53±5 years), competitive female cyclists completed 3 separate 50-repetition knee flexion/extension tests on a Biodex, separated by one-week with no familiarization. Test-retest reliability [intra-class correlation [ICC], 95% confidence intervals [CI], technical error of measurement [TEM] were calculated. **Results:** ICCs between trials exhibited excellent reliability during extension [.93–.97) and flexion [.93–.97) for all variables except time to peak torque [ICC=.35 and.45 for extension and flexion, respectively) and fatigue index [ICC=.47 for flexion). Relative TEM was minimal for extension between trial 1 and trial 2 [0.27%–0.97%) and between trial 2 and trial 3 [0.27%–1.45%) for all variables. Similar results were observed for flexion between trial 1 and trial 2 [0.87%–2.45%) and between trial 2 and trial 3 [0.54%–1.10%). No differences [Wilks Λ>.05) existed between trials, indicating no learning effect associated with the tests. **Conclusions:** There was strong test-retest reliability in masters-aged, female athletes and no learning effect was associated with the Biodex during a knee extension/flexion fatigue protocol.

Key words: Muscle Fatigue, Muscle Strength Dynamometer, Athletic Performance, Women, Athletes

INTRODUCTION

Isokinetic exercise is commonly used as a benchmark for establishing baseline strength values and tracking longitudinal performance gains (Lund, Sondergaard, Zachariasssen, Christensen, Bulow, & Henriksen, 2005). To establish trustworthy isokinetic exercise results, reliable measurement techniques are required with regard to specific devices, procedures, and participant positioning (Brown, & Weir, 2001; Caruso, Brown & Tufano, 2012). Initial studies involving isokinetic exercise have established strong test-retest reliability for devices such as the Cybex, KinCom, and Biodex dynamometers (Alvares, Rodrigues, Azevedo Franke, da Silva, Pinto, & Vaz, 2015; Gross, Huffman, Phillips, & Wray, 1991; Kramer, 1990; Tsiros, Grimshaw, Shield, & Buckley, 2011).

For the Biodex Isokinetic Dynamometer (Biodex), reliability has been previously established from various perspectives, including same-day, short-term (two consecutive days) and long-term (one week) test-retest methodological designs (Brown, Whitehurst, Bryant & Buchalter, 1993; Drouin, Valvovich-McLeod, Shultz, Gansneder, & Perrin, 2004; Lund et al., 2005). While previous literature supports the reliability of the Biodex, these studies have either utilized non-subject designs, with mechanical loads (i.e. using a standard, external weight to determine the reliability of isometric torque) or a wide range (18-55 years) of recreationally active individuals (Drouin et al., 2004; Lund et al., 2005). For aging, athletic populations (i.e. masters athletes [MA]), measuring muscular strength during fatiguing exercise is a critical factor, necessary for maximizing exercise performance in aerobic and anaerobic sports (Louis, Hausswirth, Easthope, & Brisswalter., 2012; Pearson, Young, Macaluso, Devito, Nimmo, & Cobbold, 2002). MA experience multiple acute and chronic knee injuries resulting from training, and the number of injures are significantly greater when compared to their younger counterparts (Knobloch, Yoon, &

Vogt, 2008; McKean, Manson, & Stanish, 2006). Although multiple investigations have used the Biodex to evaluate isokinetic strength performance in MA, the test-retest reliability of these measurements during a fatiguing test has not yet been established in MA (Glenn, Gray, Stewart, Moyen, Kavouras, & DiBrezzo, 2016; Wroblewski, Amati, Smiley, Goodpaster, & Wright, 2011).

Another aspect of consideration during isokinetic evaluations is the learning effect related to repeated testing. To date, only two known investigations have examined the learning effect associated with the Biodex (Lund et al., 2005; Symons, Vandervoort, Rice, Overend, & Marsh, 2005). An initial study investigated the learning effect between two subsequent testing sessions separated by 2-10 days, suggesting test-retest reliability was high (ICC range = 0.84 – 0.94) between sessions during a 5-repetition, muscular strength protocol (Symons et al., 2005). Unfortunately, this investigation did not perform a 3rd follow-up test, which would have confirmed whether a learning effect occurred between trials. As a result, the overall learning effect cannot be determined. Another study suggested there was no learning effect associated with the Biodex during knee extension/flexion, demonstrating strong reliability (ICC range = 0.89 – 0.94) between multiple measurements taken on the same day and over a longitudinal (one week) period (Lund et al., 2005). However, it is important to note that in this investigation, participants were provided a familiarization trial in which to become acquainted with the equipment and procedures prior to data collection commencing (Lund et al., 2005). The implementation of a familiarization trial eliminates the ability to detect a true learning effect and minimizes external validity of test-retest reliability for the Biodex isokinetic dynamometer. Altogether based on previous literature, it remains inconclusive whether a true learning effect exists on the isokinetic dynamometer.

Strength testing during fatiguing protocols in populations such as MA must be reliable in order to establish long-term efficacy for subsequent evaluations. Furthermore, it is imperative that the learning effect of the Biodex be evaluated without the implementation of a familiarization trial to establish testing efficacy from a clinical perspective. Therefore, the purpose of this investigation was two-fold, 1) to establish test-retest reliability of the Biodex during fatiguing exercise in MA, and 2) to determine whether a true learning effect exists with the Biodex when utilized without a familiarization.

METHODS

Particpants

This study included 22 masters-aged female cyclists from the Southern region of the United States (Table 1). Cyclists were

recruited as the push/pull nature of lower-body isokinetic exercise (i.e., knee extension/flexion) relates to muscle pattern activation utilized during cycling exercise (So, Ng, & Ng, 2005). Females were specifically recruited because they exhibit greater levels of internal motivation compared to males, which would minimize external (life-related) factors affecting testing variability (Gillet & Rosnet, 2008). MA classification requirements were determined based upon those set forth by USA Cycling and World Masters Cycling organizations. Inclusion criteria included: a) an age ≥ 35 years, b) not classified as an elite cyclist or competitor in an event based on the international cycling federation (Union Cycliste Internationale, UCI) standards, and c) not a member of a registered team under the UCI. For this investigation, MA were also required to have cycled at least 2 years for a minimum of 3 days per week (Glenn, Gray, Stewart, Moyen, Kavouras, & DiBrezzo, 2015; Glenn et al., 2016). Individuals experiencing acute or chronic lower-body musculoskeletal injuries were excluded from participation. With regard to the learning effect associated with the Biodex assessment, the rationale for using trained athletes was two-fold:

1) When determining the learning effect of a measure, the steadiness of the participant must be considered, and trained cyclists are familiar with the movement patterns associated with isokinetic knee extension/flexion (Lund et al., 2005; So et al., 2005).

2) Subjects should be well motivated when determining learning effects, and athletes participating in competitive sports exhibit greater levels of intrinsic motivation compared to non-competitive counterparts (Frederick-Recascino & Schuster-Smith, 2003; Lund et al., 2005). As previously mentioned, females were specifically recruited because of their greater levels of internal motivation compared to males (Gillet et al., 2008).

Based on these parameters, we chose to test female cyclists. As an aging population (that is more prone to knee injuries) has not yet been investigated, we chose MA. All measures and procedures were approved by the University's Institutional Review Board prior to testing and all subjects completed a health history questionnaire and signed a statement of informed consent prior to participation. Participant recruitment was completed via email, fliers, and visits to local cycling clubs and organizations.

Procedures

Food logs were distributed to all participants to record food and fluid intake for the 24 h prior to each trial. Participants were asked to replicate their 24-hour dietary intake from the first trial for all subsequent trials. To account for dietary intake affecting outcome measures on testing days, participants

Table 1. Demographic data for female masters athlete cyclists

	Age (y)	Height (cm)	Mass (kg)	Body fat (%)	Years cycling	Time cycling/week (h)	Distance cycled/week (km)
Mean	53	162.7	66.4	30.5	6.9	8.1	140.1
(SD)	(5)	(7.5)	(14.6)	(11.1)	(7.1)	(5.2)	(39.5)

All data are presented as mean±SD (*n*=22)

were required to fast for 3 h prior to each trial (Glenn et al., 2016). All participants refrained from vigorous exercise, alcohol, and caffeine during the 24 h prior to each trial. Participants verbally confirmed adherence to all controls prior to each trial. Additionally, participants were instructed to wear clothes and shoes in which they would normally exercise, and wore similar attire for all trials.

Participants reported to the laboratory for 3 visits. The initial visit included completion of an informed consent and health history questionnaire, demographic and body composition measurements, and baseline testing for the isokinetic exercise protocol (described in detail below). Body mass was assessed using a beam scale (Detecto 437 Eye-Level Weigh Beam Physician Scale, Irvington, NJ) and height was measured with a stadiometer (Detecto, Webb City, MO). Body fat and lean mass were measured via dual-energy x-ray absorptiometry (DXA; General Electric, Fairfield, CT). Prior to DXA analysis, proper calibration procedures and quality assurance analysis were followed as previously described (Glenn, Gray, & Vincenzo, 2014). In order to determine the learning effect associated with isokinetic exercise, the baseline evaluation was considered trial 1, and no familiarization was provided to the equipment or protocol. Participants were also not permitted to be in the laboratory while other evaluations were being conducted in order to ensure initial introduction to the assessment was standardized (Brown & Weir, 2001). None of the participants had ever undergone isokinetic exercise testing prior to participating in this investigation.

After baseline testing, participants reported to the lab for trials 2 and 3 and completed the same isokinetic exercise protocol. To ensure any learning effects were solely associated with the isokinetic exercise protocol, all trials were separated by exactly 1 week; no variation in this was permitted. Trials for each participant were also scheduled at the same time (± 1 hour) to ensure chronobiological control (Altamirano, Coburn, Brown, & Judelson, 2012; Mota, Stock, Carillo, Olinghouse, Drusch, & Thompson, 2015). Finally, to mask real-time performance results, participants were not permitted to see the real-time computer output during the testing procedure.

Isokinetic Exercise Testing

The Biodex system II Isokinetic Dynamometer (Biodex Medical, Inc., Shirley, NY) was used to measure isokinetic exercise variables. Once seated on the dynamometer, the participant was instructed to keep their back flat against the chair and then was stabilized using thigh, pelvic and shoulder straps. The mechanical axis of the dynamometer was aligned with the knee of the participant's dominant leg, and the lateral femoral condyle was used as the landmark for setting the axis of rotation. After trial 1, chair and dynamometer settings were recorded to ensure consistent positioning for all subsequent sessions. Before testing, all participants received specific instructions to maximally extend and flex the knee joint through the full range of motion during each individual repetition throughout the evaluation. Calibration of the Biodex isokinetic dynamometer was performed according to manufacturer-established specifications. The protocol

consisted of 50 repetitions with extension/flexion movement parameters set at 180°/240° per second, respectively (Glenn et al., 2016). To ensure maximal effort was given throughout the evaluation, strong verbal encouragement was provided during each evaluation (Glenn et al., 2016).

Variables used to determine test-retest reliability (determined a priori to testing) included the following: a) peak torque (N·m), b) relative peak torque (based on body weight [%]), c) time to peak torque (ms), d) torque generated at 30° (N·m), e) torque generated at 0.18 s (N·m), f) work completed during the highest repetition (J), g) relative work completed (based on body weight [%]), h) total work completed (J), i) work completed during the initial 3rd of exercise (J), j) work completed during the middle 3rd of exercise (J), k) work completed during the final 3rd of exercise (J), l) fatigue index (%), m) average power (W), and n) average peak torque (N·m). All variables were calculated by the Biodex software with the exception of "work completed during the middle 3rd of exercise," which was determined by subtracting the work completed during the initial and final thirds of exercise from total work completed.

Statistical Analyses

Statistical Package for the Social Sciences (SPSS, version 22) was used to conduct analyses. Normal distribution of data were assessed with histograms and boxplots.

In order to test for the degree of agreement between the trials (1 vs. 2, 2 vs. 3, and 1 vs. 3), intra-class correlation coefficients (ICC) were calculated. ICC gives a relative expression of the reliability, and general guidelines suggest an ICC ≥.75 indicates strong reliability (Little, Emery, Black, Scott, Meeuwisse, & Nettel-Aguirre, 2015; Portney & Watkins, 2000). For the purposes of this investigation, coefficients of < 0.50 indicated poor reliability between trials, 0.50 to 0.74 indicated moderate reliability, and ≥ 0.75 indicated strong reliability (Little et al., 2015). For those variables in which there was poor reliability with regard to between-trial comparisons, the 95% confidence intervals (CI) for the all between-trial ICCs were compared. For those cases, test-retest reliability was constituted if the 95% CI did not overlap for any of the between-trial comparisons (Little et al., 2015; Moyen, Ellis, Ciccone, Thurston, Cochrane, & Brown, 2014).

In conjunction with ICCs, technical error of measurement (TEM) was calculated for each variable between trials 1 vs. 2, 2 vs. 3, and 1 vs. 3. TEM is defined as the standard deviation between repeated measures and the lower the TEM obtained, the more accurate the measurement. Absolute (Equation 1) and relative (Equation 2) TEMs were calculated for each variable between trials (Perrini, Oliveira, Ornellas, & Oliveira, 2005):

Equation 1: Absolute TEM = $\sqrt{\Sigma d_i^2 / 2n}$

Where:

Σd_i^2 = the summation of deviation scores raised to the second power

n = number of participants

i = number of deviations

Equation 2: Relative TEM = (Absolute TEM)/VAV x 100

Where:

Absolute TEM = TEM calculated in equation 1

VAV = variable average value (calculated as the arithmetic mean of all subjects' mean from two trials [i.e. the mean of 22 subject means]).

Appropriate conditions to accurately measure TEM are that a) variables are always collected in the same measurement unit, b) calculations are only applied to the same measurement performed and/or the equipment utilized, c) calculations are only applied when using a similar (homogenous) population (i.e. athletes), d) measurements must include a minimum of 20 participants, and e) measurements must be performed at the same time of day (Perrini et al., 2005). The sample size (n = 22), chronobiological considerations (± 1 hour), and participant homogeneity requirements (female masters cyclists) were satisfied in this investigation. As the Biodex was utilized for all trials and variable measurement units were consistent from trial to trial, all conditions were satisfied for TEM calculations.

To determine the presence of a learning effect between testing trials, a repeated measures multivariate analysis of variance model (RM-ANOVA) was utilized for each of the Biodex variables. Greenhouse-Geisser corrections were implemented when sphericity violations occurred. When necessary (i.e. significant F score), a Bonferroni adjustment was made for multiple pairwise comparisons during post hoc analysis. A learning effect was constituted when variables exhibited a significant performance improvement between trials 1 and 2, but not trials 2 and 3 (Little et al., 2015). Where appropriate, all variables are presented as mean ± SD.

RESULTS

In order to assess the test-retest reliability of knee extension/flexion on the Biodex isokinetic dynamometer, ICC values were calculated for each extension and flexion variable between trials. For all variables, ICCs were calculated between trial 1 vs. 2, trial 2 vs. 3, and trial 1 vs. 3. ICCs between the testing trials exhibited excellent comparisons for the extension component of the protocol (Table 2); all variables demonstrated moderate to strong reliability within the 3 trial comparisons (i.e. ICC ≥.50). Only 1 variable (time to peak torque) exhibited poor reliability for trial 1 vs. 3 (ICC =.35) during the extension phase. However, the 95% CI overlapped with the trial 1 vs. 2 and 2 vs. 3 CIs, indicating there were no significant differences between ICC values for this variable. During the extension component, the highest ICC values for between trial comparisons were exhibited for peak torque (range:.93 –.96), work completed during the highest repetition (range:.94 –.96), total work completed (range:.95 –.96), and average peak torque (range:.94 –.97).

For each variable assessed during the flexion component, ICCs were calculated between trial 1 vs. trial 2, trial 2 vs. trial 3, and trial 1 vs. trial 3 (Table 3). ICCs between the trials exhibited strong comparisons for the flexion component of the protocol. All variables demonstrated moderate to strong reliability within the 3 trial comparisons (i.e., ICC ≥.50). Only 2 variables (time to peak torque and fatigue index) exhibited poor reliability between trial 1 vs. 3 (ICC =.45 and.47, respectively) during the flexion phase. However, for both variables, the 95% CIs overlapped with the trial 1 vs. 2 and 2 vs. 3 CIs, indicating there were no significant

Table 2. Intra-class correlations and limits for test-retest reliability during extension component of the 50-repetition protocol on the Biodex Isokinetic Dynamometer

	T1 – T2 ICC	95% CI	T2 – T3 ICC	95% CI	T1 – T3 ICC	95% CI
Peak torque (N·M)	0.96	0.90 – 0.98	0.97	0.92 – 0.99	0.93	0.84 – 0.97
Peak torque/body weight (%)	0.94	0.86 – 0.98	0.89	0.74 – 0.95	0.85	0.63 – 0.94
Time to peak torque (ms)	0.72	0.33 – 0.89	0.79	0.50 – 0.91	0.35	-0.56 – 0.73
Torque at 30° (N·M)	0.84	0.61 – 0.93	0.50	-0.21 – 0.79	0.59	0.02 – 0.83
Torque at 0.18 s (N·M)	0.89	0.73 – 0.95	0.95	0.87 – 0.98	0.82	0.55 – 0.92
Work completed during highest repetition (J)	0.95	0.88 – 0.98	0.96	0.91 – 0.99	0.94	0.86 – 0.98
Work/Body weight (%)	0.90	0.75 – 0.96	0.86	0.65 – 0.94	0.86	0.67 – 0.94
Total work completed during exercise (J)	0.95	0.88 – 0.98	0.96	0.91 – 0.99	0.95	0.88 – 0.98
Work completed during the initial 3rd of exercise (J)	0.95	0.87 – 0.98	0.96	0.91 – 0.98	0.94	0.86 – 0.98
Work completed during the middle 3rd of exercise (J)	0.95	0.87 – 0.98	0.95	0.88 – 0.98	0.94	0.85 – 0.97
Work completed during the final 3rd of exercise (J)	0.94	0.85 – 0.97	0.94	0.86 – 0.98	0.94	0.86 – 0.98
Rate of fatigue (%)	0.83	0.60 – 0.93	0.78	0.48 – 0.91	0.69	0.25 – 0.87
Average power (W)	0.93	0.83 – 0.97	0.97	0.92 – 0.99	0.94	0.85 – 0.97
Average peak torque (N·M)	0.95	0.88 – 0.98	0.97	0.93 – .099	0.94	0.87 – 0.98

T1=Initial testing trial, T2=Second testing trial, T3=Third testing trial, ICC=intra-class correlation, CI=Confidence interval. All data are presented as mean±SD (*n*=22)

Table 3. Intra-class correlations and limits of agreement for test-retest reliability during the flexion component of the 50-repetition protocol completed on the Biodex Isokinetic Dynamometer

	T1 – T2 ICC	95% CI	T2 – T3 ICC	95% CI	T1 – T3 ICC	95% CI
Peak torque (N·M)	0.75	0.39 – 0.90	0.86	0.66 – 0.94	0.81	0.55 – 0.92
Peak torque/body weight (%)	0.69	0.25 – 0.87	0.76	0.43 – 0.90	0.66	0.18 – 0.86
Time to peak torque (ms)	0.65	0.15 – 0.85	0.80	0.51 – 0.92	0.45	−0.32 – 0.77
Torque at 30° (N·M)	0.74	0.38 – 0.89	0.94	0.85 – 0.97	0.81	0.54 – 0.92
Torque at 0.18 s (N·M)	0.75	0.40 – 0.90	0.92	0.81 – 0.97	0.76	0.42 – 0.90
Work completed during highest repetition (J)	0.83	0.59 – 0.93	0.96	0.91 – 0.98	0.85	0.64 – 0.94
Work/body weight (%)	0.80	0.52 – 0.92	0.93	0.83 – 0.97	0.77	0.44 – 0.90
Total work completed during exercise (J)	0.81	0.54 – 0.92	0.94	0.85 – 0.97	0.80	0.52 – 0.92
Total work during the initial 3rd of exercise (J)	0.83	0.59 – 0.93	0.95	0.88 – 0.98	0.83	0.58 – 0.93
Total work during the middle 3rd of exercise (J)	0.78	0.47 – 0.91	0.91	0.79 – 0.96	0.71	0.31 – 0.88
Total work during the final 3rd of exercise (J)	0.70	0.28 – 0.88	0.88	0.72 – 0.95	0.71	0.30 – 0.88
Rate of fatigue (%)	0.65	0.15 – 0.85	0.86	0.66 – 0.94	0.47	−0.27 – 0.78
Average power (W)	0.84	0.61 – 0.93	0.94	0.84 – 0.97	0.80	0.51 – 0.92
Average peak torque (N·M)	0.73	0.35 – 0.89	0.92	0.80 – 0.97	0.84	0.62 – 0.93

T1=Initial testing trial, T2=Second testing trial, T3=Third testing trial, ICC=intra-class correlation, CI=Confidence interval. All data are presented as mean±SD (n=22)

differences between ICC values for this variable. The highest ICC values between all trials were exhibited for peak torque (range:.93 –.96), work completed during the highest repetition (range:.94 –.96), total work completed (range:.95 –.96), and average peak torque (range:.94 –.97).

Absolute and relative TEMs were calculated for all variables. Relative TEM exhibited minimal measurement error between trial 1 vs. trial 2 (range: 0.27% – 0.97% for all variables), trial 2 vs. trial 3 (range: 0.27% – 1.45% for all variables), and trial 1 vs. trial 3 (range: 0.32% – 1.30% for all variables) during the extension component of the isokinetic exercise protocol (Table 4). The flexion component of the protocol (Table 5) also exhibited low relative TEM between trial 1 vs. trial 2 (range: 0.87% – 2.45% for all variables), trial 2 vs. trial 3 (range: 0.54% – 1.10% for all variables), and trial 1 vs. trial 3 (range: 0.71% – 2.26% for all variables).

Raw values from the extension and flexion components of the 50 repetition protocol are displayed in Tables 6 and 7, respectively. For the extension component of the protocol, RM-MANOVA indicated no significant differences (Wilks Λ >.05) between the trials for any of the isokinetic exercise variables measured. These non-significant results were mirrored when evaluating the flexion component of the protocol (Wilks Λ >.05). This indicates that there was no learning effect with the Biodex knee extension/flexion for female MA cyclists.

DISCUSSION

The purpose of this investigation was two-fold, 1) to establish test-retest reliability of the Biodex isokinetic dynamometer in female MA, and 2) to determine whether there is a learning effect associated with the Biodex isokinetic dynamometer when utilized without a familiarization. For reliability in MA, the results from this study indicate the Biodex exhibits strong test-retest consistency between trials.

Most all variables exhibited moderate to strong reliability (as defined by ICC ≥.50) indicating strong test-retest reliability. There were also no performance improvements for any measured variables during knee extension/flexion between trials, suggesting there is no learning effect with the Biodex in female MA cyclists.

Based on the ICCs and 95% CI, there is a very high test-retest reliability on the Biodex isokinetic dynamometer in female MA cyclists. Additionally, measurement errors between trials were extremely low (relative TEM ≤ 2.5%) for all extension (Table 4) and flexion (Table 5) variables. Previous investigations have examined test-retest reliability in young, healthy males and females, pediatrics, and untrained older males; however, these are the first data demonstrating these results in MA and an all-female subject sample (Brown, Whitehurst, Gilbert, & Buchalter, 1995; Feiring, Ellenbecker, & Derscheid, 1990; Symons et al., 2005; Tsiros et al., 2011). Not only are MA at a greater risk for lower-extremity injury when compared to younger, trained individuals, females are also at a greater risk for knee injury compared to males (Dugan, 2005; McKean et al., 2006). As a result, it is important that baseline testing results are accurate when used as an outcome measure for a training program or in rehabilitation from a knee injury. In non-research settings, it may take considerable time and financial resources to schedule on-site evaluations in clinics or performance facilities and as a result, initial familiarization to the equipment/procedures may not be feasible. If a test is not reliable between visits, it would make tracking longitudinal performance gains and recovery from injury difficult in MA, as measurement sensitivity may not be appropriate to detect minor improvements. Reliable measurements from trial to trial are critical for these athletes in order to determine minute changes in strength and evaluate agonist/antagonist ratios between the quadriceps and hamstrings musculature (Mota et al., 2015). It is also im-

Table 4. Absolute and relative technical error of measurement calculations during the extension component of the 50-repetition protocol completed on the Biodex Isokinetic Dynamometer between testing trials

	Absolute TEM			Relative TEM		
	T1 – T2	T2 – T3	T1 – T3	T1 – T2	T2 – T3	T1 – T3
Peak torque (N·M)	3.43	3.74	5.60	0.32	0.33	0.50
Peak torque/body weight (%)	2.59	3.35	4.13	0.33	0.42	0.52
Time to peak torque (ms)	41.67	38.31	53.83	0.70	0.65	0.92
Torque at 30° (N·M)	5.25	7.87	7.22	0.97	1.45	1.30
Torque at 0.18 s (N·M)	4.38	3.59	5.82	0.45	0.35	0.58
Work completed during highest repetition (J)	5.10	4.85	6.33	0.35	0.32	0.42
Work/body weight (%)	5.01	5.44	5.03	0.48	0.51	0.47
Total work completed during exercise (J)	155.24	150.21	170.55	0.29	0.28	0.32
Work completed during the initial 3rd of exercise (J)	85.14	73.29	100.28	0.38	0.32	0.44
Work completed during the middle 3rd of exercise (J)	54.40	53.94	58.96	0.31	0.30	0.33
Work completed during the final 3rd of exercise (J)	43.78	44.30	43.95	0.34	0.35	0.34
Rate of fatigue (%)	5.56	3.91	6.45	0.64	0.43	0.75
Average power (W)	7.15	6.11	7.98	0.34	0.29	0.38
Average peak torque (N·M)	2.08	2.17	2.91	0.27	0.27	0.37

T1=Initial testing trial, T2=Second testing trial, T3=Third testing trial, TEM=technical error of measurement. All data are presented as mean±SD (n=22)

Table 5. Absolute and relative technical error of measurement calculations during the flexion component of the 50-repetition protocol completed on the Biodex Isokinetic Dynamometer between testing trials

	Absolute TEM			Relative TEM		
	T1 – T2	T2 – T3	T1 – T3	T1 – T2	T2 – T3	T1 – T3
Peak Torque (N·M)	5.17	4.09	3.84	0.93	0.71	0.71
Peak Torque/body weight (%)	3.87	3.55	3.04	0.95	0.87	0.79
Time to peak torque (ms)	133.61	99.67	159.35	1.46	1.07	1.83
Torque at 30° (N·M)	6.02	3.23	5.77	2.45	1.10	2.26
Torque at 0.18 s (N·M)	6.90	4.07	7.41	2.16	1.08	2.18
Work completed during highest repetition (J)	7.06	3.23	6.51	1.28	0.55	1.18
Work/Body weight (%)	4.60	2.49	4.73	1.16	0.60	1.20
Total work completed during exercise (J)	240.11	128.09	226.74	1.36	0.69	1.29
Work completed during the initial 3rd of exercise (J)	118.83	58.45	111.39	1.58	0.71	1.48
Work completed during the middle 3rd of exercise (J)	81.49	48.25	84.07	1.37	0.79	1.41
Work completed during the final 3rd of exercise (J)	59.59	35.65	52.99	1.44	0.84	1.29
Rate of fatigue (%)	14.66	8.57	16.90	1.80	0.94	2.05
Average power (W)	10.79	6.35	11.20	1.35	0.74	1.39
Average peak torque (N·M)	3.54	2.21	2.62	0.87	0.54	0.65

T1=Initial testing trial, T2=Second testing trial, T3=Third testing trial, TEM=technical error of measurement. All data are presented as mean±SD (n=22)

portant to note that the MA cyclists utilized in this investigation would be a population likely to demonstrate the least amount of testing variability, based on familiarity with muscle recruitment patterns that mimic those used in sport-based settings and high intrinsic motivation to give maximal efforts each time (Frederick-Recascino & Schuster-Smith, 2003; So et al., 2005). Thus, these results cannot be extrapolated to an untrained population, which might display more variability between trials.

The Biodex is a multifaceted tool providing numerous outcome performance variables. Nevertheless, when determining test-retest reliability of the Biodex, peak torque is commonly used as the outcome variable associated with measurement consistency (Bagley, McLeland, Arevalo, Brown, Coburn, & Galpin, 2016; Lund et al., 2005; McLeland, Ruas, Arevalo, Bagley, Ciccone, Brown, Coburn, Galpin, & Malyszek, 2016; Tsiros et al., 2011). These are the

Table 6. Raw values calculated during the extension component of the 50-repetition protocol completed on the Biodex Isokinetic Dynamometer

	T1	T2	T3	p - value
Peak Torque (N·M)	50.7±10.4	53.0±11.5	56.6±11.0	0.20
Peak Torque/body weight (%)	36.2±6.7	37.9±7.5	39.2±7.3	0.38
Time to peak torque (ms)	280.5±59.8	284.1±69	280.5±64.4	0.98
Torque at 30° (N·M)	27.1±10.0	26.4±10.2	26.6±9.4	0.97
Torque at 0.18 s (N·M)	45.7±9.0	47.4±10.1	50.1±9.0	0.29
Work completed during highest repetition (J)	70.8±16.7	72.2±17.0	74.7±17.8	0.74
Work/Body weight (%)	50.2±9.7	50.5±9.0	51.5±10.9	0.90
Total work completed during exercise (J)	2548.4±524.4	2544.8±516.0	2615.3±579.3	0.89
Work completed during the initial 3rd of exercise (J)	1052.7±252.5	1094.7±251.4	1124.7±271.7	0.65
Work completed during the middle 3rd of exercise (J)	863.5±168.1	841.9±166.7	864.0±182.0	0.89
Work completed during the final 3rd of exercise (J)	632.2±126.7	608.3±115.8	626.6±140.0	0.81
Rate of fatigue (%)	38.8±9.5	43.7±6.9	43.6±6.5	0.06
Average power (W)	99.0±19.4	100.5±20.6	104.6±21.7	0.65
Average peak torque (N·M)	36.6±6.3	37.5±7.1	39.4±7.1	0.39

T1 = Initial testing trial, T2 = Second testing trial, T3 = Third testing trial. All data are presented as mean ± SD (n = 22)

Table 7. Raw values calculated during the flexion component of the 50-repetition protocol completed on the Biodex Isokinetic Dynamometer

	T1	T2	T3	p - value
Peak torque (N·M)	25.8±6.3	28.5±8.9	27.2±7.3	0.50
Peak torque/body weight (%)	18.6±4.2	20.6±6.3	18.8±4.5	0.39
Time to peak torque (ms)	409.7±206.9	457.2±155.2	414.5±179.4	0.64
Torque at 30° (N·M)	10.5±7.7	14.4±9.4	15.1±9.5	0.19
Torque at 0.18 s (N·M)	13.8±10.1	17.7±10.5	19.8±9.9	0.15
Work completed during highest repetition (J)	25.7±12.4	29.3±12.7	29.8±12.0	0.49
Work/body weight (%)	18.5±8.2	20.5±7.3	20.5±6.8	0.59
Total work completed during exercise (J)	826.0±420.6	921.0±415.8	920.2±342.6	0.66
Work completed during the initial 3rd of exercise (J)	346.4±201.7	409.8±213.7	413.0±178.5	0.46
Work completed during the middle 3rd of exercise (J)	284.3±142.1	301.3±133.2	302.9±111.0	0.87
Work completed during the final 3rd of exercise (J)	195.3±89.4	209.9±88.1	204.3±69.9	0.84
Rate of fatigue (%)	35.9±21.1	43.3±17.5	44.6±17.5	0.26
Average power (W)	36.6±19.2	42.1±19.9	42.8±17.0	0.49
Average peak torque (N·M)	19.3±4.5	20.1±6.2	19.9±5.4	0.88

T1 = Initial testing trial, T2 = Second testing trial, T3 = Third testing trial. All data are presented as mean ± SD *(n = 22)*.

first data, in any population, to evaluate test-retest reliability of the following outcome variables (Tables 2 and 3): a) time to peak torque, b) torque generated at 30°, c) torque generated at 0.18s, d) work completed during the highest repetition, e) relative work completed (based on body weight), f) total work completed, g) work completed during the initial 3rd of exercise, h) work completed during the middle 3rd of exercise, i) work completed during the final 3rd of exercise, j) fatigue index, k) average power, and l) average peak torque. In our study, the ICCs for peak torque were consistently high (>.75), indicating strong test-retest reliability. Additionally, most other variables demonstrated moderate to strong reliability (ICC ≥.50). Only 1 variable in extension (time to peak

torque) and 2 variables during flexion (time to peak torque and fatigue rate) exhibited poor reliability for one of the between-trial comparisons (trial 1 vs. 3). Still, for these variables, the 95% CI overlapped with the CI for the other trials (i.e. trial 1 vs. 2 CI overlapped with trial 2 vs. 3 CI overlapped with trial 1 vs. 3 CI). This indicates that although the ICC was low for those variables, values were not significantly different from ICC values in the other 2 trial comparisons. Additionally, it has been shown that the effect of the leg flexors on the outcome of the isokinetic fatigue test is minimal (Mota et al., 2015). Ensuring that all variables calculated by the Biodex software demonstrate strong test-retest reliability is important because different populations may have different goals associated with the Biodex evaluation. For example, an endurance athlete attempting to improve finishing speed during a race would require reliable measurements of 'work completed during the final 3rd of exercise' to successfully track changes associated with training. Our study indicates that the Biodex can be considered a reliable tool for all of these measures.

Previously, the presence of a learning effect associated with the Biodex remained unclear, as only two studies had evaluated this concept with conflicting results (Lund et al., 2005; Symons et al., 2005). Although the work by Lund et al. (2005) suggested there is no learning effect associated with the evaluation, the incorporation of a familiarization trial inherently invalidates these claims. The other investigation examining the learning effect of the Biodex suggested test-retest reliability was high (ICC = 0.84 – 0.94) during a 5-repetition, muscular strength protocol (Symons et al., 2005). However, as the work by Symons et al. (2005) only examined an initial test-retest design and did not account for additional follow-up assessments (i.e. a 3rd evaluation to determine changes in variability from initial testing), an overall learning effect cannot be determined. Results from the current investigation suggest there is not a learning effect associated with the Biodex isokinetic dynamometer (based on non-significant $Wilks\ \Lambda$, $p > 0.05$) when tested at 3 separate time points, 1 week apart.

While the outcomes of this investigation are novel and important for future research, there are certain constraints associated with the results that must be addressed. This investigation included athletes (specifically females) who were comfortable with the exercise patterns recruited, and it cannot be assumed untrained individuals would exhibit similar results because these individuals tend to have lower intrinsic motivation and therefore, may not give a maximal effort each time (Frederick-Rescascino & Schuster-Smith, 2003). These data were also collected in trained, healthy, athletic individuals free from lower-extremity injury; thus these results may not be valid for untrained or individuals undergoing a rehabilitation program based on a potential increase in measurement variability. Finally, this investigation allotted exactly 1 week between testing trials, where participants were required to come at the same time each day. This chronobiological control may not always be feasible in a clinical setting, and could lead to augmented measurement variability between testing.

In this investigation, we present the first data exhibiting strong test-retest reliability of the Biodex isokinetic dynamometer in MA. Additionally, this is the first investigation to demonstrate strong test-retest reliability in an all-female subject population. Furthermore, we demonstrate that there is no learning effect associated with either the extension or flexion component of isokinetic knee exercise on the Biodex. When used in clinical or research settings, a familiarization protocol does not appear necessary before undergoing isokinetic exercise testing. The removal of a familiarization trial to the Biodex can save time and minimize financial requirements for athletes tracking longitudinal performance gains. However, these results only pertain to a highly trained, older female population, and these results cannot be extrapolated to injured or non-athlete populations. Future investigations are required in lesser-trained and/or individuals in clinical

settings to further elucidate whether there is a learning effect associated with the Biodex isokinetic dynamometer.

CONCLUSIONS

There was strong test-retest reliability in masters-aged, female athletes. No learning effect was associated with the Biodex during a knee extension/flexion fatigue protocol, indicating that a familiarization protocol is not necessary for isokinetic testing.

ACKNOWLEDGEMENTS

The authors would like to thank Rodger Stewart, Mikaila Davis, Aaron Martinez, Lauren Wethington, Carly Arnold, and Landon Lavene for their assistance during the data collection and input process. We would also like to thank the participants for their cooperation and effort.

REFERENCES

Altamirano K.M., Coburn J.W., Brown L.E., Judelson D.A. (2012). Effects of warm up on peak torque, rate of torque development, and electromyographic and mechanomyographic signals. *Journal of Strength and Conditioning Research,* 26(5), 1296-1301. https://doi.org/10.1519/JSC.0b013e31822e7a85

Alvares J., Rodrigues R., Azevedo Franke R., da Silva B., Pinto R., Vaz M., et al. (2015). Inter-machine reliability of the Biodex and Cybex isokinetic dynamometers for knee flexor/extensor isometric, concentric, and eccentric tests. *Physical Therapy in Sport,* 16(1), 59-65. https://doi.org/10.1016/j.ptsp.2014.04.004

Bagley J.R., McLeland K.A., Arevalo J.A., Brown L.E., Coburn J.W., Galpin A.J. (2016). Skeletal muscle fatigability and myosin heavy chain fiber type in resistance trained men. *Journal of Strength and Conditioning Research,* 31(3), 602-607. https://doi.org/10.1519/JSC.0000000000001759

Brown L.E. (2000). *Isokinetics in Human Performance.* Champaign, IL: Human Kinetics.

Brown L.E., Weir J.P. (2001). ASEP procedures recommendation I: Accurate assessment of muscular strength and power. *JEPonline,* 4(3), 1-21. http://dx.doi.org/10.4236/ojmip.2013.32014

Brown L.E., Whitehurst M., Bryant J.R., Buchalter D.N. (1993). Reliability of the Biodex System 2 isokinetic dynamometer concentric mode. *Isokinetics and Exercise Science,* 3(3), 160-163. http://dx.doi.org/10.3233/IES-1993-3307

Brown L.E., Whitehurst M., Gilbert R., Buchalter, D.N. (1995). The effect of velocity and gender on load range knee extension and flexion exercise on an isokinetic device. *Journal of Orthopaedic & Sports Physical Therapy,* 21(2), 107-112. https://doi.org/10.2519/jospt.1995.21.2.107

Caruso J.F., Brown L.E., Tufano J.J. (2012). The reproducibility of isokinetic dynamometry data. *Isokinetics and Exercise Science,* 20(4), 239-253. http://dx.doi.org/10.3233/IES-2012-0477

Drouin J.M., Valovich-McLeod T.C., Shultz S.J., Gansneder B.M., Perrin D.H. (2004). Reliability and validity of the Biodex System 3 pro isokinetic dynamometer velocity, torque, and position measurements. *European Journal of Applied Physiology*, 91(1), 22-29. https://doi.org/10.1007/s00421-003-0933-0

Dugan S.A. (2005). Sports-related knee injuries in female athletes: what gives? *American Journal of Physical Medicine & Rehabilitation*, 84(2), 122-130. http://dx.doi.org10.1097/01.PHM.0000154183.40640.93

Feiring D.C., Ellenbecker T.S., Derscheid G.L. (1990). Test-retest reliability of the Biodex isokinetic dynamometer. *Journal of Orthopaedic & Sports Physical Therapy*, 11(7), 298-300.

Frederick-Recascino C.M., Schuster-Smith H. (2003). Competition and intrinsic motivation in physical activity: a comparison of two groups. *Journal of Sport Behavior*, 26(3), 240-254.

Gillet N., Rosnet E. (2008). Basic need satisfaction and motivation in sport. *The Online Journal of Sport Psychology*, 10(3), 1-3.

Glenn J., Gray M., Stewart R., Moyen N.E., Kavouras S., DiBrezzo R., et al. (2015). Incremental effects of 28 days of beta-alanine supplementation on high-intensity cycling performance and blood lactate in masters female cyclists. *Amino Acids*, 47(12), 2593-2600. https://doi.org/10.1007/s00726-015-2050-x

Glenn J., Gray M., Stewart R., Moyen N.E., Kavouras S.A., DiBrezzo R., et al. (2016). Effects of longitudinal beta-alanine supplementation on isokinetic exercise performance and body composition in female masters athletes. *Journal of Strength and Conditioning Research*, 30(1), 201-207. https://doi.org/10.1519/JSC.0000000000001077

Glenn J., Gray M., Vincenzo J. (2014). Differences in regional adiposity, bone mineral density, and physical exercise participation based on exercise self-efficacy among senior adults. *The Journal of Sports Medicine and Physical Fitness*, 55(10), 1166-1173.

Gross M.T., Huffman G.M., Phillips C.N., Wray J.A. (1991). Intramachine and intermachine reliability of the Biodex and Cybex® II for knee flexion and extension peak torque and angular work. *Journal of Orthopaedic & Sports Physical Therapy*, 13(6), 329-335. http://dx.doi.org/10.2519/jospt.1991.13.6.329

Knobloch K., Yoon U., Vogt P.M. (2008). Acute and overuse injuries correlated to hours of training in master running athletes. *Foot & Ankle International*, 29(7), 671-676. https://doi.org/10.3113/FAI.2008.0671

Kramer J.F. (1990). Reliability of knee extensor and flexor torques during continuous concentric-eccentric cycles. *Archives of Physical Medicine and Rehabilitation*, 71(7), 460-464.

Little C.E., Emery C., Black A., Scott S.H., Meeuwisse W., Nettel-Aguirre A., et al. (2015). Test-retest reliability of KINARM robot sensorimotor and cognitive assessment: in pediatric ice hockey players. *Journal of NeuroEngineering and Rehabilitation*, 12(78), 1-18. https://doi.org/10.1186/s12984-015-0070-0

Louis J., Hausswirth C., Easthope C., Brisswalter J. (2012). Strength training improves cycling efficiency in master endurance athletes. *European Journal of Applied Physiology*, 112(2), 631-640. https://doi.org/10.1007/s00421-011-2013-1

Lund H., Søndergaard K., Zachariassen T., Christensen R., Bulow P., Henriksen M., et al. (2005). Learning effect of isokinetic measurements in healthy subjects, and reliability and comparability of Biodex and Lido dynamometers. *Clinical Physiology & Functional Imaging*, 25(2), 75-82. https://doi.org/10.1111/j.1475-097X.2004.00593.x

McKean K.A., Manson N.A., Stanish W.D. (2006). Musculoskeletal injury in the masters runners. *Clinical Journal of Sports Medicine*, 16(2), 149-154.

McLeland K.A., Ruas C.V., Arevalo J.A., Bagley J.R., Ciccone A.B., Brown L.E., Coburn J.W., Galpin A.J., Malyszek K.K. (2016). Comparison of knee extension concentric fatigue between repetition ranges. Isokinetics and Exercise Science, 24(1), 33-38. http://dx.doi.org/10.3233/IES-150595

Mota J.A., Stock M.S., Carillo E.C., Olinghouse K.D., Drusch A.S., Thompson B.J. (2015). Influence of hamstring fatigue on the estimated percentage of fast-twitch muscle fibers for the vastus lateralis. *Journal of Strength and Conditioning Research*, 29(12), 3509-3516. https://doi.org/10.1519/JSC.0000000000000996

Moyen N.E., Ellis C.L., Ciccone A.B., Thurston T.S., Cochrane K.C., Brown L.E., et al. (2014). Increasing relative humidity impacts low-intensity exercise in the heat. *Aviation, Space, and Environmental Medicine*, 85(2), 112-119.

Pearson S.J., Young A., Macaluso A., Devito G., Nimmo M.A., Cobbold M., et al. (2002). Muscle function in elite master weightlifters. *Medicine & Science in Sports & Exercise*, 34(7), 1199-1206.

Perini T.A., Oliveria G. L.d., Ornellas J.d.S., Oliveira F.P.d. (2005). Technical error of measurement in anthropometry. *Rev Bras Med Esporte*, 11(1), 81-85. http://dx.doi.org/10.1590/S1517-86922005000100009

Portney L.G. & Watkins M.P. (2000). Foundations of clinical research: applications to practice. (3rd ed.). New Jersey: Prentiss Hall.

So R.C., Ng J.K., Ng G.Y. (2005). Muscle recruitment pattern in cycling: a review. *Physical Therapy in Sport*, 6(2), 114-119. https://doi.org/10.1016/j.ptsp.2005.02.004

Symons T.B., Vandervoort A.A., Rice C.L., Overend T.J., Marsh G.D. (2005). Reliability of a single-session isokinetic and isometric strength measurement protocol in older men. *The Journals of Gerontology. Series A, Biological Sciences and Medical Sciences*, 60(1), 114-119.

Tsiros M.D., Grimshaw P.N., Shield A.J., Buckley J.D. (2001). Test-retest reliability of the Biodex System 4 isokinetic dynamometer for knee strength assessment in paediatric populations. *Journal of Allied Health*, 40(3), 115-119

Wroblewski A.P., Amati F., Smiley M.A., Goodpaster B., Wright V. (2011). Chronic exercise preserves lean muscle mass in masters athletes. *The Physician and Sportsmedicine*, 39(3), 172-178. https://doi.org/10.3810/psm.2011.09.1933

23

Prediction of 3000-m Running Performance Using Classic Physiological Respiratory Responses

Thiago F. Lourenço[1]*, Fernando O. C. da Silva[1], Lucas S. Tessutti[1], Carlos E. da Silva[1], Cesar C. C. Abad[2]

[1]*Biochemistry Department, State University of Campinas, Cidade Universitária Zeferino Vaz, Campinas, SP, 13083-970, Brazil*

[2]*Department of Phyical Education, SENAC University, Av. Eng.Eusébio Stevaux São Paulo, SP 04696-000, Brazil*

Corresponding Author: Thiago F. Lourenço, E-mail: thiago.fernando.lourenco@outlook.com
The research was not funded.

ARTICLE INFO

Conflicts of interest: None
Funding: None

ABSTRACT

Introduction: Knowing which physiological variables predict running performance could help coaches to optimize training prescription to improve running performance. **Objective:** The present study investigated which physiological respiratory responses could predict 3000-m running performance. **Methods:** Seventeen amateur runners (29.82 ± 7.1years; 173.12 ± 9.0cm; 64.59 ± 9.3kg) performed a maximal graded running test on a treadmill. The ventilatory threshold (VT), respiratory compensation point (RCP), and maximal oxygen consumption (VO2max) were assessed, as well as the respective velocities (vVT, vRCP, vVO2max). After 72 to 96 hours the runners performed the 3000-m running field test. The relationships between variables were performed using Pearson product momentum correlations. Thereafter, simple and multiple regression models were applied. The significance level adopted was 5% ($p<0.05$). **Results:** The majority of physiological responses were positive and well related to each other ($r\geq0.70$; $p<0.05$). Despite vVT, vRCP, and vVO2max demonstrating a higher and inverse relationship with 3000-m time ($r=-0.92$; $r=-0.96$; $r=-0.89$; $p<0.05$), the multiple regression model indicated that vRCP and vVO2max are the best variables to predict 3000-m performance in experienced amateur road runners ($R2=0.94$). The equation proposed by the model was: 3000-m(s)=1399.21–[31.65*vRCP(km.h-1)]–[12.06*vVO2max (km.h-1)]. **Conclusion:** The vRCP and vVO2max may be used to predict 3000-m performance using only a maximal running test on a treadmill. In practical terms, coaches and physical conditioners can use performance in the 3000-m to select different exercise running intensities to prescribe exercise training intensities.

Key words: Running, Athletes, Exercise, Athletic Performance

INTRODUCTION

The number of road runners has increased greatly in recent years. In the USA, for example, there was an increase of 57% in road runners in the last decade. Moreover, there are estimated to be 50 million road runners in the USA and almost 14 million US road race participants in 2011 alone (Hryvniak, Dicharry, & Wilder, 2014). The total number of US running events reached 26,370 in 2012. Similar events are held annually worldwide. For instance, the City to Surf in Sydney attracts 60,000 participants, and the Women's Mini Marathon in Dublin has over 40,000 participants, while the BUPA sponsored Great Run series attracts several hundred thousand participants across 15 events (Murphy, Lane, & Bauman, 2015). In São Paulo, the most important economical Brazilian city (South America), from 2001 to 2015, road races increased from 11 to 415 with over 724,000 participants in 2015. This represents an increase of 10.87% in comparison to 2014 (Atletismo, 2016). Finally, in 2016, the International Association of Athletics Federation (IAAF) included 88 road races worldwide in their official calendar (IAAF,

2017). Hence the trend in the number of competitions and practitioners looks likely to continue to increase in the near future. Due to the increase in road races worldwide, knowing the responses of physiological variables during some physical fitness tests, as well their relationship with simple, low-cost, fast, trustable, reproducible, easy, and valid field tests for running training prescription could help personal trainers, physical conditioners, coaches of amateurs, and sports scientists to prescribe better running training intensities and volumes, aiming to improve the physical fitness, pacing, wellbeing, health, and running performance of amateur runners (Maron, Douglas, Graham, Nishimura, & Thompson, 2005; Starkoff, Eneli, Bonny, Hoffman, & Devor, 2014).

Previous studies have reported that classic physiological respiratory variables such as those related to maximal aerobic power [i.e.; maximal oxygen uptake (VO2max), ventilatory threshold (VT), respiratory compensation point (RCP), and the velocity at which VO2max occurs (vVO2max) present significant relationships with running performance (Arrese, Izquierdo, & Serveto Galindo, 2006; Bellar & Judge, 2012; Duffield, Bishop, & Dawson, 2006; S, Craig, Wilson, &

Aitchison, 1997). Therefore, these variables have frequently been used to evaluate, prescribe, and monitor running training programs (Bragada et al., 2010; Bunc, Heller, Leso, Šprynarová, & Zdanowicz, 1987; Esfarjani & Laursen, 2007; Esteve-Lanao, Foster, Seiler, & Lucia, 2007; Esteve-Lanao, Juan, Earnest, Foster, & Lucia, 2005; Muñoz et al., 2014). However, the majority of these studies were conducted with elite or well-trained athletes and the relationship between these physiological variables and simplified field tests such as the 3000-m running test remain undescribed in amateur athletes. Therefore, the aim of the present study was to investigate the relationships between VT, RCP, VO2max, vVT, vRCP, and vVO2max assessed in a maximal running test on a treadmill until exhaustion and the 3000-m running field test. The hypothesis was that the running velocities related to these classic respiratory physiological responses would predict 3000-m running performance.

MATERIAL AND METHODS

The present work may be described as a descriptive cross-sectional study. All volunteers were informed of the procedures and signed the informed consent form. The procedures were conducted in accordance with the Helsinki Declaration for studies with humans, approved by the Ethics Committee of the Faculty of Medical Sciences of the State University of Campinas (n° 523/2010).

Participants

Seventeen amateur road runners (age: 29.82 ± 7.10 years; body height: 173.12 ± 9.02 cm; body weight: 64.59 ± 9.39 kg; BMI: 21.57 ± 2.81; training experience: 8.34 ± 3.16 years) participated in this study. All participants competed at regional level and were tested during their pre-competitive period. The volunteers were required to maintain their routines concerning fluid, food, sleep, physical activity, and recovery. At least 24-h before the tests, the volunteers were required to suspend their physical training.

Maximal Graded Test

The runners underwent a maximal incremental running test to determine the ventilatory threshold (VT), respiratory compensation point (RCP), and maximal oxygen uptake (VO2max). After a 3-min warm-up at $8 - 8.5$ km·h⁻1, the treadmill (Inbrasport Super-ATL, Porto Alegre, RS, Brazil) was set at 9 km·h⁻1 and a fixed slope of 1% and after each 25-sec interval, the running speed was increased by 0.3 km·h⁻1 until volitional exhaustion according to Lourenço, Martins, Tesutti, Brenzikofer, & Macedo (2011). Oxygen uptake (VO2), carbon dioxide output (VCO2), breathing frequency (Bf), and tidal volume (Vt) were continuously collected with an automated breath-by-breath system (CPX/D Med Graphics, St. Paul, MN) using a Nafion filter tube and a turbine flow meter (opto-electric). Minute ventilation (Ve) was calculated as the product of Bf by VT, respectively. To analyze the data and decrease the variability in breath-by-breath acquisition we used the average of each 25-s of exercise as recommend-

ed by Robergs, Dwyer, & Astorino (2010). Prior to each test, the analyzer was calibrated using a known gas mixture (12% O2 and 5% CO2), and the volume sensor was calibrated using a 3-L syringe. The laboratory temperature was maintained at 21 ± 1°C and the relative air humidity between 45-50%. The VT and RCP were determined by non–invasive gas exchange measurements using the V-Slope method (Beaver, Wasserman, & Whipp, 1986). The VT was detected by the loss of linearity of VCO2 as a function of VO2 during the incremental test. RCP was detected as the point of departure from linearity of the Ve vs. VCO2 relationship. The software supplied by Medical Graphics Breeze SuiteTM 6.4 MediGraphicsTM was used, supported by visual inspection from three independent and experienced researchers. The VO2max were considered as the value related to the last completed stage with a respiratory exchange ratio (RER) greater than 1.10 (Poole, Wilkerson, & Jones, 2008).

3000-m Running Test

From 72 to 96 hours after the maximal graded test the runners performed, individually, a 3000-m time trial on a 400-m outdoor track. The test began at 9 A.M. and after a standardized warm-up consisting of 15 minutes of jogging at a low speed (about 50% of maximal 6-20 RPE scale), 10 to 15 minutes of active and ballistic stretching, and three 30- to 50-m sprints at increasing speeds, the athletes performed the 3000-m running test. All participants were instructed to run as fast as possible at a self-selected pace and the total race time was measured using a stopwatch. The mean temperature was 24.2 ± 2.2°C and the air humidity 47.4 ± 1.8%. The runners were allowed ad libitum hydration during the trial. Each subject was verbally encouraged to perform at maximum effort and could not use any kind of time device during the test.

Statistical Analysis

The normality of the data was checked using the Shapiro Wilk test. Data were described as mean (X) and standard deviation (SD). Pearson product–moment correlation coefficients (r) and simple linear regression (R^2) were used to determine the relationships between parameters. A multiple regression analysis (stepwise) was also used to evaluate the overall relationship between physiological (VT, RCP, VO2max), mechanical (vVT, vRCP, vVO2max), and 3000-m running test performance. The magnitudes of correlation (90 % confidence limits) between test measures were assessed as follows: < 0.1, trivial; < 0.1–0.3, small; < 0.3–0.5, moderate; < 0.5–0.7, large; < 0.7– 0.9, very large; and < 0.9–1.0, almost perfect. If the 90 % confidence intervals overlapped small positive and negative values, the magnitude was deemed unclear; otherwise the magnitude was deemed to be the observed magnitude (Hopkins, Marshall, Batterham, & Hanin, 2009).

RESULTS

The results of the maximal running test until exhaustion on the treadmill are described in Table 1.

The results of the relationship between VT, RCP, VO2max, vVT, vRCP, vVO2max, and 3000-m are described in Table 2. The Pearson product–moment correlation coefficients (r) and simple linear regression (R^2) showed very large (r ≤ 0.7–0.9) and almost perfect (r ≤ 0.9–1.0) correlations between all mechanical variables analyzed (vVT, vRCP, vVO2max) and 3000-m running test performance. The relationship between vVT and 3000-m running test performance was almost perfect (r=-0.92; R^2=0.85; P<0.05) as was found for vRCP and 3000-m running test performance (r=-0.96; R2=0.91; P<0.05).

The linear regression to predict the 3000-m running test performance is reported in Figure 1.

Table 1. Individual, average (X) and standard deviation (SD) of physiological responses and running velocity of a maximal running test until exhaustion on a treadmill and 3000-m time and velocity.

Athlete	VT Vel (km.h⁻¹)	VT VO₂ (L.min⁻¹)	VT VO₂ (ml.kg⁻¹.min⁻¹)	RCP Vel (km.h⁻¹)	RCP VO₂ (L.min⁻¹)	RCP VO₂ (ml.kg⁻¹.min⁻¹)	VO₂ max Vel (km.h⁻¹)	VO₂ max VO₂ (L.min⁻¹)	VO₂ max VO₂ (ml.kg⁻¹.min⁻¹)	3000-m Time (s)	3000-m Vel (km.h⁻¹)
1	13.0	2.5	35.3	13.5	3.2	45.0	17.9	3.6	50.3	742.0	14.6
2	12.1	2.3	35.4	13.0	1.7	34.4	17.9	2.0	42.1	763.0	14.2
3	11.2	1.9	30.5	12.7	2.4	38.7	15.0	2.8	47.3	870.0	12.4
4	13.8	2.5	35.3	16.4	3.2	45.0	22.2	3.6	55.9	619.0	17.4
5	13.0	2.0	39.8	15.0	2.3	46.1	19.9	2.6	53.7	692.0	15.6
6	14.7	2.5	31.4	17.3	2.5	35.4	22.8	3.6	55.6	606.0	17.8
7	11.8	1.9	30.2	13.2	2.2	34.7	17.0	2.4	43.6	764.0	14.1
8	11.5	1.7	36.0	12.7	1.9	38.6	15.6	2.0	42.1	814.0	13.3
9	12.1	2.0	33.2	13.8	2.4	40.7	19.3	2.6	49.5	714.0	15.1
10	11.8	2.4	29.9	13.0	2.5	32.2	15.8	3.1	39.6	770.0	14.0
11	13.0	2.5	32.8	14.7	2.9	38.3	18.7	3.3	42.8	710.0	15.2
12	13.2	1.8	28.4	15.0	2.2	34.8	18.4	2.6	40.0	721.0	15.0
13	14.7	2.3	39.7	17.4	2.6	44.7	20.4	3.5	60.2	545.5	19.8
14	17.7	2.4	40.0	19.2	2.5	42.2	21.9	3.2	54.4	537.3	20.1
15	14.7	2.8	45.4	17.1	3.9	63.1	19.2	4.1	67.2	631.6	17.1
16	15.9	1.7	30.4	17.7	2.1	37.5	19.2	2.6	46.4	596.7	18.1
17	16.8	2.1	42.4	19.2	2.4	49.4	21.6	2.9	60.0	540.0	20.0
X	13.6	2.2	35.1	15.3	2.5	41.2	19.0	3.0	50.0	684.5	16.1
SD	1.9	0.3	4.9	2.3	0.5	7.5	2.3	0.6	8.1	100.0	2.4

Legend: VT – Ventilatory Threshold; RCP – Respiratory Compensation Point, VO₂ max – Maximal Oxygen Consumption

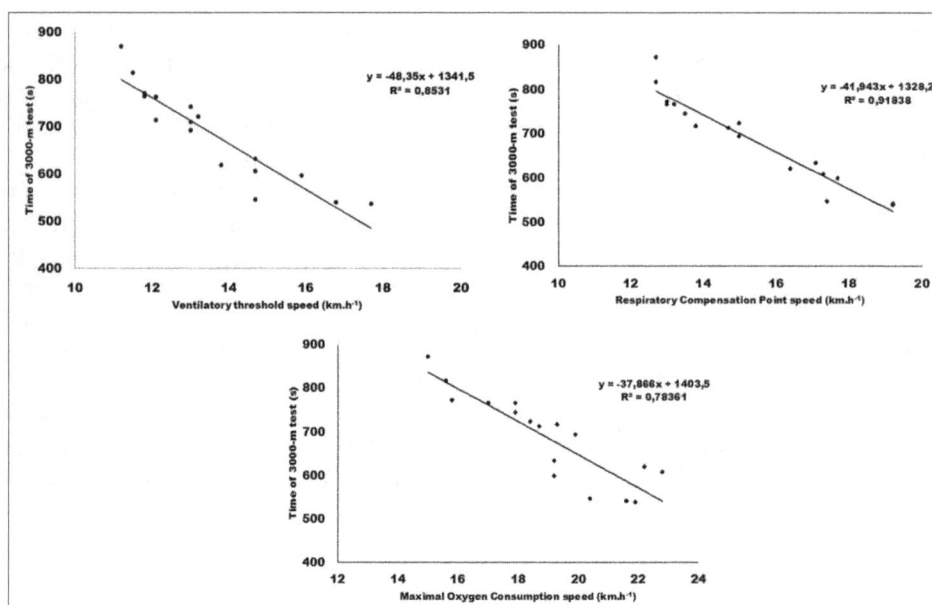

Figure 1. Linear regression of velocity of ventilatory threshold (Panel A), respiratory compensation point (Panel B), and maximal oxygen consumption (Panel C) to predict 3000-m running field test performance.

Table 2. Relationships between physiological responses, mechanical variables, and the 3000-m running field test

Variables (km.h^{-1})	VT Vel (km.h^{-1})	VT VO$_2$ (L.min^{-1})	VT VO$_2$ (ml.kg^{-1}.min^{-1})	RCP Vel (km.h^{-1})	RCP VO$_2$ (L.min^{-1})	RCP VO$_2$ (ml.kg^{-1}.min^{-1})	VO$_2$max Vel (km.h^{-1})	VO$_2$max VO$_2$ (L.min^{-1})	VO$_2$max VO$_2$ (ml.kg^{-1}.min^{-1})	3000-m Time (s)	3000-m Vel (km.h^{-1})
VT Vel (km.h^{-1})	-		0.24*	0.97*	0.22	0.41	0.77*	0.41*	0.61	-0.92*	0.94*
VO$_2$ (L.min^{-1})		-		0.25	0.76*	0.44	0.39	0.82*	0.49*	-0.32	0.29
VO$_2$ (ml.kg^{-1}.min^{-1})			-	0.52*	0.40	0.86*	0.42	0.36	0.79*	-0.52*	0.54*
RCP Vel (km.h^{-1})				-	0.27	0.46	0.83*	0.47	0.70*	-0.96*	0.97*
VO$_2$ (L.min^{-1})					-	0.70*	0.27	0.91*	0.60*	-0.28	0.24
VO$_2$ (ml.kg^{-1}.min^{-1})						-	0.34	0.57*	0.85*	-0.43	0.42
VO2peak Vel (km.h^{-1})							-	0.47	0.66*	-0.89*	0.85*
VO$_2$ (L.min^{-1})								-	0.68*	-0.49*	0.47
VO$_2$ (ml.kg^{-1}.min^{-1})									-	-0.70*	0.70*
3000-m Time (s)										-	0.99*
Vel (km.h^{-1})											-

Legend: VT – Ventilatory Threshold; RCP – Respiratory Compensation Point, VO$_2$ max – Maximal Oxygen Consumption; * - P<0.05

The multiple regression model is reported in Table 3.

The model indicates that the vRCP and vVO2max demonstrate better prediction of 3000-m running performance than the individual linear models (F = 114.87; r = 0.97; R^2 = 0.94; P<0.05). The effect of vVT (P>0.05) and ventilatory responses (F = 0.07; r = 0.63; R^2 = 0.40; P>0.05) on 3000-m performance were not significant and were not included in the final model. The equation proposed by the model is described as follows:

3000-m (s) = 1399.21 – (31.65 * vRCP) – (12.06 * vVO2max)   (Equation 1)

DISCUSSION

The present study aimed to investigate the relationships between physiological respiratory responses of a graded maximal running test on a treadmill and 3000-m running field performance in amateur male runners. We hypothesized that running speeds related to the classic physiological responses such as vVT, vRCP, and vVO2max would demonstrate good to strong relationships to predict 3000-m running performance. The main finding of the present study was that, as expected, the physiological variables were well related to each other. Furthermore, the multiple regressions showed that vRCP and vVO2max were the most important variables to predict 3000-m running performance. Although widely used in practice as an evaluative test, to our knowledge no work has investigated the relationship between 3000-m running performance and physiological responses in experienced amateur male runners. The results were according to our prior hypothesis since the Pearson product–moment correlation coefficients (r) and simple linear regression (R2) showed very large (r ≤ 0.7– 0.9) and almost perfect (r ≤ 0.9–1.0) correlations, with vRCP presenting the best relationship found (r=-0.96; R^2=0.91; P<0.05) followed by vVT (r = 0.94; R^2 = 0.85; P<0.05) and vVO2max (r = 0.85; R^2 = 0.78; P<0.05). These data are, in part, in agreement with those found by Yoshida et al. (1993), who found that 3000m running performance of female athletes in distance runners (10000 m) was closely associated with blood variables such as lactate threshold (r = 0.73), onset blood lactate accumulation (r = 0.78), and VO2max (r = 0.52). In addition, when performing the stepwise multiple regression, the authors also found that variables related to blood lactate contributed significantly to performance in the 3000-m. More recently, Bragada et al. (2010) showed similar results, indicating that vVO2max and running speed at 4 mmol L^{-1} were strongly correlated to 3000-m performance in well-trained middle-distance runners. However, in the present study, although we observed that the vVT, which corresponds to the lactate threshold, showed a higher correlation than these studies, when the stepwise multiple regression was performed it had no contribution to the 3000-m running performance. This may be due to the protocol used in other studies as whereas Bragada et al. (2010) used a fixed blood lactate concentration protocol which has been previously strongly questioned (see review of Faude, Kindermann, & Meyer, 2009). Herein, we used a validated and reproducible protocol for the studied population (Lourenço et al., 2011).

Table 3. Multiple regression model to predict 3000-m running test performance.

Variable	Coefficient	Standard error	t-Stat	P-value	95% lower CI	95% upper CI
Intersection	1399.21	52.40	26.70	0.00	1286.82	1511.60
vRCP (km.h^{-1})	-31.65	5.08	-6.22	0.00	-42.55	-20.74
vVO$_{2\,max}$ (km.h^{-1})	-12.06	4.97	-2.43	0.03	-22.72	-1.41

vPCR=respiratory compensation point velocity, vVO$_2$ max=maximal oxygen consumption velocity

Yoshida, Udo, Iwai, & Yamaguchi (1993) used a protocol with higher stage times (5 minutes) to highlight the quantification of serum lactate concentration. Stage protocols lasting > 3 minutes result in lower VO2max without consistency for vVT and vRCP determinations through gas analysis (Bentley, Newell, & Bishop, 2007). It seems that smaller speed increments are more appropriate for determining vVT, vRCP, and vVO2max due to the mild adjustment of oxidative and glycolytic enzymes to compensate for the new adenosine triphosphate (ATP) demands (Bentley et al., 2007). Traditionally, lactate production/removal kinetics and ventilatory threshold are considered strong predictors of running performance ranging from 5-km running to marathon (Faude et al., 2009; McLaughlin, Howley, Bassett, Thompson, & Fitzhugh, 2010). This is in line with Billat, Binsse, Petit, & Koralsztein (1998) and Lima-Silva et al. (2010) who considered that the ability to maintain running speed above VT represents one of the best predictors of 10-km running performance. It is already known that exercises performed above vVT induce greater removal of lactate and hydrogen (H$^+$) from the musculature, which may lead to a decrease in blood pH (Juel, 2008), reinforcing the importance of vRCP in the 3000-m performance, since RCP indicates the limit of blood buffering capacity (Wasserman, Beaver, Sun, & Stringer, 2011). Furthermore, Noakes, Myburgh, & Schall (1990) suggest that peak treadmill running velocity during the VO2max test alone predicts running performance. According to Billat, Renoux, Pinoteau, Petit, & Koralsztein (1994) and Jones (1998), 3000-m running velocity ranged between 97 and 101% vVO2peak (mean 100%), which suggests that the 3000-m race pace utilizes approximately 100% of the VO2peak. Instead, in the present study, we found that amateur runners performed the 3000-m at velocities located between vRCP and vVO2max, that is, at training intensity zone 3. They performed at 105% of vRCP and at 84% of vVO2max, which reinforces the importance of plasma buffer capacity for endurance athletes. Theoretically, running speeds or exercise intensities above sRCP induce decreases in bpH and acidosis is detected by sensory feedback from working skeletal muscle, inducing hyperventilation to control blood pH (Amann et al., 2013; Bhambhani, Malik, & Mookerjee, 2007). As a consequence, hyperventilation serves to reduce the arterial pressure of CO$_2$ which has a direct effect on cerebral blood flow, and may decrease arterial oxygenation in the frontal cortex reducing/modifying the neural motor drive to protect the system and thereby choosing the exercise intensity slightly above vRCP (Amann et al., 2013; Bhambhani et al., 2007; Wasserman et al., 2011). Furthermore, as we found, the amateur runners performed the 3000-m at a slightly higher exercise intensity than vRCP, suggesting the possibility of using the mean running speed of 3000-m as a parameter to prescribe different exercise training intensities for this population. Although the data revealed high correlations between 3000-m performance and a "gold standard" measure, the main limitation of the present study was the lack of control for wind speed, dehydration status, and convection load. It is already known that when running outdoors, air flows across the body at a speed equivalent to forward motion, which can aid heat loss through convection and evaporation and improve or impair running performance (Stevens & Dascombe, 2015). Other studies should be designed to examine the influence of wind speed, dehydration, and convection load on the relationship between 3000-m and mechanical variables (vVT, vRCP, and vVO2max). Furthermore, we did not investigate any physiological parameters during the 3000-m time trial which opens the way for further studies to include these variables in their design. From a practical point of view, we can suggest that exercise intensities below the mean running speed of 3000-m would represent metabolic conditions similar to those found in zones 1 and 2 and, above this would represent zone 3. These results can be useful to coaches and athletes as they involve a single exercise protocol, with minimal disturbance of the training routine and decreased recovery time, fatigue, and risk of injury, since they are amateur runners. Furthermore, the 3000-m is a protocol that reproduces a situation close to the daily reality experienced by athletes.

CONCLUSION

We conclude that the vRCP and vVT showed the strongest relationship with 3000-m running performance. In practical terms, coaches and physical conditioners can use performance in the 3000-m to select different exercise running intensities which may be similar to those found in zone 1 (above vLT), zone 2 (between vVT and vRCP), and zone 3 (above vRCP).

ACKNOWLEDGMENTS

I thank all the athletes and coaches who participated in the study, highlighting the results found here.

REFERENCES

Amann, M., Venturelli, M., Ives, S. J., McDaniel, J., Layec, G., Rossman, M. J., & Richardson, R. S. (2013). Peripheral fatigue limits endurance exercise via a sensory feedback-mediated reduction in spinal motoneuronal output. *Journal of Applied Physiology, 115*(3), 355–364. https://doi.org/10.1152/japplphysiol.00049.2013

Arrese, A. L., Izquierdo, D. M., & Serveto Galindo, J. (2006). Physiological measures associated with marathon running performance in high-level male and female homogeneous groups. *International Journal of Sports Medicine, 27*(4), 289–95.

Atletismo, F. P. de. (2016). Estatística 2016. Retrieved January 1, 2017, from http://www.atletismofpa.org.br/estatistica-2016.html,67

Beaver, W. L., Wasserman, K., & Whipp, B. J. (1986). A new method for detecting anaerobic threshold by gas exchange. *Journal of Applied Physiology, 60*(6), 2020–7.

Bellar, D., & Judge, L. (2012). Modeling and relationship of respiratory exchange ratio to athletic performance. *Journal of Strength & Conditioning and Research, 26*(9), 2484–9.

Bentley, D. J., Newell, J., & Bishop, D. (2007). Incremental exercise test design and analysis: implications for performance diagnostics in endurance athletes. *Sports Medicine, 37*(7), 575–86.

Bhambhani, Y., Malik, R., & Mookerjee, S. (2007). Cerebral oxygenation declines at exercise intensities above the respiratory compensation threshold. *Respiratory Physiology and Neurobiology, 156*(2), 196–202. https://doi.org/10.1016/j.resp.2006.08.009

Billat, V., Binsse, V., Petit, B., & Koralsztein, J. (1998). High level runners are able to maintain a VO2 steady-state below VO2peak in an all-out run over their critical velocity. *Archieves of Physiology and Biochemistry, 38–45*(106), 1.

Billat, V., Renoux, J. C., Pinoteau, J., Petit, B., & Koralsztein, J. P. (1994). Reproducibility of running time to exhaustion at VO2peak in subelite runners. *Medicine and Science in Sports and Exercise, 26*(2), 254–257.

Bragada, J., Santos, P. J., Maia, J. A., Colaço, P. J., Lopes, V. P., & Barbosa, T. M. (2010). Longitudinal study in 3,000m male runners: relationship between performance and selected physiological parameters. *Journal of Sports Science and Medicine, 9*, 439–444.

Bunc, V., Heller, J., Leso, J., Šprynarová, Š., & Zdanowicz, R. (1987). Ventilatory threshold in various groups of highly trained athletes. *International Journal of Sports Medicine1, 8*(4), 275–280.

Duffield, R., Bishop, D., & Dawson, B. (2006). Comparison of the VO2 response to 800-m, 1500-m and 3000-m track running events. *Journal of Sports Medicine and Physical Fitness, 46*(3), 353–60.

Esfarjani, F., & Laursen, P. B. (2007). Manipulating high-intensity interval training: Effects on, the lactate threshold and 3000-m running performance in moderately trained males. *Journal of Science and Medicine in Sport, 10*(1), 27–35.

Esteve-Lanao, J., Foster, C., Seiler, S., & Lucia, A. (2007). Impact of training intensity distribution on performance in endurance athletes. *The Journal of Strength & Conditioning Research, 21*(3), 943–949.

Esteve-Lanao, J., Juan, A. F. S., Earnest, C. P., Foster, C., & Lucia, A. (2005). How do endurance runners actually train? Relationship with competition performance. *Medicine & Science in Sports & Exercise, 496–504*(37), 3.

Faude, O., Kindermann, W., & Meyer, T. (2009). Lactate threshold concepts: how valid are they? *Sports Medicine, 39*(6), 469–90.

Hopkins, W., Marshall, S., Batterham, A., & Hanin, J. (2009). Progressive statistics for studies in sports medicine and exercise science. *Medicine & Science in Sports & Exercise, 41*(1), 3–13.

Hryvniak, D., Dicharry, J., & Wilder, R. (2014). Barefoot running survey: Evidence from the field. *Journal of Sport and Health Science, 3*(2), 131–136.

IAAF. (2017). Calendar 2017. Retrieved January 1, 2017, from https://www.iaaf.org/competition/calendar

Jones, A. M. (1998). A five year physiological case study of an Olympic runner. *British Journal of Sports Medicine, 32*(1), 39–43.

Juel, C. (2008). Regulation of pH in human skeletal muscle: Adaptations to physical activity. *Acta Physiologica, 193*(1), 17–24. https://doi.org/10.1111/j.1748-1716.2008.01840.x

Lima-Silva, A. E., Bertuzzi, R. C. M., Pires, F. O., Barros, R. V., Gagliardi, J. F., Hammond, J.,… Bishop, D. J. (2010). Effect of performance level on pacing strategy during a 10-km running race. *European Journal of Applied Physiology, 108*(5), 1045–1053. https://doi.org/10.1007/s00421-009-1300-6

Lourenço, T. F., Martins, L. E., Tesutti, L. S., Brenzikofer, R., & Macedo, D. V. De. (2011). Reproducibility of an incremental treadmill VO(2)max test with gas exchange analysis for runners. *Journal of Strength and Conditioning Research, 25*(7), 1994–9.

Maron, B., Douglas, P., Graham, T., Nishimura, R., & Thompson, P. (2005). Task Force 1: preparticipation screening and diagnosis of cardiovascular disease in athletes. *J Am Coll Cardiol, 45*, 1322–1326.

McLaughlin, J. E., Howley, E. T., Bassett, D. R., Thompson, D. L., & Fitzhugh, E. C. (2010). Test of the classic model for predicting endurance running performance. *Medicine & Science in Sports & Exercise, 42*(5), 991–7.

Muñoz, I., Seiler, S., Bautista, J., España, J., Larumbe, E., & Esteve-Lanao, J. (2014). Does polarized training improve performance in recreational runners? *International Journal of Sports Physiology and Performance, 9*(2), 265–272.

Murphy, N., Lane, A., & Bauman, A. (2015). Leveraging mass participation events for sustainable health legacy. *Leisure Studies, 34*(6), 758–766.

Noakes, T. D., Myburgh, K. H., & Schall, R. (1990). Peak treadmill running velocity during the VO2 max test predicts running performance. *Journal of Sports Sciences, 8*(1), 35–45.

Poole, D. C., Wilkerson, D. P., & Jones, A. M. (2008). Validity of criteria for establishing maximal O2 uptake during ramp exercise tests. *European Journal of Applied Physiology, 102*(4), 403–10.

Robergs, R. A., Dwyer, D., & Astorino, T. (2010). Recommendations for improved data processing from expired gas analysis indirect calorimetry. *Sports Medicine, 40*(2), 95–111.

S, G., Craig, I., Wilson, J., & Aitchison, T. (1997). The relationship between 3 km running performance and selected physiological variables. *Journal of Sports Sciences*, *15*(4), 403–410.

Starkoff, B. E., Eneli, I. U., Bonny, A. E., Hoffman, R. P., & Devor, S. T. (2014). Estimated Aerobic Capacity Changes in Adolescents with Obesity Following High Intensity Interval Exercise. *International Journal of Kinesiology & Sports Science*, *2*(3), 1–8.

Stevens, C. J., & Dascombe, B. J. (2015). The Reliability and Validity of Protocols for the Assessment of Endurance Sports Performance: An Updated Review. *Measurement in Physical Education and Exercise Science*, *19*(4), 177–185.

Wasserman, K., Beaver, W. L., Sun, X. G., & Stringer, W. W. (2011). Arterial H+ regulation during exercise in humans. *Respiratory Physiology and Neurobiology*, *178*(2), 191–195. https://doi.org/10.1016/j.resp.2011.05.018

Yoshida, T., Udo, M., Iwai, K., & Yamaguchi, T. (1993). Physiological characteristics related to endurance running performance in female distance runners. *Journal of Sports Sciences*, *11*(1), 57–62.

24

The Impact of Different Game Types and Sports on College Students' Physical Activity and Motivation in Basic Instruction Program Settings

Yang Song[1]*, Stephen Harvey[2], James Hannon[3], Karen Rambo-Hernandez[4], Emily Jones[5], Sean Bulger[6]

[1]*The Division of Liberal Studies and Education, Lane College, Jackson, Tennessee, United States*

[2]*Patton College of Education, Department of Recreation and Sport Pedagogy, Ohio University Athens, Ohio, United States*

[3]*College of Education, Health and Human Services, Kent State University Kent, Ohio, United States*

[4]*College of Education and Human Services, West Virginia University Morgantown, West Virginia, United States*

[5]*College of Applied Science and Technology, Illinois State University Normal, Illinois, United States*

[6]*College of Physical Activity and Sport Sciences, West Virginia University Morgantown, West Virginia, United States*

Corresponding Author: Yang Song, E-mail: ysong@lanecollege.edu

ARTICLE INFO

Conflicts of interest: None
Funding: None

ABSTRACT

Background: Although Basic Instruction Program (BIP) or Higher Education Physical Activity Program (HEPAP) classes within university/colleges are founded on the rationale of providing students with opportunities to be physically active, little is known about the physical activity (PA) accrual and/or motivation levels in these classes. **Objective:** The purpose of the present study was to investigate college students' Moderate to Vigorous Physical Activity (MVPA) and motivation levels while playing different games types (modified games/MGs, small-sided games/SSGs, and full-sided games/FSGs) in badminton and soccer classes. In addition, the study examined the extent to which motivation levels predicted students MVPA. **Method:** Participants were seventy-one college students (14 females) from a rural Mid-Atlantic university in the United States (U.S.). Triaxial accelerometers were used to collect MVPA data and the Intrinsic Motivation Inventory (IMI) to measure student motivation. **Results:** Students in soccer classes had statistically significant more MVPA than those in badminton. Students in soccer and badminton classes had most MVPA in FSGs and SSGs, respectively. Although students reported similar scores in the three IMI subscales when data were aggregated, soccer students reported higher levels of competence and effort in MGs, whereas badminton students reported higher levels of competence and effort in SSGs. Interest was the only statistically significant predictor of MVPA in MGs whereas perceived competence statistically significantly predicted MVPA in both SSGs and FSGs. **Conclusion:** PE and sport practitioners should utilize the different game types to find the optimal balance between MVPA and student motivation and realize lesson objectives.

Key words: Universities, Students, Exercise, Motivation, Soccer, Racquet sports, Accelerometry

INTRODUCTION

Healthy People (2020) provides the physical activity guidelines for adults in aerobic physical activity (at least 150 minutes/week at moderate intensity or 75 minutes/week at vigorous intensity) and in muscle-strengthening activity (two or more days a week). However, only about 20% of adults meet the guidelines for both aerobic and muscle-strengthening activity (Healthy People, 2020). With about 20 million students served in U.S. colleges and universities (American College Health Association, 2012), college/university students, a major source of future generations of parents and policy-makers, should be a research targeted population for enhancing the proportion of adults achieving the Healthy People 2020 physical activity goals. Fortunately, most col-

leges/universities provide their students with physical activity (PA) opportunities in the form of a Basic Instruction Program (BIP) or Higher Education Physical Activity Program (HEPAP) (Stapleton, Taliaferro, & Bulger, 2017). It is crucial for adult learners to develop the appreciation for physical activity in BIPs or HEPAP because physical activity behaviors established during the college years will persist into adulthood (Sparling & Snow, 2002). To encourage student participation in BIP or HEPAP classes, many colleges/universities offer a variety of classes in activities and sports that students will have previously participated in, either recreationally or within a competitive context, during high school. However, despite BIP and HEPAP classes being founded on the rationale of providing college students with opportunities to be physically active during their time at university, little is known about how these classes assist students in meeting slated PA goals. In addition, although the Institute of Medicine (IOM, 2013) has recommended k-12 students engage in moderate to vigorous physical activity (MVPA) levels for at least 50 percent of PE class time, no such stipulations have been afforded to university BIP/HEPAP classes. Moreover, it is clear that the nature of the activity being conducted within these BIP/HEPAP classes could affect the amount of PA accumulation during one session. Emerging research in sport and physical education research, for example, suggests that using a variety of smaller-sided games (SSG's), and/ or modified games (MGs) as opposed to full-sided games (FSGs) may affect participant PA levels. For the purpose of the study, the definitions of the following terms were taken from Roberts & Fairclough (2012). *Modified games (MGs)*: the class is engaged in a modified game. Modification of the game includes rules (e.g., the ball or the projectile is not allowed over a certain distance, height), conditions and equipment (e.g., throw-catch badminton, alternative scoring zones). The game reduces the dominance of skills and techniques. The numbers in the team must be equal for it to be considered a game (1 vs. 1, 2 vs. 2, 3 vs. 3, 4 vs. 4) and not an overload practice. *Small-sided games (SSGs)*: the class is engaged in SSGs with no conditions. For example, a 1 vs. 1 half-court game of badminton, which uses regulation size rackets/shuttlecocks and there is no restriction on the skills and techniques, i.e. smashing; or, a 6 vs. 6 small-sided soccer game with no conditions other than the numbers on the playing area and adaptations to the pitch/court size. *Full-sided games (FSGs)*: the class is involved in a full version of the game including numbers and pitch/court size.

In contrast to the benefits of MGs and SSGs, physical education (PE) researchers have demonstrated that frequent usage of FSGs would result in low MVPA. For example, Roberts and Fairclough (2011) found that students were mostly inactive during class time. They believed that the overuse of FSGs (21% of class time), compared to 4% class time of MGs, led to the low PA levels. Sport researchers have previously investigated the effects of the number of players and pitch sizes on students'/players' PA levels (e.g., Bell, Johnson, Shimon, & Bale, 2013; Rampinini et al., 2007). In general, these studies have demonstrated that game formats with fewer players elicit more PA levels than the game format with more players. For example, Rampinini et al. (2007) found that soccer players in a 3-a-side game could achieve 87-90% heart rate (HR) max range, whereas, players in a 5-a-side game could only achieve 82-87 % HR max range. Based on the findings of those studies, students are more active in MGs and SSGs than they are in FSGs. Despite these trends in PE and sport research, little to no previous research in BIP/HEPAP contexts has examined PA accumulations, exclusively in game play period.

Previous research (e.g., Carroll & Loumidis, 2001) has demonstrated the strong correlations between students' propensity to engage in PA in PE and their motivation. Understanding students' motivation for PE and sport is helpful for PE and sport practitioners so they can adjust session to meet participant needs, thus, enhance their motivation, and therefore PA levels. Self-determination theory (SDT; Deci &

Ryan, 1985) is a general psychology theory to explain human behaviors and it provides a valuable framework to understand students' motivation in PE. SDT assumes that when the three basic needs are met: autonomy (having choices), competence (abilities to control outcomes), and relatedness (involvement and connection with others), students are more likely to demonstrate higher levels of self-determined motivation, which would lead to positive intentions to participate in PE (e.g., Sun & Chen, 2010).

SDT posits that behaviors are driven by both intrinsic motivations and extrinsic motivations. The core of SDT is the provisions to satisfy the three psychological needs and the progressions from amotivation, extrinsic motivation, to intrinsic motivation. Intrinsic motivation refers to the engagement in a behavior for the sake of the behavior itself. Extrinsic motivation refers to the engagement in a behavior for the sake of other benefits. For example, when a boy chooses to play soccer, he is intrinsically motivated if he does so for the love of playing soccer, but he is extrinsically motivated if he treats playing soccer only as a way to get involved with his friends. The last form of motivation is amotivation, which means that a person is neither intrinsically nor extrinsically motivated. Based on SDT, the quality of motivation is on a continuum ranging from amotivation all the way up to intrinsic motivation.

Many instruments have been designed to measure participants perceived levels of self-determined motivation related to a target activity in experimental psychology research. The Intrinsic Motivation Inventory (IMI; Ryan, 1982) is one such instrument. The original IMI includes six subscales. They are: (1) interest/enjoyment, (2) perceived competence, (3) effort, (4) value/usefulness, (5) pressure and tension, and (6) perceived choice. A seventh subscale, relatedness, was subsequently added. The IMI subscale items have been shown to be valid through factorial analysis studies (Deci & Ryan, 2003). The authors of the current study only focused on the first three subscales. Some of the subscales were not selected since they did not fit the current study purposes. For example, students were assigned to play three games that were pre-determined by the researchers, thus, the perceived choice subscale does not fit. The authors also did not put students in a situation where they would experience significant pressures during any of the games.

Even though researchers have conducted numerous studies concerning students' PA or MVPA in Game-Centered Approach interventions (Harvey et al., 2016), to our knowledge, no studies have examined university students' PA levels and motivations when they participate in different game types (SSGs, MGs, and FSGs) across two different sports – badminton and soccer. Badminton and soccer are one of the most popular net/wall games and invasion games in the world, respectively (Almond, 1986). Although Ainsworth et al. (2011) previously found that adults would get more MVPA from soccer than badminton it is still necessary to investigate MVPA differences in the current study. First, Ainsworth and colleagues utilized subjective self-reported questionnaires to collect PA data, while in this current study accelerometers will be used. Heyward and Gibson (2014) stated that accelerometers are the best devices to measure

PA levels objectively because of their ability to monitor PA minute-by-minute, differentiate intensity levels, are feasible with people of all ages, are accurate with static and dynamic behaviors, and hold large amounts of data memory. Second, Ainsworth and colleagues only collected PA data only in regular games abiding by the official rules and court sizes rather than across different game types (SSGs, MGs, and GSGs) which may affect MVPA differently. The purpose of this study was to investigate college-aged students' PA levels and motivation in different game types (i.e., MGs, SSGs, and FSGs) and in different sports (badminton and soccer). The current study will answer the following three research questions: a) how do students' MVPA levels differ in the different game types and sports; b) how do students' motivation levels differ in different game types and sports; and, c) to what extent do motivation levels predict PA levels. The findings of this study will provide PE and sport practitioners with knowledge about the likely MVPA levels derived from MGs, SSGs, and FSGs, and with knowledge about students' motivations toward the different game types so they can be judiciously applied in their respective instructional settings.

METHOD

Participants and Setting

One hundred and twelve students from a rural mid-Atlantic University in the U.S. initially participated the study. Seventy-one students between the ages of 18 and 39 years old ($M = 19.6$, $SD = 3.1$) completed MVPA data collection, and 67 of them finished the MVPA and IMI data collection. The students were from three soccer classes (40 males and 8 females) and two badminton classes (17 males and 6 females). This sample size was verified based on power calculations for a significant effect ($p =.05$) at an effect size of 0.35, with a repeated measures, within-between interaction, F test MANOVA conducted for 5 groups (five classes), with three repetitions (types of games were played) using the G-Power 3.0.10 software (Erdfelder, Faul, & Buchner, 1996). The activity classes were general electives and open to the whole university community. All the classes lasted five weeks and classes met either three times a week (75 minutes per class) or twice a week (100 minutes per class). Before recruiting participants, the University Institutional Review Board (IRB) protocol was submitted and approved. All participants signed consent forms and received a data collection schedule. Students did not receive extra credit or penalties for choosing to participate or not participate in the study. A Graduate Teaching Assistant (GTA) taught all three soccer classes. A different GTA taught the two badminton classes.

Research Design

The study was a cross-sectional quasi-experimental design. It was a cross-sectional design since both MVPA data and IMI data were collected from three soccer classes and two badminton classes in three-game type conditions: modified-games (MGs), small-sided games (SSGs), and full-sided games (FSGs). It was a quasi-experimental design because students chose the classes on their own, and, therefore, were not randomly assigned to the two sports. Participants played the three game types in a fixed order. They played the MGs first, SSGs second, and FSGs third. Participants played each of the games for 15 minutes on three different days of class.

Procedure

No badminton classes were available for a pilot study; thus, a pilot study was conducted only in soccer MGs and SSGs. However, the purpose of familiarizing the researchers with the data collection instruments was achieved. When it was the time for the formal study, the lead researcher held meetings with the two GTAs to inform them about the data collection schedules and the game types. Moreover, the researcher stressed the importance to the two GTAs that researchers would not intervene in how they teach the classes except for embedding the three games on data collection days. GTAs of the university used the Sport Education model to teach activity classes (Meeteer, Housner, Bulger, Hawkins, & Wiegand, 2012). Thus, using games in activity classes was a part of their already existing teaching repertoire. The request of having students play the three games on different days was a natural fit for the class schedule. Moreover, GTAs were required not to provide any instructions, feedback, or encouragement when students were playing the games. Researchers found that interactions between coaches with players would positively enhance players' MVPA (e.g., Coutts et al., 2004; Hoff et al., 2002;). The non-interaction requirement would eliminate this influence.

Given the fact that GTAs spend most of the first class in administration duties, the researchers attended the second class to request the students' participation in the current study. After students received and signed consent forms, researchers collected necessary anthropometric data to assign accelerometers to them. The required data for programming accelerometers was: gender, date of birth, weight (measured a bioimpedance scale OMRON HBF-516B), height (measured by a portable stadiometer CHARDERHM-200P Portstad), dominant side, and race.

On the specific data collection days, participants put their accelerometers on at the beginning of the class. After the warm-up, GTAs introduced the game types to students by explaining the games and having them play the game type (i.e., MGs, SSGs, and FSGs) for five minutes for familiarity purposes. Immediately after playing, GTAs provided opportunities for participants to ask questions about the games. GTAs taught content in accordance with their planning for the rest of the class before having students play the official non-stop 15-minute games. To keep students playing the whole time, the GTAs granted students a two-minute water break right before the official gameplay. The researcher utilized a digital stopwatch to record the time. The researcher reminded the participants of the remaining game time at 10-minute, 5-minute, 3-minute and 1-minute time points.

Participants in the badminton classes played the MGs and SSGs using half of the court with the middle line as one sideline and the doubles sideline as another sideline (white or grey part of Figure 1). The only difference between the badminton MGs and SSGs was that students were *not* allowed to utilize smashes

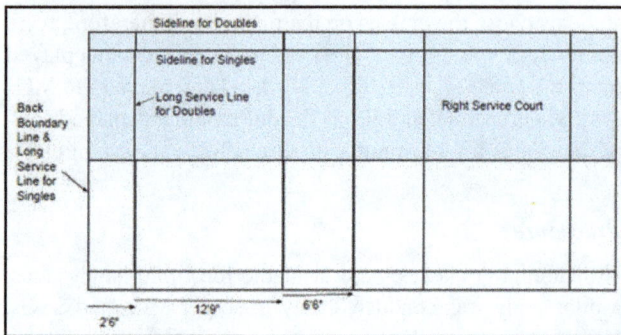

Figure 1. Badminton MSGs, SSGs, and FSGs

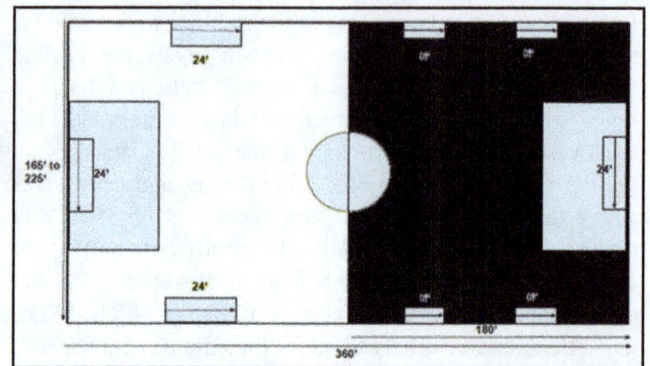

Figure 2. Soccer MSGs, SSGs, and FSGs

in MGs, whereas, they were permitted to utilize all the skills they could perform in SSGs. Four students played the MGs and SSGs at the same time. In other words, two games happened simultaneously on a court. To reduce the time to retrieve shuttlecocks, three shuttlecocks were stood on the outer sidelines, but far away from the court, so as not to cause injury. Participants played a regulation full-court singles game as FSGs.

Participants in the soccer classes played the 6 vs. 6 MGs and 7 vs. 7 SSGs on a pitch size of 50 yards x 40 yards (black or white half of Figure 2), which is the medium size of the recommend field size for US youth soccer 6 vs. 6 (US Youth Soccer, 2012). Another reason for choosing this size was the ability to have two MGs or SSGs arranged at the same time. In the soccer MGs, tall cones made up two small goals placed evenly on the sidelines. Each of the goals was six feet wide. In the SSGs, one regular size goal was placed in the center of each of the sideline. The main differences between MGs and SSGs in soccer were that no goalkeepers were present in MGs, but one goalkeeper defended a goal in SSGs. To keep 6 vs. 6 formats in both MGs and SSGs, even though it was 7 vs.7 in SSGs, researchers did not collect data from goalkeepers in the SSGs. Participants played the FSGs on a pitch size of 120 yards x 73 yards, which was the marked size on the field. Similar to placing extra shuttlecocks on the badminton sidelines, two soccer balls were placed evenly on each of the sidelines on the soccer field.

Immediately after playing each of the game types, participants were provided with the IMI paper questionnaires and pencils to fill out the questionnaires, which were originally created by the Qualtrics system. The first author brought paper versions of the questionnaire to each of the classes to avoid the situation where some students may not have been able to complete the questionnaire electronically. The first author collected the paper questionnaires, immediately transferring these paper versions of the IMI data to the Qualtrics system. After the initial data input, the researcher double-checked the accuracy of the transfer of paper records to the online system by exporting the each of the electronic datasets and double checking these against the initial paper records.

Instrumentation

Physical activity data.

Actigraph GT3X triaxial accelerometers (validated by Kelly et al., 2013) were used to collect students' PA data. Follow-

ing procedures outlined by Harvey et al., (2016), on data collection days, accelerometers were placed in a clear plastic bag that had the participants' ID number written on the outside, which corresponded with the ID number of the accelerometer inside the bag. Before the start of the session all participants attached the accelerometers around the waist of the dominant side of their body. Assistance was provided by researchers where required. This procedure was tested during a previous session before the study began. Once the data collection session was completed, each device was placed back into the correct bag and taken back to the lead researcher's office where the data on the devices were downloaded onto a laptop computer via the Actigraph software. The utilization of the Actigraph software permitted GT3X activity counts for each game at a 1-second epoch (Harvey et al., 2016). Data were extracted by applying a filter with the specific times of the lesson, which had previously been noted during data collection. This enabled the mean percentage of time spent in MVPA to be calculated using the Troiano et al. (2008) cut-off points for adults (2020 counts per minute) housed within the Actigraph software. These MVPA data were imported into Version 21 of SPSS (SPSS Inc, Chicago, IL) for statistical analyses.

Intrinsic motivation inventory

The IMI is a multidimensional measurement instrument designed for assessing participants' subjective experience related to a specific activity (e.g. Ryan, Mims, & Koestner, 1983; Deci, Eghrari, Patrick, & Leone, 1994). McAuley, Duncan, and Tammen (1989) validated the use of the IMI in PE settings. The original IMI includes six subscales, and include: (a) interest/enjoyment, (b) perceived competence, (c) effort, (d) value/usefulness, (e) pressure and tension, and (f) perceived choice. A seventh subscale, relatedness, was later added. Data were collected on the scales of interest/enjoyment (7 items), perceived competence (6 items), and effort/importance (5 items). The IMI data were collected on a 7-point Likert scale ranging from 1 = "not true at all" to 7 = "very true". There are two steps in scoring the IMI. First, items that were reverse scored were recoded. Second, subscale scores were calculated by averaging the scores across all the items on that subscale for each participant. The subscale scores were then used in the analyses of relevant questions. Reliability tests were conducted for each of the subscales, with results showing high reliability on each of the three sub-scales: interest/enjoyment ($\alpha = .93$), perceived/competence ($\alpha = .94$), effort/importance ($\alpha = .91$).

Data Analyses

A two-way repeated measures ANOVA was utilized to test whether statistically significant MVPA differences existed among students from soccer classes and badminton classes (the main effect of sports on MVPA) and whether statistically significant MVPA differences existed among the three different game types (the main effect of game types on MVPA). The dependent variable was MVPA. The two independent variables were sports and game types. Interactions between the sports and game types are also reported if the interactions were statistically significant. Based on Green-Geisser Correction, $F (1.84, 126.95) = 3.02$, $p = .06$, two separate one-way repeated measures ANOVA with Bonferroni correction ($p = .03$) were also utilized to test whether MVPA differed in the three games forms for each sport (i.e., badminton and soccer). A two-way repeated measures MANOVA was utilized to test whether statistically significant differences existed in the three IMI sub-scales between the two sports and the three different game types. The dependent variables were the three IMI subscales (enjoyment, perceived competence, and effort), while the two independent variables were sports and game types. Statistically significant interactions are also reported.

Multiple regressions (where the grand mean centering technique was employed) were used to investigate the extent to which IMI scores and sports predicted MVPA, with one regression performed for each game form. The dependent variable was MVPA and the independent variables were IMI motivation (enjoyment/interest, perceived competence, and effort) and sports (badminton and soccer). All regression tests were conducted in two steps. The first step (Model 1) was completed by entering only the sports variable (badminton or soccer) and the second step (Model 2) involved entering both the sports variable and the three motivation subscale variables concurrently. With the addition of the motivation variables, the change of predicted variance of the dependent variables brought by the motivation data can be explained.

RESULTS

In this section, results pertaining to each of the three different research questions will be reported.

Research question 1. How do students' MVPA levels differ in the different game types and sports?

Based on findings from a split plot ANOVA ($F(1,69)=29.1$; $p <.01$), on average, students had statistically significantly more MVPA in soccer ($M = 51.17$; $SD = 1.81$) than they did in badminton ($M = 34.04$; $SD = 2.61$) (Figure 3). Moreover, when data from the two sports were combined, students attained similar MVPA in the three-game types (Figure 4). However, the interaction between game types and sports was

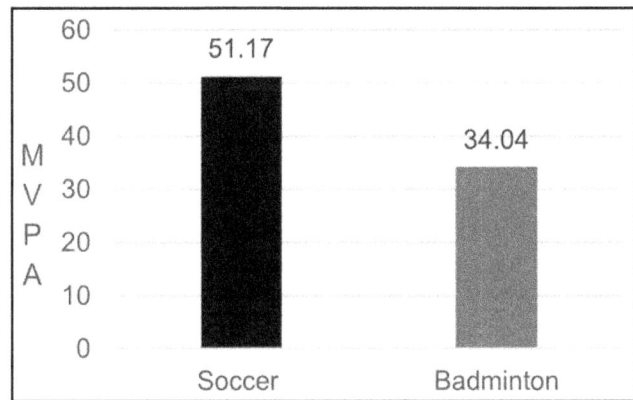

Figure 3. Aggregated MVPA data in soccer and badminton classes

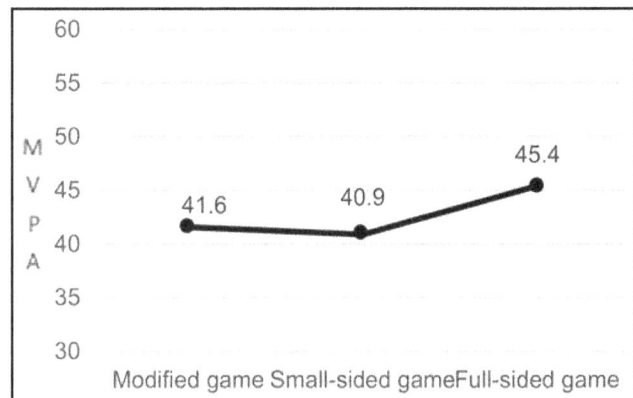

Figure 4. Aggregated MVPA data in different game types

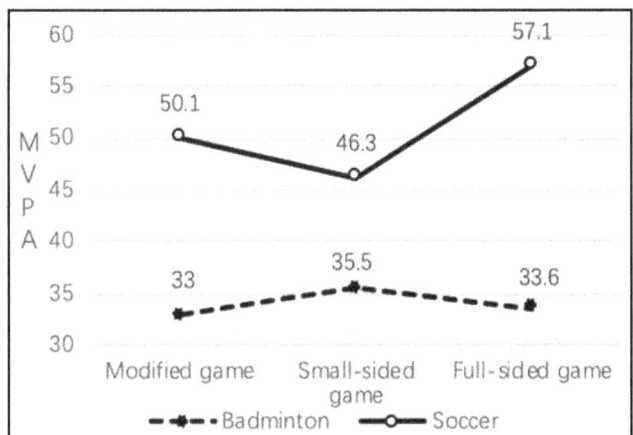

Figure 5. Badminton and soccer MVPA data in different game types

statistically significant ($p <.05$). For example, students in soccer classes attained the most MVPA in FSGs and the least MVPA in SSGs. In contrast, students in badminton classes attained the most MVPA in SSGs and the least MVPA in MGs (Figure 5).

Based on findings from a one-way repeated measures ANOVA, students in the badminton classes had similar MVPA in the three games ($F(2,44)=.461$, $p>.05$). However, students in the soccer classes had similar MVPA in MGs and SSGs, but statistically significantly more MVPA in FSGs ($F(1.715,80.594)=10.60$, $p<.001$) when compared to MGs and SSGs.

Research question 2. How do students' motivation levels differ in different game types and sports?

Findings from the two-way repeated measures MANOVA revealed there were no statistically significant differences in motivation between the two sports (Table 1). For example, students from both classes viewed the games as interesting, with students scoring more than 5.2 points in the interest/enjoyment scale. Moreover, there were no statistically significant differences in interest/enjoyment and perceived competence among the games. However, students perceived that they put statistically significantly more effort in SSGs and FSGs than that they did in MGs (Table 1).

Despite there being no statistically significant motivation differences between the two sports, the interaction patterns between the games and sports were statistically significant in the perceived competence subscale ($F(2,130)=4.3$; $p<.05$). Students in badminton classes felt the most competent in SSGs games and the least competent in MGs. In contrast, students in soccer classes felt the most competent in MGs and the least competent in FSGs (Figure 6). In addition, the interaction between the games and sports was significant in terms of effort/importance ($F(2,130)=8.6$; $p<.01$), with the interaction patterns the same as those seen in the perceived competence subscale. Students in badminton classes perceived they put the greatest effort into SSGs and least effort in MGs. Students in soccer classes perceived they put the greatest effort in MGs and least effort in FSGs (Figure 7).

Research question 3. To what extent do motivation levels predict PA levels?

Three multiple regressions were conducted to answer the research question with a regression for each of the game types (Table 2, Table 3, and Table 4). All the regressions were conducted with two steps. The first step was entering only the sports variable (badminton or soccer, Model 1) and the second step was entering both the sports variable and the three grand-mean centered motivation variables at the same time (Model 2).

The two-step entering helped detect the R square change brought by the addition of the three motivation variables. Collinearity statistics Variance Inflation Factors (VIF) ranged from 1.03 to 2.46, which was below the multicollinearity criterion (10), thus all the variables were maintained for subsequent analysis. In the regression models for MGs (Table 2), Sports was a statistically significant variable at $p=.01$ level, and it accounted for 20% of the variance of the dependent variable-MVPA. Based on the model, students in soccer

classes had 17.63 units MVPA more than those in badminton classes (dummy coded as 0). When the three motivation variables were added into the model, the whole model accounted for 29% of the variance of the dependent variable. However, the addition of the motivation data did not make the change statistically significant. The interest/enjoyment variable was a statistically significant variable at a $p=.05$ level to predict MVPA. Based on the model, while holding all the other variables constant, every unit increase in interest/enjoyment would decrease 5.76 units MVPA. Sports was a statistically significant variable ($p<.01$) in the regression models for SSGs (Table 3) and it accounted for 12% of the variance of dependent variable-MVPA. Based on the model, students in soccer classes had 12.17 units MVPA more than those in badminton classes. When the three motivation variables were added into the model, the whole model accounted for 36% of the variance of the dependent variable. Moreover, the addition of the motivation variables made the change statistically significant at the $p=.01$ level. In the whole model (model 2), both the sports and perceived competence variables were sta-

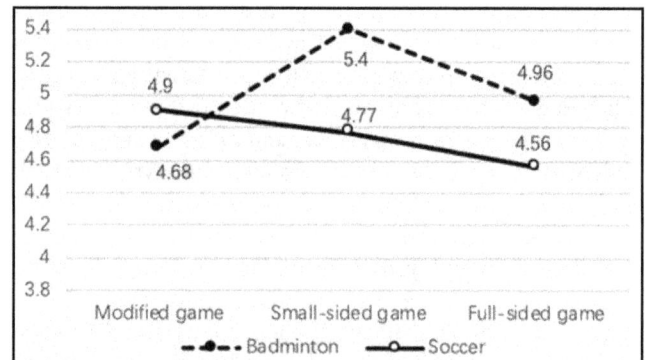

Figure 6. Perceived competence in game types and sports

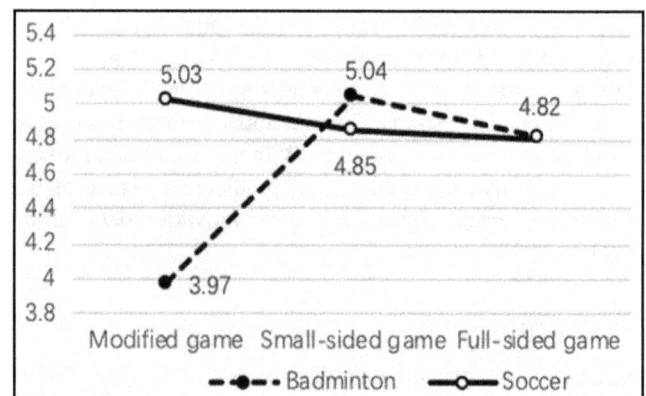

Figure 7. Effort/importance in game types and sports

Table 1. Motivation Data in Different Sports and Different Game Types

| Motivation | Sports | | | | Game Types | | | | | |
| | Badminton | | Soccer | | MGs | | SSGs | | FSGs | |
	Mean	SD	Mean	SD	Mean	SD	Mean	SD	Mean	SD
Interest	5.40	0.20	5.21	0.14	5.26	1.13	5.39	1.12	5.16	1.28
Competence	5.01	0.25	4.74	0.17	4.83	1.18	4.97	1.31	4.69	1.48
Effort	4.61	0.22	4.90	0.15	4.50	1.17	4.91*	1.28	4.81	1.31

*$p<0.05$

Table 2. Summary of Hierarchical Regression Analysis for Variables Predicting MVPA in MGs (N=67)

Variable	Model 1			Model 2		
	B	SE B	*β*	*B*	SE B	*β*
Constant	32.93	3.58		38.11	4.24	
Sports	17.63	4.32	0.45**	10.06	5.49	0.26
Interest/Enjoyment				-5.76	2.45	-0.36*
Competence				2.49	1.84	0.16
Effort				4.21	2.62	0.27
R^2		0.20			0.29	
F for change in R^2		16.66**			2.36	

Sports was represented as one dummy variable with badminton serving as the reference group; Interest, competence, and effort were centered at their means; *p < 0.05. **p < 0.01

Table 3. Summary of Hierarchical Regression Analysis for Variables Predicting MVPA in SSGs (N=67)

Variable	Model 1			Model 2		
	B	SE B	*β*	*B*	SE B	*β*
Constant	35.05	3.37		32.36	3.00	
Sports	12.17	4.06	0.35**	16.12	3.66	0.46**
Interest/Enjoyment				-1.05	2.06	-0.07
Competence				6.56	1.44	0.53*
Effort				-0.35	1.86	-0.27
R^2		0.12			0.36	
F for change in R^2		8.98**			7.53**	

Sports was represented as one dummy variable with badminton serving as the reference group; Interest, competence, and effort were centered at their means; *p < 0.05. **p < 0.01

Table 4. Summary of Hierarchical Regression Analysis for Variables Predicting MVPA in FSGs (N=67)

Variable	Model 1			Model 2		
	B	SE B	*β*	*B*	SE B	*β*
Constant	33.70	3.15		32.82	3.08	
Sports	23.35	3.81	0.61**	24.65	3.73	0.64**
Interest/Enjoyment				-1.29	1.88	-0.09
Competence				3.28	1.47	0.27*
Effort				0.93	1.77	-0.07
R^2		0.37			0.44	
F for change in R^2		37.6*			2.48	

Sports was represented as one dummy variable with badminton serving as the reference group; Interest, competence, and effort were centered at their means; *p < 0.05. **p < 0.01

tistically significant predictor variables (*p<.01*). Based on the model, students in soccer classes had 16.12 units MVPA more than those in badminton classes. While holding all the other variables constant, every unit increase in the competence would increase MVPA by 6.56 units. For FSGs (Table 4), the patterns of the regression models were similar with those in SSGs. Sports was a statistically significant variable (*p<.01*) and it accounted for 37% of the variance of the dependent variable-MVPA. Students in soccer classes had 23.35 units MVPA more than those in badminton classes did. The whole model accounted for 44% of the variance of the dependent variable. However, the addition of the variables did not make

the change statistically significant. Both the sports (*p<.01*) and perceived competence variables (*p<.05*) were statistically significant predictor variables. Based on the model, students in soccer classes had 24.65 units MVPA more than those in badminton classes. While holding all the other variables constant, every unit increase in perceived competence will increase MVPA by 3.28 units.

DISCUSSION

The discussion will be in accordance with the sequence of the three research questions. These were related to: MVPA differences, motivation differences, and using motivation qualities to predict students MVPA in the three different game types within each of the two sports. Students in badminton classes had statistically significantly less MVPA than those in soccer classes. The result aligns with previous studies (e.g., Ainsworth et al., 2011). The previous studies were conducted in regular games abiding by the official rules. Whereas, participants in the current study played the MGs, SSGs, and FSGs in each of the sports. Data in the current study showed that the different game types did not change the overall MVPA pattern in badminton and soccer that players have more MVPA in soccer than they do in badminton. With similar motivation qualities (Table 1), the MVPA difference between the two sports was due to the different nature of the sports. Students at the beginning badminton level have difficulty maintaining longer rallies and they need to retrieve shuttlecocks when the shuttlecocks land. Moreover, students play the game at a relatively slow pace, and they have to wait for the return of shuttlecocks to continue to play. The time associated with frequently retrieving and waiting for the return of shuttlecocks restricted students in the current study from achieving higher MVPA. However, students at the beginning soccer level can keep moving most of the time either for guiding opponents defensively or for moving off the ball offensively. While the soccer players do need to retrieve the balls when they go out of play, this occurred at a much lower frequency because soccer game play is more continuous.

The MVPA results demonstrated that the college students in badminton classes fell short of having more than 50% MVPA during gameplay even though the counterparts in soccer classes barely achieved the goal (see Figure 1). The findings were not commensurate with previous studies (e.g., Arnett, 2001; Van Acker et al., 2010) where students' MVPA was greater than this recommendation (about 60% MVPA). Moreover, the participants in the two previous studies accumulated those high MVPA levels from the whole class time. However, the college students in this current study only had their MVPA measured when they played each of the three game types for a continuous 15-minute period. The MVPA that the college students had in the current study was much lower than the MVPA collected during gameplay in other studies (e.g., McCormick et al., 2012; Slingerland et al., 2014). For example, Slingerland et al. (2014) found that boys achieved 74% MVPA and girls achieved 64% MVPA during twenty-five-minute small-sided basketball games.

Compared with MVPA findings in other studies, the relatively lower MVPA in the current study may be a result of several differences. First, Van Acker et al. (2010) and Slingerland et al. (2014) collected MVPA data by heart rate monitors, whereas the data for the current study were collected by accelerometers, which have been suggested to be more accurate devices for measuring MVPA (e.g., Heyward & Gibson, 2014). Second, the participants of the two previous studies were middle school students, whereas the participants in the current study were college students. That said, it is not clear whether these age differences lead to the MVPA differences. After all, adult learners are less active than younger learners (e.g., Douglas et al., 1997; Grunbaum et al., 2002).

The MVPA attained in the three badminton classes was not significantly different. This suggests that PE and sport practitioners can utilize a mixture of MGs, SSGs and/or FSGs when teaching badminton without compromising MVPA. However, it is necessary to point out that badminton students demonstrated the statistically significant better quality of perceived competence and effort/importance in SSGs than they did in MGs and FSGs. When combining both MVPA and motivation data, SSGs were the most optimal game types for badminton classes.

Contrary to the findings by Mallo and Navarro (2008) that students would get significant PA levels when no goalkeepers were present, the university students in the soccer classes had similar MVPA in MGs where no goalkeepers were used as they had in SSGs where goalkeepers were employed. Additionally, and contrary to previous findings in invasion games with middle school students (e.g. Roberts & Fairclough, 2011), the university students in the soccer classes had the highest MVPA in FSGs. However, they also reported the lowest motivation quality in FSGs. In terms of motivation data, students from badminton classes and soccer classes shared a similar quality of interest/enjoyment, perceived competence, and effort and importance when the data were aggregated across the three game types. It is interesting to find that students demonstrated similar interaction patterns between game types and sports in the perceived competence and effort/importance subscales. In other words, perceived competence and effort/importance are highly associated. For example, students from badminton felt the most competent in SSGs and they made the greatest effort in SSGs. They felt the least competent in MGs and they made the least effort in MGs.

Even though students played the MGs and SSGs on the same sized court, the rules of the MGs prevented students from using smash shots, whereas, in SSGs, students were permitted to use all techniques and tactics. In addition, by the time students played the MGs, the GTA leading the class had not taught the smash shot, thus, it was reasonable to design the MGs without smashes. To have students understand the MGs and to have them more involved, PE and sport practitioners need to emphasize why the specific MGs are necessary and beneficial for the development of techniques and tactics when they first introduce MGs (e.g., Alfieri, Brooks, Aldrich, & Tenenbaum, 2011). With the stipulations of the importance of MGs, students are more likely to see the objective of the MGs. A good example of using MGs to emphasize the usage of clears and drop shots in badminton is when PE and sport practitioners can explicitly state the focus of the MGs is for the students to use clears to move their opponents to the deep corners of the court and, subsequently, follow this shot with a drop shot to the front of the court near the net. The purpose of the badminton MGs is to, therefore, find the correct moments to employ drop shots after the clear. Students in the badminton classes reported less quality of perceived competence and effort/importance in FSGs. Based on the first author's previous BIP teaching experience, most students in badminton classes were beginners and this was probably the same for those students in the badminton classes used in this current study. Even though they felt the most comfortable in SSGs, it was likely they found it much harder to utilize the techniques and tactics in FSGs with an almost doubled-size playing area. It was also likely that in FSGs students found it harder to place the shuttlecocks accurately on areas close to the sidelines without overhitting the shuttlecocks and to defend their spaces without missing the oncoming shuttlecocks.

Students from soccer classes reported the highest score in perceived competence and effort/importance in MGs where two goals were placed, and no goalkeepers existed. Even though no studies were found on the impact of one extra goal on students' playing behaviors, students were expected to be more involved with the presence of two goals. It was likely that in using two goals they found they could play more offensively and, consequently, found it easier to score. When students scored more points, they felt that they were competent, and they would, as a result, try harder to score. This was also a potential reason why perceived competence data aligned well with effort/importance.

Data showed that students in the soccer classes felt the least competent and perceived they put in the least effort in FSGs even though they had the most MVPA in FSGs. Werner, Bunker, and Thorpe (1996) emphasized that games should be taught sequentially from the least tactical complexity (target games) to the most tactical complexity (invasion games). As one of the most popular invasion games, soccer is one of the most complicated sports in the world (Almond, 1986). Players need to keep running to track the ball and other players to set up offensive opportunities or defensive strategies. Players with the ball also need to keep dribbling it at high speed or use skilled footwork to avoid being tackled by defensive players. This was probably the case for the students in the soccer classes when they played the game on a 120 yards x 73 yards pitch size, which is on the slightly bigger side for a recommended full-size soccer pitch. The game was set at this size because there were markers signifying the size of the full-size pitch on the specific field that was used. Consequently, it was interesting that students in the soccer classes reported the lowest scores in the perceived competence and effort/import scales, but they had the most MVPA in FSGs. Due to the size of the FSGs field, students had longer distance sprints on the field to chase opponents defensively and chase the ball offensively. This was the reason they accumulated more MVPA. At the same time, the field was so large that they found it was much harder to use skills competently and why they presented lower quality of motivation data.

As for the multiple regression analyses, it is not surprising to find that sports is a statistically significant predictor of MVPA in all the models because students in soccer classes had statistically significant more MVPA than those in badminton classes. After adding the motivation data to the model, the full model did explain more variance in MVPA. However, the change of explained variance of the dependent variable was only statistically significant in the SSGs. In the SSGs and FSGs, perceived competence was a statistically significant predictor of MVPA. In other words, students who perceived themselves as more competent in both the SSGs and FSGs were likely to possess greater MVPA in those two game types.

From a motivation perspective, our current results suggest that having students feel competent is the key to enhancing their MVPA. Given the characteristics of students such as current levels of technique and tactical development, gender, social compatibility, and ethnicity, PE and sport practitioners should make continuous modifications to accommodate those characteristics. When students make progress, the games should be harder. When students struggle, the games should be easier. Constant adjustment is the key. For example, Van Acker et al. (2010) utilized the same-gender defense rules in their korfball units, and they believed this rule contributed to the girls possessing higher MVPA levels. The same-gender defense may also work for other games like basketball, soccer, and hockey. In addition, playing badminton against someone of more or less equal skill-level may also result in higher MVPA as rallies will last longer.

To our knowledge, no studies have investigated college students' MVPA and motivation for different sports and different game types systematically. The current study helps PE and sport practitioners develop an increased understanding of the potential influences of sport and game types on students' MVPA and their motivations. Thus, PE and sport practitioners can accordingly adjust the use of the three game types to balance students' MVPA and motivations. Conflicting with previous findings that students had low MVPA when FSGs were utilized the most, students in soccer classes had the most MVPA in FSGs. Researchers found that adult learners were less active than younger learners (e.g., Douglas et al., 1997; Grunbaum et al., 2002). With the participants in the previous studies middle-school students (e.g., Roberts & Fairclough, 2011) and the participants in the current studies adult learners, it is not clear whether the MVPA difference is caused by the age disparity.

The three IMI motivation subscales were utilized to predict students' MVPA. It was surprising to find that interest/importance was a statistically significant negative predictor of MVPA in MGs and a negative predictor in SSGs and FSGs. Since the overall reported scores for the interest/enjoyment were over 5.2 out of 7, the assumption for this situation is that students who had less MVPA also viewed the games were interesting. Further studies are needed to verify this claim. Effort/importance was not a statistically significant predictor in all the three-game types. However, perceived competence was a statistically significant predictor of MVPA in both SSGs and FSGs. A student with higher perceived competence was predicted to gain greater MVPA. Moreover, a student who reported higher perceived competence was likely to put in greater effort when playing the games. Even though students in soccer classes attained the most MVPA in FSGs, it does not mean that PE and sport practitioners should mainly utilize FSGs as the main learning organizer for soccer, after all, the students also demonstrated the lowest motivation qualities across all subscales in FSGs. The principle of exaggeration (i.e., Bunker & Thorpe, 1986) rationalized the utilization of MGs, which stated that changing game structures, such as rules, equipment, and play space, to promote and exaggerate a particular aspect of a game. The principle of representation (i.e., Bunker & Thorpe, 1986) provided the theoretical support for using SSGs, which stated that SSGs structured to suit the age and/or experience of the players. The SSGs are developed to contain the same tactical structures of the adult game but are played with adaptations to suit players' characteristics. We must realize that PE classes are not only about MVPA, they are also about motivation. Even though students in the soccer classes had the most MVPA in FSGs, they also reported the lowest motivation qualities at the perceived competence and effort/importance. Thus, we should refute the idea that PE and sport practitioners should mainly use FSGs as the main learning organizer. It is clearer to refute the idea when it comes to badminton classes, given the fact that students in badminton had the best MVPA (even though not statistically significant) and the best motivation qualities in the perceived competence and effort/importance subscales in SSGs instead of FSGs. Even though students in soccer may not have the most MVPA in MGs and SSGs, they could perform more technical requirements in MGs and SSGs when the pitches were reduced (Bell et al., 2013; Platt et al., 2001).

The current study had several strengths. First, accelerometers were utilized to objectively measure MVPA. Second, the quasi-experimental design enables the researchers to conduct the study in a non-interference and natural teaching and learning environment. Finally, the researchers systematically investigated the MVPA and motivation not only in different game types but also in two sports from different game categories.

There were several limitations in the study. First, while the current study adds to the literature on BIP/HEPAP studies, further research with adult learners is needed to further confirm the results of the study. Second, the badminton and soccer classes were general elective classes, and there were no levels of skill differentiation in any of the classes studied. Therefore, it may have been possible there were more intermediate players in one class than in another class. Gender effects were not examined even though the ratio of genders were almost equal since six of the 23 participants in the badminton classes were females and eight of 48 participants in the soccer classes were female. Third, no student learning data were included in this study. Future studies could include authentic assessment data to demonstrate that students learned in addition to gaining MVPA and increasing the quality of their motivation. Finally, due to the quasi-experimental design, we did not manipulate the game sequence, which was fixed in the order of MGs-SSGs-FSGs.

CONCLUSION

The key findings of the study were that PE and sport practitioners should find the most parsimonious balance between MVPA and motivation through adjusting games to ensure they meet the developmental needs to their students. One way this can be done according to the results of this current study is to manipulate the field/court size and dimensions for MGs and SSGs. Additional ways could be to consider player numbers (i.e., 1 vs. 1, 2 vs. 1, 2 vs. 2, 3 vs. 2, 3 vs. 3, and so on) and specific game rules (i.e., players assigned to specific zones, using different goals, using target zones for winning shots in badminton, etc.).

REFERENCES

Ainsworth, B. E., Haskell, W. L., Herrmann, S. D., Meckes, N., Bassett Jr, D. R., Tudor-Locke, C., & Leon, A. S.(2011). 2011 Compendium of physical activities: a second update of codes and MET values. *Medicine and Science in Sports and Exercise, 43*(8), 1575-1581.

Alfieri, L., Brooks, P. J., Aldrich, N. J., & Tenenbaum, H. R. (2011). Does discovery-based instruction enhance learning?.*American Psychological Association, 103*(1), 1-18

Almond, L. (1986). Reflecting on themes: A games classification. Rethinking games teaching. (D. Bunker, R. Thorpe, & L. Almond, Eds.). England: University of Technology, Loughborough, Department of Physical Education and Sports Science.

American College Health Association. (2012, June). Healthy Campus 2020. Retrieved from http://www.acha.org/HealthyCampus/index.cfm

Arnett, M. G. (2001). The effect of sport-based physical education lessons on physical activity. *Physical Educator,58*(3), 158-167.

Bell, K., Johnson, T. G., Shimon, J., & Bale, J. (2013). The effects of game size on the physical activity levels and ball touches of elementary school children in physical education. *Journal of Kinesiology and Wellness. 1,* 1-5

Bunker, D., & Thorpe, R. (1982). A model for the teaching of games in secondary schools. *Bulletin of Physical Education, 18*(1), 5–8.

Bunker, D., & Thorpe, R. (1986).The curriculum mode. Rethinking games teaching. (R. Thorpe, D. Bunker, & L. Almond, Eds.). Loughborough, UK: University of Technology, Department of Physical Education and Sports Science.

Carroll, B., & Loumidis, J. (2001). Children's perceived competence and enjoyment in physical education and physical activity outside of school. *European Physical Education Review, 7*(1), 24-43.

Coutts AJ. Murphy AJ. Dascombe BJ. (2004). The effect of direct supervision of a strength coach on measures of muscular strength and power in young rugby league players. *The Journal of Strength and Conditioning Research, 18*(2), 157-164.

Crouter, S. E., Schneider, P. L., Karabulut, M., & Bassett Jr, D. R. (2003). Validity of ten electronic pedometers for measuring steps, distance, and kcals. *Medicine and Science in Sports and Exercise, 35*(5), 283-288

Deci, E. L., Eghrari, H., Patrick, B. C., & Leone, D. R. (1994). Facilitating internalization: The self-determination theory perspective. *Journal of Personality, 62*(1), 119–142

Deci, E. L., & Ryan, R. M. (1985). The general causality orientations scale: Self-determination in personality. *Journal of Research in Personality, 19*(2), 109-134.

Deci, E. L., & Ryan, R. M. (2003). Intrinsic motivation inventory. *Self-determination theory.* 267

Douglas, K. A., Collins, J. L., Warren, C., Kann, L., Gold, R., Clayton, S., & Kolbe, L. J. (1997). Results from the 1995 national college health risk behavior survey. *Journal of American College Health, 46*(2), 55-67.

Eston, R. G., Rowlands, A. V., & Ingledew, D. K. (1998). Validity of heart rate, pedometry, and accelerometry for predicting the energy cost of children's activities. *Journal of Applied Physiology, 84*(1), 362-371.

Erdfelder, E., Faul, F., & Buchner, A. (1996). GPOWER: A general power analysis program. *Behavior Research Methods, Instruments, and Computers, 28*(1), 1-11.

Gabbett, T. J. (2002). Training injuries in rugby league: an evaluation of skill-based conditioning games. *The Journal of Strength and Conditioning Research, 16*(2), 236-241.

Grunbaum, J. A., Kann, L., Kinchen, S. A., Williams, B., Ross, J. G., Lowry, R., & Kolbe, L. (2002). Youth risk behavior surveillance—United States, 2001. *Journal of School Health, 72*(8), 313-328.

Hannon, J. C., & Ratliffe, T. (2005). Physical activity levels in coeducational and single-gender high school physical education settings. *Journal of Teaching in Physical Education, 24*(2), 149-164.

Harvey, S., & Jarrett, K. (2014). A review of the game-centered approaches to teaching and coaching literature since 2006. *Physical Education and Sport Pedagogy, 19*(3), 278–300.

Harvey, S., Smith, M. L., Song, Y., Robertson, D., Brown, R., & Smith, L. R. (2016). Gender and School-Level Differences in Students' Moderate and Vigorous Physical Activity Levels When Taught Basketball Through the Tactical Games Model. *Journal of Teaching in Physical Education, 35*(4), 349-357.

Harvey, S., Song, Y., Baek, J. H., & van der Mars, H. (2015). Two sides of the same coin: Student physical activity levels during a game-centered soccer unit. *European Physical Education Review, 22*(4), 411-429

Healthy People 2020. Retrieved from https://www.healthypeople.gov/2020/topics-objectives/topic/physical-activity

Heyward, V. H., & Gibson, A. (2014). Advanced fitness assessment and exercise prescription 7th edition. In A.N. Tocco; K.Matz; & S.Huls (Eds), Using technology to promote physical activity (pp.63-68).Champaign, IL: Human kinetics.

Institute of Medicine. (2013). Educating the student body: Taking physical activity and physical education to school. In H.W.Kohl III & H.D. Cook (Eds.), Status and trends of physical activity behaviors and related school policies (pp.32-65). Washington, D.C. The National Academies Press

Mallo, J., & Navarro, E. (2008). Physical load imposed on soccer players during small-sided training games. *Journal of Sports Medicine and Physical Fitness, 48*(2), 166-171.

McAuley, E., Duncan, T., & Tammen, V. V. (1989). Psychometric properties of the Intrinsic Motivation Inventoryin a competitive sport setting: A confirmatory factor analysis. *Research Quarterly for Exercise and Sport, 60*(1), 48-58.

Meeteer, W., Housner, L., Bulger, S., Hawkins, A., & Wiegand, R. (2012). Applying Sport Education in university basic instruction courses. In P. Hastie (Eds.), Sport Education international perspectives (pp.58-72). NewYork, NY: Routledge

Miller, A., Christensen, E. M., Eather, N., Sproule, J., Annis-Brown, L., & Lubans, D. R. (2015).The PLUNGE randomized controlled trial: Evaluation of a games-based physical activity professional learning program in primary school physical education. *Preventive Medicine, 74*, 1-8.

Moore, L. L., Lombardi, D. A., White, M. J., Campbell, J. L., Oliveria, S. A., & Ellison,R. C. (1991). Influence of parents' physical activity levels on activity levels of young children. *The Journal of pediatrics, 118*(2), 215-219.

Platt, D., Maxwell, A., Horn, R., Williams, M., & Reilly, T. (2001). Physiological and technical analysis of 3 vs. 3 and 5 vs. 5 youth football matches. *Insight, 4*(4), 23-24.

Rampinini E. Impellizzeri FM. Castagna C. Abt G. Chamari K. Sassi A. Marcora SM. (2007). Factors influencing physiological responses to small-sided soccer games. *Journal of Sports Sciences, 25*(6), 659-666.

Reilly, T., & White, C. (2005). Small-sided games as an alternative to interval training for soccer players. *Science and football V,* 355-358

Ryan, R. M. (1982). Control and information in the intrapersonal sphere: An extension of cognitive evaluation theory. *Journal of Personality and Social Psychology, 43*(3), 450-462.

Roberts, S., &Fairclough, S. (2011). Observational analysis of student activity modes, lesson contexts and teacher-interactions during games classes in high school (11—16 years) physical education. *European Physical Education Review, 17*(2), 255–268.

Sparling, P. B., & Snow, T. K. (2002). Physical activity patterns in recent college alumni.Research Quarterly for Exercise & Sport, 73, 200-205.doi:10.1080/02701367.2002.10609009

Stapleton, D. T., Taliaferro, A. R., & Bulger, S. M. (2017). Teaching an old dog new tricks: Past, present, and future priorities for higher education physical activity programs. *Quest,* 1-18.

Sun, H., & Chen, A. (2010). A pedagogical understanding of the self-determination theory in physical education. *Quest, 62*(4), 364-384.

Van Acker, R., Carreiro da Costa, F., De Bourdeaudhuij, I., Cardon, G., & Haerens, L. (2010). Sex equity and physical activity levels in coeducational physical education: exploring the potential of modified game forms. *Physical Education and Sport Pedagogy, 15*(2), 159-173.

Werner, P., Thorpe, R., & Bunker, D. (1996). Teaching games for understanding: Evolution of a model. *Journal of Physical Education, Recreation and Dance, 67*(1), 28-33.

Yelling, M., Penney, D., & Swaine, I. L. (2000). Physical activity in physical education: A case study investigation. *European Journal of Physical Education, 5*(1), 45–66.

25

Quantifying Forearm Soft Tissue Motion from Massless Skin Markers following Forward Fall Hand Impacts

Danielle L. Gyemi[1], Don Clarke[1], Paula M. van Wyk[1], William J. Altenhof[2], David M. Andrews[1]*

[1]*Department of Kinesiology, University of Windsor, 401 Sunset Avenue, Windsor, ON, Canada, N9B 3P4*

[2]*Department of Mechanical, Automotive and Materials Engineering, University of Windsor, 401 Sunset Avenue, Windsor, ON Canada, N9B 3P4*

Corresponding Author: David M. Andrews, E-mail: dandrews@uwindsor.ca

This research was funded by the Natural Sciences and Engineering Research Council of Canada (NSERC).

ARTICLE INFO

Conflicts of interest: None
Funding: NSERC

ABSTRACT

Background: Investigating soft tissue motion related to impact events is important for understanding how the body mitigates potentially injurious forces through shock attenuation. **Objectives:** The aims of this study were to: 1) quantify displacement and velocity of the forearm soft tissues following forward fall impacts; and 2) compare two massless skin marker designs (single layer, uniform (SLU) design; stacked, non-uniform (SNU) design) in terms of how well they could be tracked over varying skin pigmentations using automated motion capture software. **Methods:** Two participant groups (skin pigmentation: light – 9F, 8M; dark – 9F, 6M) underwent simulated forward fall hand impacts for each marker design using a torso-release apparatus. Marker positions associated with planar motion of forearm soft tissues during impact were automatically tracked (ProAnalyst®) in the proximal-distal and anterior-posterior axes from high speed recordings (5000 f/s). Mean peak displacements and velocities for eight forearm regions were then calculated (LabVIEW®). **Results:** Overall, soft tissue displacement and velocity increased from distal to proximal forearm regions. The greatest displacement (1.47 cm) and velocity (112.8 cm/s) occurred distally toward the wrist. Soft tissue impact responses between sexes did not differ, on average ($p > 0.05$). The SLU and SNU markers produced different kinematic values ($p < 0.05$); however, the magnitudes of, and consequently meaningfulness of these statistical differences for automatically tracking soft tissue motion, were negligible (displacement: ≤ 0.05 cm; velocity: ≤ 2.5 cm/s). **Conclusions:** Forearm soft tissue motion was successfully quantified for forward fall hand impacts; both marker designs were deemed functionally equivalent.

Key words: Upper Extremity, Forearm, Accidental Falls, Biomechanical Phenomena, Pattern Recognition, Automated

---

INTRODUCTION

Impacts to the hands and wrists resulting from forward falls, whether accidental in nature or due to recreational sporting activities, are problematic in both young and older adult populations because of the high incidence of upper extremity injuries (e.g., sprains, dislocations, fractures) associated with them (Nevitt & Cummings, 1993; Idzikowski, Janes & Abbott, 2000; Palvanen et al., 2000; Mirhadi, Ashwood & Karagkevrekis, 2015). Research concerning the injury mechanisms of a forward fall onto the hands of outstretched arms has largely focused on the in vitro impact response of the distal radius and its ability to dissipate high levels of mechanical energy (Myers et al., 1991; Muller, Webber & Bouxsein, 2003; Burkhart, Andrews & Dunning, 2012). However, the movement of soft tissue masses (muscle, fat, skin) relative to bone also plays a protective role in mitigating the injurious effects of impact through shock attenua-

tion (Cole, Nigg, van den Bogert & Gerritsen, 1996; Pain & Challis, 2002; Gittoes, Brewin & Kerwin, 2006; Pain & Challis, 2006). Compared to impact events involving the lower extremity (e.g., running, drop landings) (Cole et al., 1996; Gittoes et al., 2006; Pain & Challis, 2006), very limited information exists regarding soft tissue shock attenuation for upper extremity impacts to date (Pain & Challis, 2002).

Various motion tracking techniques have been employed to quantify soft tissue motion (predominantly in the lower extremity) for human movement analysis, including 3D optoelectronic systems (Fuller, Liu, Murphy & Mann, 1997; Gao & Zheng, 2008; Akbarshahi et al., 2010; Wolf & Senesh, 2011), magnetic resonance imaging (Sangeux, Marin, Charleux, Dürselen & Ho Ba Tho, 2006), as well as radiological methods such as X-ray and video fluoroscopy (Sati, Guise, Larouche & Drouin, 1996; Südhoff, Van Driessche, Laporte, de Guise & Skall, 2007; Wrbaškić & Dowling,

2007; Akbarshahi et al., 2010; Kuo et al., 2011). A noted major limitation across each of these methods is the need to affix external devices (e.g., accelerometers, active or passive surface markers) to the body segment in order to track soft tissue motion; an action shown to alter natural physiological soft tissue movement following impact (Leardini, Chiari & Croce, 2005; Stefanczyk, Brydges, Burkhart, Altenhof & Andrews 2013). Thus, utilizing motion tracking techniques that do not require external devices is key to prevent interference with the soft tissue impact response.

One such technique was presented in studies by Stefanczyk et al. (2013) and Brydges, Burkhart, Altenhof and Andrews (2015), in which position and velocity data of leg soft tissue motion following pendulum and drop landing heel impacts was quantified using massless skin markers and motion capture software with automatic feature tracking capabilities (ProAnalyst®; Xcitex, Cambridge, MA, USA). The marker design (2 x 2 cm grid of 0.5 cm diameter black dots) required no mechanical interaction with the leg, and was applied using flexible plastic stencils and a permanent black marker pen. Overall, Brydges et al. (2015) reported good to acceptable reliability for this technique. Nonetheless, modifications to marker shape and contrast might help to further improve its capacity to automatically track soft tissue motion and reduce measurement error (Haddadi & Belhabib, 2008; Crammond, Boyd & Dulieu-Barton, 2013), especially across different skin pigmentations.

Therefore, the aims of this study were to: 1) quantify planar displacement and velocity of the forearm soft tissues following a forward fall impact, and assess if there were differences between sexes or as a function of forearm region measured; and 2) determine if a stacked, non-uniform (SNU) marker design (non-uniform, ~0.5 cm diameter black dots overlaid on top of a grid of contrasting ~1 cm diameter white dots; 2 cm inter-marker distance) produced significantly different kinematic results and/or improved automated marker tracking across different skin pigmentations compared to the single layer, uniform (SLU) marker design (grid of uniform, 0.5 cm diameter black dots; 2 cm inter-marker distance) previously established by Stefanczyk et al. (2013) and Brydges et al. (2015).

METHODS

Participants and Study Design

The repeated-measures design of the present experimental study involved thirty-two (18 female, 14 male) healthy, young adult participants (mean [SD] age, height, and body mass of 22.3 [2.8] years, 1.73 [0.09] m, and 71.2 [14.0] kg, respectively), who were right hand dominant and free of upper extremity pain or injury over the previous year (as indicated on a general health questionnaire). Prior to testing, all aspects of the study were communicated and informed consent was obtained from each participant. All methods and experimental procedures were approved by the participating university.

A modified Fitzpatrick Skin Type Questionnaire (i.e., a numerical classification system for human skin color found-

ed on genetic disposition and the reaction of different skin types to ultraviolet light (Fitzpatrick, 1988)) was used to categorize participants into either a light (Type I–III: 9 female, 8 male) or dark (Type IV–VI: 9 female, 6 male) skin pigmentation group. Effort was made to match participants between groups according to height (m), body mass (kg), age (17–30 years), and sex.

Impact Apparatus

Bilateral hand impacts consistent with a forward fall onto the hands of outstretched arms were applied using a torso-release apparatus (Figure 1). Wearing a fitted safety harness connected to a tether, participants stood on an elevated platform (72 x 9 x 4 cm), which helped prevent ankle plantarflexion during the fall (Kim & Ashton-Miller, 2003). Each participant started the impact trials in a slight forward lean (approximately 10°) with their shoulders flexed to 90° and arms outstretched in front of their body. A manually-controlled quick release device securely affixed to a heavy, steel frame acted as an attachment point for the tether to support the participant's body weight. Across all impact trials, a distance of approximately 30 cm was maintained between the thenar regions of participants' palms and two force plates, which were mounted rigidly to a vertical steel structure attached to the steel framing of the laboratory wall. The force plates were positioned side-by-side at a 20° angle from vertical to simulate the positions of the wrist (~45° extension) and forearm (~75° with respect to the ground), characteristic of a forward fall (Myers et al., 1991; Greenwald, Janes, Swanson & McDonald, 1998; Burkhart et al., 2012; Burkhart, Quenneville, Dunning & Andrews, 2014). Targets were also outlined on the force plates to help standardize the impact postures for each participant. From the start position, participants were manually quick-released by the investigator after a random time delay between 0 and 5 seconds. Participants were instructed to maintain vertical alignment of their head, trunk, and lower extremities for the

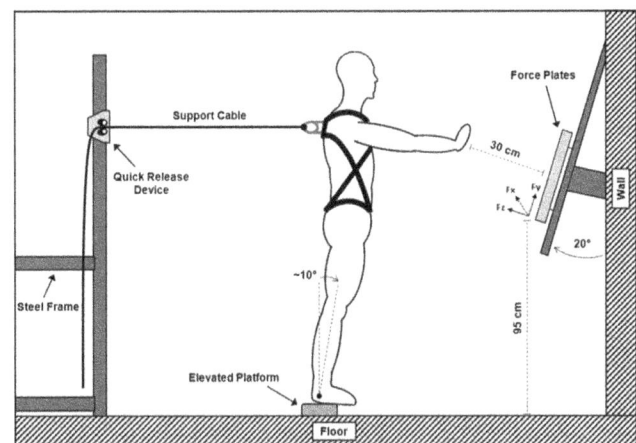

Figure 1. An illustration of the experimental test set-up from a lateral view showing the torso release apparatus and location of the force plates. The diagram depicts the positioning of the participant prior to initiating the forward fall simulation. Note that there were two force plates mounted side-by-side, one for each hand to impact.

entirety of the impact trial by imitating the fall of a broom-stick (Kim & Ashton-Miller, 2003; Hwang, Kim, Kaufman, Cooney & An, 2006), and arrest the fall with their arms in full elbow extension (i.e., stiff-arm landing) (Robinovitch & Chiu, 1998; DeGoede & AstonMiller, 2002a).

Instrumentation

Force data for each hand during the impact trials were collected using two force plates (AMTI-OR6–6-1000, A-Tech Instruments Ltd., Scarborough, ON, Canada; 1000 Hz natural frequency) (Figure 2). A high speed camera (FAST-CAM SA4, Photron USA, Inc., San Diego, CA, USA; 5000 frames/s, 1024 x 800 pixels^2 resolution, shutter speed 0.2 ms) was used to record planar soft tissue motion of the lateral aspect of the pronated right forearm. Two industrial-grade spot lights (T1 Fresnel, ARRI, Munich, Germany; 1000W, 120V) were positioned above and below the forearm to ensure ample lighting for video capture. A non-contact laser displacement transducer (AR700-50, Acuity®, Schmitt Measurement Systems, Inc., Portland, OR, USA; sampling rate 9 kHz), configured along the same plane as the force plates, was used to trigger and synchronize the collection of force and video data during the impact trials, such that the participants' hands would cross the laser beam approximately 1 cm before contacting the surface of the force plates.

Procedures

The SLU marker design was tested first (Figure 3a and b). With the right forearm in pronation, a flexible plastic stencil was wrapped around the posterior and lateral surface of each participant's forearm and the markers were applied using a black permanent marker pen. A designated row along the midline of the posterior forearm (first marker just lateral to the styloid process of the ulna) was used to maintain consistent marker placement between participants; the number of marker columns depended on the forearm length from the wrist to the elbow joint. The SNU marker design was tested second (Figure 3c and d), and was manually drawn over top of the SLU marker design on the right forearm using white and black water-based paint marker pens. The same investigator applied both marker designs for all participants. If necessary, any hair interfering with the marker application was shaved.

Each participant then underwent a minimum of three impact trials per marker design; a total of six trials were used for subsequent analyses (SLU: impact trials 1-3; SNU impact trials 4-6). Three-dimensional impact forces (F_x, F_y, and F_z: see coordinate system in Figure 1 for orientation) were recorded at each hand. However, based on the bilateral symmetry of the impact forces and small magnitudes of F_x and F_y, only mean peak F_z at the right hand was reported. To ensure consistent impacts between marker designs, the variability of the impact forces across all six impact trials was limited to a range of 10% to 15% of each participant's body weight. Trials that fell outside of this range were mostly attributable to improper body postures at impact (e.g., elbow flexion), and thus, were repeated. The to-

tal number of trials executed did not exceed more than six per marker design.

Video Analysis

Videos of forearm soft tissue motion were imported into Pro-Analyst® motion tracking software and were subjected to the same calibration process to set the scale and coordinate system for automated tracking. To convert pixels to centimetres

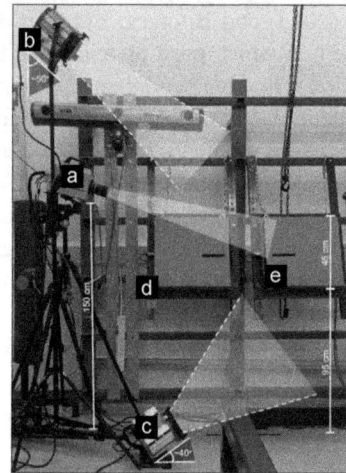

Figure 2. Schematic diagram of the experimental test set-up: a) high-speed camera; b) primary flood light; c) secondary flood light; d) left hand force plate; e) right hand force plate

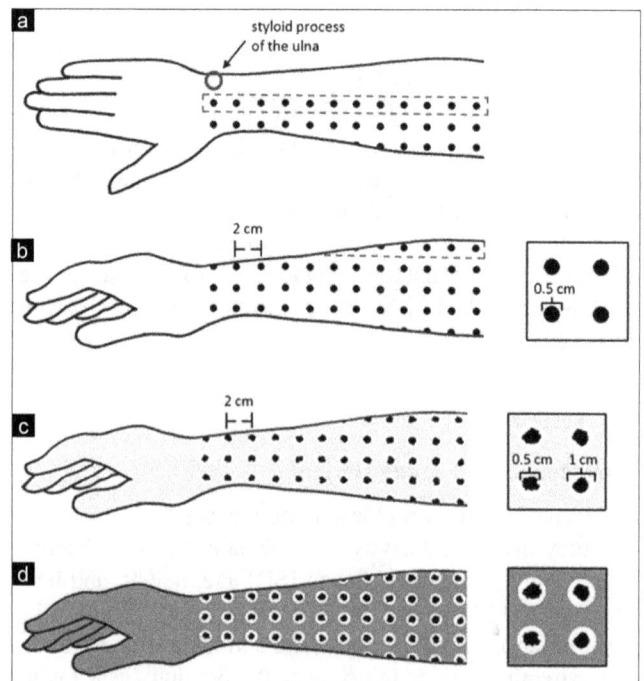

Figure 3. Schematic diagram of the SLU marker design (2 x 2 cm square grid of 0.5 cm diameter circular black dots) on the forearm from (a) posterior and (b) lateral views; schematic diagram of the SNU marker design (2 x 2 cm square grid of ~1 cm diameter circular white dots with ~0.5 cm diameter random black dots overlaid on top) on the forearm demonstrating the contrast for (c) light and (d) dark skin pigmentations.

a calibration unit of 6 cm was applied between four adjacent markers (in the same row) that were directly distal to the elbow (Stefanczyk et al., 2013; Brydges et al., 2015); the planar (2D) axes of the coordinate system were aligned in two directions (x-axis: parallel with the long axis of the radius and ulna, running in the proximal-distal direction; y-axis: perpendicular to the long axis of the radius and ulna, running in the anterior-posterior direction of the forearm) (Figure 4). A single image filter (Convolve: Sharpening (3 x 3 Center)) was applied using the default settings to slightly enhance the overall sharpness of the raw video footage for better contrast and marker edge detection.

The grid of markers on the forearm was segmented into four zones, similar to Brydges et al. (2015) for the leg, wherein two columns of markers (A and B) were selected at 0 %, 25 %, 50 %, and 75 % of the distance from the styloid process of the ulna to the elbow joint (Figure 4). Each marker location was manually selected by the investigator, ensuring that the rectangular boundary of the defined search region was as close to the marker edge as possible. Following appropriate marker selection, automated motion tracking was performed in ProAnalyst® (search region multiplier – 125%; threshold tolerance – 0.75) for each impact trial, in which the centre point of all defined regions (i.e., selected markers) was tracked, and the x and y position coordinates were subsequently outputted. The search parameters were held the same for all markers that were automatically tracked. Analysis of the markers began just prior to the right palm impacting the force plate and continued until forearm soft tissue motion following impact had ceased; a duration of approximately 100 to 230 ms (500 to 1150 frames) across all participants.

Data Analysis

Marker position coordinates from ProAnalyst® were imported into a custom LabVIEW program (LabVIEW® 2016, National Instruments, Austin, TX, USA) where they were converted to displacement data and filtered using a dual-pass, fourth-order Butterworth low-pass digital filter (Stefanczyk et al., 2013; Brydges et al., 2015) with a cut-off frequency of 60 Hz, determined by residual analysis (Winter, 2005). Velocity data were calculated using a 2nd order central differentiation method (Equation 1). Overall, 10 impact response parameters were assessed in relation to the planar movement of forearm soft tissue following forward fall hand impacts: peak displacement (cm) and velocity (cm/s) in the proximal-distal and anterior-posterior directions, as well as two additional variables of proximal and posterior rebound distance (cm) (i.e., the distance the marker rebounded from peak displacement in the distal and anterior directions, respectively). To account for potential differences in these impact responses due to soft tissue distribution, each of the four zones (0%, 25%, 50%, 75%) were further split into anterior and posterior regions by visually dividing the forearm in half, creating a total of eight separate regions along the forearm to be analyzed and ensuring that a relatively equal number of markers were allocated to both sides (Figure 5). For each

participant, a single marker was randomly selected within each of these regions for soft tissue kinematic analyses; the same marker was used for both the SLU and SNU marker designs.

$$\frac{dx}{dt} = \frac{x_{i+1} - x_{i-1}}{2\Delta t} \qquad \text{(Eq. 1)}$$

for $i = 0, 1, 2,..., n - 1$
where n is the number of samples.

In order to isolate forearm soft tissue motion caused by impact consistently across all trials and participants, a specific onset point was selected at which to start the analysis of the filtered kinematic data. The onset point was specified as the moment the right palm fully contacted the force plate and the forearm ceased the "free-fall" phase of the fall simulation. The onset point corresponded to a "knee point" in the proximal-distal velocity curve where the velocity in the distal direction began to rapidly decrease from a relatively constant value. For each participant, the onset point was based on the kinematic data from the most distal marker closest to the site of impact (i.e., the thenar region of the palm), which was then subsequently used for all remaining markers.

Statistical Analysis

Statistical analyses were executed using SPSS 24.0 (IBM SPSS Statistics, IBM Corporation, Somers, NY, USA). Independent samples t-tests were used to compare differences

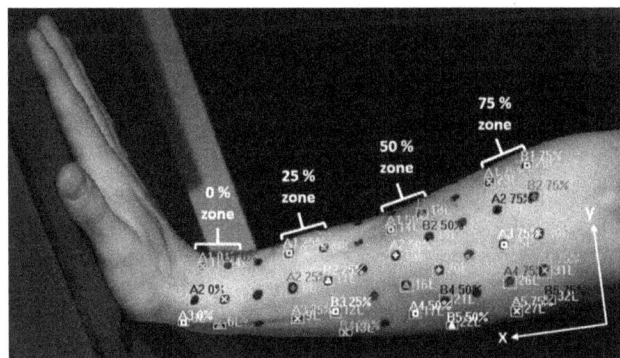

Figure 4. Screenshot from ProAnalyst® (zoomed in) showing the two columns of markers (A and B) selected for the 0%, 25%, 50%, and 75% zones.

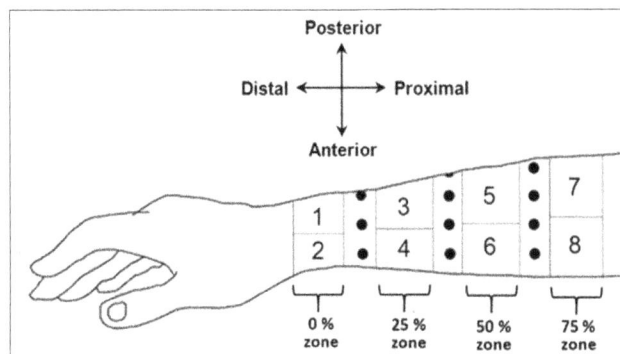

Figure 5. Schematic diagram of the marker grid (2 x 2 cm squares of dots) and the eight regions within the four analysis zones (0%, 25%, 50%, and 75%) on the forearm.

in age, height, and body mass between skin pigmentation groups. Mean peak values for each impact response parameter (displacement, velocity, rebound distance) were obtained by averaging participants' peak values across the three impact trials from the SLU marker design in the proximal-distal and anterior-posterior directions for each region. Two-way mixed ANOVAs (between-subject factor: sex (female, male); within-subject factor: forearm region (1–8)) were used to examine if the impact responses (from the SLU impact trials) differed between sexes depending on the region of the forearm being tracked. Two-way mixed ANOVAs (between-subject factor: skin pigmentation (light, dark); within-subject factor: marker design (SLU, SNU)) were also performed to examine if the impact responses differed between the light and dark skin pigmentation groups depending on the marker design applied to the skin; data were collapsed across the eight forearm regions and the mean peak soft tissue impact responses of the three impact trials for each marker design (SLU and SNU) were used.

A value of alpha as 0.05 was implemented for all statistical comparisons. Normality of all soft tissue impact responses was assessed using Shapiro-Wilk tests and Q-Q Plots. Variance assumptions for between- and within-subject factors were assessed using Levene's Test for Equality of Variance and Mauchly's Test of Sphericity, respectively. Bonferroni Post Hoc tests for pairwise comparisons were performed for any significant main effects that were found, and if any significant interactions were revealed, simple effects tests were conducted.

RESULTS

Preliminary screening of the forearm impact responses revealed that two male participants in the light pigmentation group had extreme outliers (z-score > 3.29) with respect to anterior soft tissue displacement. Visual inspection of the automated motion tracking recordings in ProAnalyst® veri-

fied that these values were not representative of genuine soft tissue motion, but rather, downward movement of the entire forearm due to moderate elbow flexion after impact. Since this violated the impact protocol guidelines, their data were excluded from all subsequent analyses.

No significant differences were found between the two skin pigmentation groups in terms of age, height, and body mass across all participants, and when split by sex ($p > 0.05$). All impact responses were approximately normally distributed, as assessed by Shapiro-Wilk tests ($p > 0.05$) and QQ Plots, with the exception of mean peak proximal and posterior displacement. Automated tracking of the soft tissue motion showed that the majority of markers did not return past the onset point in these two directions (see Figure 6), producing frequent zero values. This resulted in very positively skewed distributions with mean peak displacements

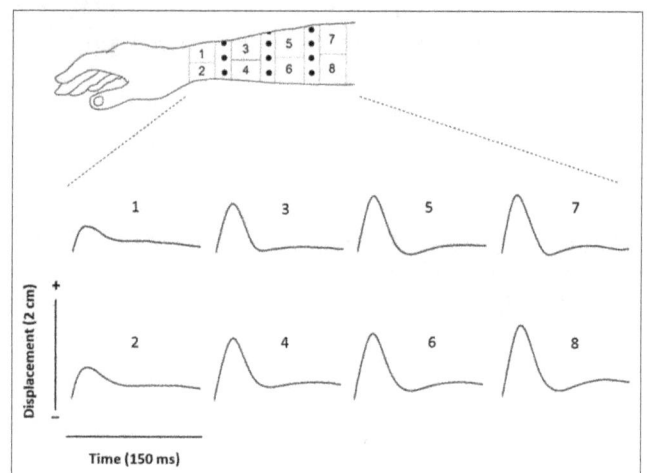

Figure 6. Sample displacement/time responses (proximal-distal axis) for each of the eight regions across the forearm for a single trial from one participant. The responses from each region have been aligned in time and displacement in order to show the relative differences.

Table 1. Mean (±SD) overall female and male peak soft tissue displacement (cm) in the proximal, distal, anterior, and posterior directions for each of the four zones (0%, 25%, 50%, 75%) and eight regions.

Direction	Regions							
	(0%)		(25%)		(50%)		(75%)	
	1	2	3	4	5	6	7	8
Female								
Distal	0.67 (0.12)	0.78 (0.15)	1.14 (0.15)	1.29 (0.17)	1.16 (0.17)	1.37 (0.18)	1.12 (0.18)	1.52 (0.18)
Proximal	0.03 (0.05)	0.01 (0.03)	0.11 (0.15)	0.03 (0.09)	0.13 (0.15)	0.07 (0.11)	0.07 (0.12)	0.05 (0.13)
Anterior	0.18 (0.08)	0.18 (0.08)	0.52 (0.16)	0.47 (0.19)	0.91 (0.28)	0.77 (0.35)	1.29 (0.46)	1.07 (0.51)
Posterior	0.09 (0.09)	0.06 (0.10)	0.05 (0.09)	0.06 (0.10)	0.06 (0.12)	0.06 (0.13)	0.07 (0.14)	0.08 (0.15)
Male								
Distal	0.61 (0.13)	0.71 (0.11)	1.05 (0.25)	1.10 (0.24)	1.07 (0.26)	1.23 (0.28)	1.06 (0.23)	1.39 (0.30)
Proximal	0.07 (0.11)	0.04 (0.09)	0.05 (0.09)	0.03 (0.07)	0.05 (0.10)	0.02 (0.06)	0.03 (0.08)	0.01 (0.03)
Anterior	0.33 (0.13)	0.30 (0.13)	0.60 (0.14)	0.53 (0.19)	1.00 (0.38)	0.90 (0.40)	1.36 (0.45)	1.13 (0.53)
Posterior	0.07 (0.08)	0.07 (0.09)	0.05 (0.09)	0.06 (0.09)	0.04 (0.08)	0.05 (0.08)	0.04 (0.08)	0.06 (0.11)

Distal=soft tissue motion toward the wrist; Proximal=soft tissue motion toward the elbow; Anterior=downward soft tissue motion perpendicular to the long axis of the forearm; Posterior=upward soft tissue motion perpendicular to the long axis of the forearm of ≤ 0.1 cm (Table 1), which provided little information on the actual soft tissue motion occurring in the proximal and posterior directions. Consequently, proximal and posterior rebound distances were also analyzed. Variances of the soft tissue impact responses between females and males for all regions of the forearm were homogeneous ($p > 0.05$), apart from proximal displacement in regions 1 ($p = 0.08$) and 2 ($p = 0.07$), anterior displacement in region 1 ($p = 0.023$), and posterior rebound distance in regions 6 ($p = 0.027$) and 8 ($p = 0.033$). Within these regions, the variances for the males were approximately double that of the females, consistently. Mauchly's Test of Sphericity was found to be significant ($p < 0.05$) for each soft tissue impact response, therefore, corrected Greenhouse-Geisser estimates were used for all the following analyses.

Displacement

No significant sex differences in mean peak displacement were found in any of the directions (proximal, distal, anterior, posterior) analyzed when compared across the eight regions of the forearm ($p > 0.05$) (Table 1). With respect to the proximal-distal axis, the greatest peak displacement occurred in region 8 in the distal direction toward the wrist (1.47 cm); the greatest peak displacement along the anterior-posterior axis was in region 7 in the anterior direction (1.32 cm). In these two directions, a general trend of increasing displacements was observed moving from distal to proximal regions of the forearm (i.e., 0% to 75% zone) (Figure 7a and c). In contrast, peak displacements in both the proximal and posterior directions had very small magnitudes (≤ 0.10 cm and ≤ 0.08 cm, respectively) across all regions (Figure 7b and d).

Based on the forearm region measured, significant differences in peak displacement were found. For peak distal displacement, significant consecutive increases in displacement

were seen across all anterior regions of the forearm (2, 4, 6, and 8) ($p < 0.05$), whereas posterior regions only showed one significant increase from region 1 to regions 3, 5, and 7 ($p < 0.05$) (Figure 7a). Peak distal displacements demonstrated the greatest increase from the 0% zone (0.70 cm) to the 25% zone (1.16 cm) of approximately 66%. On average, peak distal displacement in the anterior regions of the forearm was 19% greater than the posterior regions. Peak anterior displacement in anterior and posterior regions of the forearm, also showed significant increases, moving distally to proximally ($p < 0.05$) (Figure 7c). No significant differences were observed between anterior and posterior regions for multiple pairs (regions 1 and 2, regions 3 and 4, regions 5 and 8) ($p > 0.05$). Posterior forearm regions had 16% greater peak anterior displacement than anterior regions, on average, however.

Rebound Distance

A significant interaction was present between sex and forearm region for proximal rebound distance [$F(3.111, 87.115) = 6.724$, $p < 0.001$, partial $\eta^2 = 0.194$], in which females demonstrated significantly more soft tissue rebound proximally toward the elbow for regions 3 through 8 compared to males ($p < 0.05$) (Figure 8a). Simple main effects showed that both sexes demonstrated similar patterns across forearm region: regions 1 and 2 had significantly lower magnitudes than the remaining regions (3–8), resulting in an approximate increase in proximal rebound distance of 81% and 56% for females and males, respectively, from the 0% to 25% zone. No interactions were found between sex and forearm region for peak posterior rebound distance, although the magnitudes of regions 1 and 2 were also significantly lower than all other regions of the forearm ($p < 0.05$) (Figure 8b).

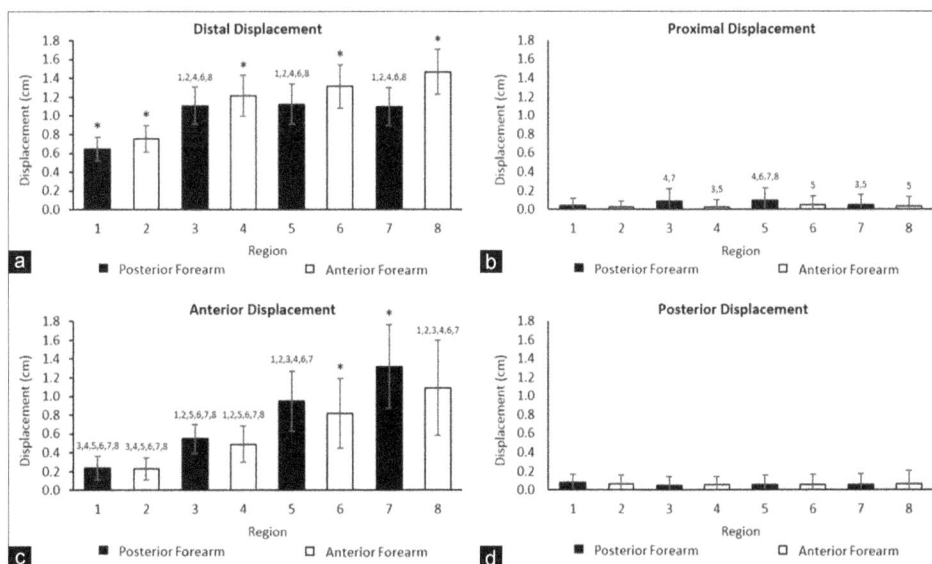

Figure 7. Mean (SD) peak soft tissue displacement (cm) in the (a) distal, (b) proximal, (c) anterior, and (d) posterior direction for all forearm regions (1–8). Note. * = significant difference from all regions ($p < 0.05$); each number represents a significant difference from that specific region ($p < 0.05$).

Velocity

Mean peak velocities paralleled the displacement results (Table 2): no significant sex differences were found across the eight forearm regions in any of the directions analyzed ($p > 0.05$), and a general pattern of increasing velocities was observed when moving from distal to proximal regions (Figure 9). The greatest peak velocities occurred along the proximal-distal axis in the distal direction (≥ 90.9 cm/s), with region 7 having the highest magnitude of 112.8 cm/s. For the anterior-posterior axis, region 7 also possessed the greatest peak velocity in the anterior direction, although, the magnitude was approximately half that of the highest distal velocity (61.2 cm/s). The smallest peak velocities collectively occurred in the posterior direction (≤ 27.6 cm/s).

With respect to forearm region, peak distal velocities in region 1 and region 7 had significantly lower and higher magnitudes than all other regions, respectively ($p < 0.05$), while the remaining regions demonstrated no significant differences across multiple pairs ($p > 0.05$) (Figure 9a). The effect of region on peak proximal velocity was comparable to proximal rebound distance, as proximal velocities in the 0% zone were also significantly lower than regions 3 through 8 ($p < 0.05$) (Figure 9b), resulting in an approximate increase of 85% when transitioning to the 25% zone. A significant interaction

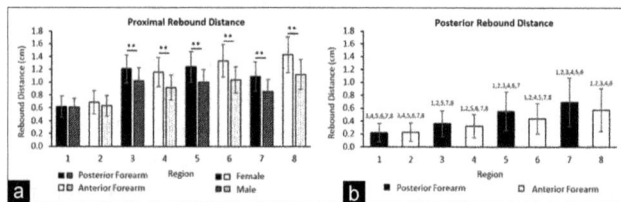

Figure 8. Mean (SD) peak soft tissue rebound distance (cm) in the (a) proximal and (b) posterior direction for all forearm regions (1–8). Note. ** = significant difference between females and males ($P < 0.05$); each number represents a significant difference from that specific region ($P < 0.05$).

between sex and forearm region [$F(2.556, 71.566) = 3.023$, $p = 0.043$, partial $\eta^2 = 0.097$] for peak anterior velocity revealed significantly different regional comparisons across the forearm for females and males ($p < 0.05$), but no significant differences between the sexes for any regions ($p > 0.05$). Similar to anterior displacement, the peak anerior velocities in the posterior regions were increasingly higher than the anterior regions within the same zone moving proximally along the forearm (e.g., 25% zone: + 3%; 50% zone: + 16%; 75% zone: + 24%) (Figure 9c). For peak posterior velocity, no significant differences were observed in the distal half of the forearm (regions 1–4), however, in the proximal half of the forearm (regions 5–8), region 7 (27.6 cm/s) had the significantly greatest posterior velocity compared to all other regions, except region 5 (24.2 cm/s) (Figure 9d).

Massless Skin Marker Designs

Variances of all soft tissue impact responses between light and dark skin pigmentation groups for each marker design were homogeneous ($p > 0.05$). A significant interaction was found between skin pigmentation and marker design on peak distal displacement [$F(1.000, 28.000) = 4.530$, $p = 0.042$, partial $\eta^2 = 0.139$]. For the dark skin pigmentation group, distal displacement for the SLU marker design was 0.05 cm greater than the SNU marker design ($p < 0.05$); the light skin pigmentation group showed no significant differences ($p > 0.05$). A cross-over interaction for peak proximal displacement [$F(1.000, 28.000) = 5.554$, $p = 0.026$, partial $\eta^2 = 0.166$] showed that the SLU marker design resulted in higher proximal displacement for the light skin pigmentation group and lower for the dark skin pigmentation group, compared to the SNU marker design, though, these differences were not significant ($p > 0.05$). A significant main effect of marker design on peak proximal rebound distance revealed that the SLU marker design (1.02 cm) had significantly greater soft tissue rebound in relation to the SNU marker design (0.98 cm) ($p < 0.05$). Peak velocities in the distal,

Table 2. Mean (±SD) overall female and male peak soft tissue velocity (cm/s) in the proximal, distal, anterior, and posterior directions for each of the four zones (0%, 25%, 50%, 75%) and eight regions.

Direction	Regions							
	(0%)		(25%)		(50%)		(75%)	
	1	2	3	4	5	6	7	8
Female								
Distal	88.9 (13.4)	96.6 (12.8)	100.6 (12.4)	103.4 (12.6)	105.5 (14.4)	104.3 (13.1)	110.3 (14.7)	107.6 (13.4)
Proximal	32.7 (10.3)	29.7 (9.7)	61.2 (11.5)	55.3 (6.9)	57.0 (9.8)	57.5 (7.8)	45.9 (11.0)	59.8 (10.9)
Anterior	32.1 (8.5)	34.3 (9.5)	42.8 (10.4)	43.2 (10.7)	58.9 (12.9)	48.3 (13.0)	63.8 (15.7)	49.3 (15.5)
Posterior	20.3 (8.7)	15.6 (7.0)	15.1 (6.1)	16.8 (7.7)	25.9 (10.4)	18.0 (7.3)	30.4 (11.3)	19.8 (8.8)
Male								
Distal	94.0 (14.0)	103.6 (12.9)	108.7 (15.2)	110.3 (14.0)	112.9 (17.4)	111.7 (14.9)	116.6 (18.4)	113.4 (15.0)
Proximal	35.4 (10.2)	33.4 (12.5)	68.9 (16.6)	56.0 (12.5)	62.2 (16.6)	61.4 (12.7)	52.0 (15.9)	62.9 (13.8)
Anterior	38.4 (11.3)	38.8 (11.5)	44.9 (8.8)	41.7 (9.7)	52.9 (13.5)	49.1 (12.3)	57.3 (13.2)	49.3 (10.9)
Posterior	11.8 (5.5)	11.3 (6.4)	16.6 (9.6)	13.9 (8.0)	21.5 (11.9)	19.1 (10.1)	23.4 (12.1)	17.8 (11.5)

Distal=soft tissue motion toward the wrist; Proximal=soft tissue motion toward the elbow; Anterior=downward soft tissue motion perpendicular to the long axis of the forearm; Posterior=upward soft tissue motion perpendicular to the long axis of the forearm

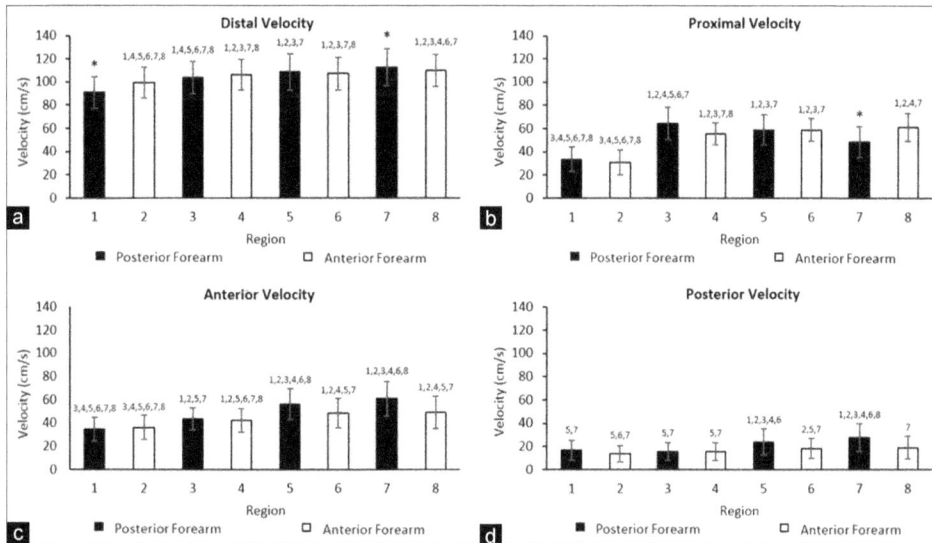

Figure 9. Mean (SD) peak soft tissue velocity (cm/s) in the (a) distal, (b) proximal, (c) anterior, and (d) posterior direction for all forearm regions (1–8). Note. * = significant difference from all regions ($p < 0.05$); each number represents a significant difference from that specific region ($p < 0.05$).

proximal, and anterior directions also demonstrated similar trends in which the SLU marker design produced significantly higher velocities than the SNU marker design of 2.5 cm/s, 1.5 cm/s, and 1.5 cm/s, respectively ($p < 0.05$).

During automated motion tracking in ProAnalyst®, one case occurred in which the defined region surrounding a SLU marker jumped to an adjacent marker mid-way through the automated tracking process; no tracking discrepancies occurred with the SNU markers. SLU markers located near the anterior and posterior edges of the forearm were found to be slightly more susceptible to marker drop out compared to the SNU markers, especially where minor shadowing underneath the forearm reduced the contrast on the anterior edge. Additionally, higher rates of marker drop out during automated tracking were observed for SLU markers located distally and posteriorly in the 0% zone of the forearm, as the smaller sized SLU markers (0.5 cm diameter) were more easily lost where the skin compressed near the wrist joint due to hyperextension; the larger sized SNU markers (~1 cm diameter) proved to be slightly more resilient to this issue.

DISCUSSION

In the present study, forearm soft tissue motion following forward fall hand impacts was able to be recorded and analyzed successfully using massless skin markers and automated motion tracking software. On average, the greatest peak soft tissue displacements and velocities occurred distally toward the wrist compared to all other directions, consistent with the findings by Stefanczyk et al. (2013) for leg soft tissue motion following heel impacts. The greatest distal displacement along the long axis of the forearm (1.47 cm) was slightly less than the maximum marker motion (1.7 cm) previously determined by Pain and Challis (2002), though, this is most likely attributable to the different impact scenarios utilized (e.g., simulated forward fall and active downward palm striking task, respectively). While no comparable velocity data currently exists for the upper extremity, the greatest distal velocity of leg soft

tissue reported by Brydges et al. (2015) was found to be moderately lower or higher than that of the forearm (112.8 cm/s) depending on the impact technique: horizontal pendulum impacts (95.2 cm/s) and vertical drop tests (137.5 cm/s).

Peak proximal (and posterior) displacements observed in this study were very limited given that the motion pathways of the selected markers (and thus the underlying forearm soft tissues) often did not return past the onset point (Figure 6). This is in contrast to the underdamped oscillatory response seen by Pain and Challis (2002). Despite providing both a practical and reputable method for simulating real-life forward fall events that has been frequently used in past literature (Kim & Ashton-Miller, 2003; Hwang et al., 2006; Lattimer et al., 2016; Lattimer et al., 2017), the design of the torso-release apparatus, in combination with the effects of gravity, may have contributed to these results since the final orientation of the forearm at impact was relatively horizontal. This would likely pull the soft tissues towards the ground (i.e., anteriorly), limiting soft tissue recovery in the proximal and posterior directions.

Despite clear differences in upper extremity soft and rigid tissue masses between females and males (Maughan, Abel, Watson & Weir, 1986; Mazess, Barden, Bisek & Hanson, 1990), the general lack of sex differences across the impact responses in this study suggests that forearm soft tissue motion associated with forward fall hand impacts may not be driven by tissue composition, but rather, the distribution of soft tissues along the forearm. Only proximal rebound distance showed significant differences between sexes, where females had approximately 25% greater proximal rebound in intermediate and distal forearm regions (3–8) compared to males. However, due to insufficient space for marker placement on the hand, palm deformation could not be measured in the current study as Brydges et al. (2015) did for the heel pad, to verify its contribution to the impact responses between females and males. To date, palm soft tissue thickness has only been quantified by ultrasound for young women (Choi & Robinovitch, 2011). Therefore, assuming that the palmar soft tissues for males are thicker than for females, similar to what has been shown for the heel pad of the foot (Prichasuk, 1994), this would help explain the reduced proximal motion of the forearm soft tissues for males, as more impact shock would be absorbed at the hand as the palm compresses.

The increase in regional impact responses observed moving distally to proximally further supports the notion that the movement of the forearm soft tissues after a forward fall hand impact is, to some degree, a function of tissue distribution along the segment, especially with the greatest impact responses commonly occurring in regions 7 and 8 where the most tissue is located. In addition, notably sharp increases from the 0% to 25% zones for distal displacement, proximal rebound distance, and proximal velocity highlight the potential importance of this section of the distal forearm when analyzing shock attenuation in the body related to forward falls. Given the high incidence of distal radius fractures occurring at or near this location (Nellans, Kowalski & Chung, 2012), more research is needed to better understand the protective mechanisms of the underlying tissues occurring here.

Overall, the magnitudes of the statistical differences between the soft tissue impact responses for the SLU and SNU marker designs were extremely small (displacements: ≤ 0.05 cm; rebound distances: ≤ 0.04 cm; velocities: ≤ 2.5 cm/s). As a result, for the purpose of automatically tracking soft tissue motion across varying skin pigmentations, it is suggested that the overall precision of each marker design is functionally equivalent. The greater shape variation of the SNU markers did not have as beneficial of an effect as what has been previously reported for other non-contact motion tracking methods, such as digital image correlation (Haddadi & Belhabib, 2008; Crammond et al., 2013), and enhancements to marker contrast offered only minimal improvements to the automatic tracking process (i.e., marker drop out) when minor shadowing and marker placement were taken into account. Therefore, based on the practicality of each approach, the SLU marker design may prove to be superior since it was more time- and cost-effective than the SNU marker design (i.e., applying only one layer compared to two; using a standard permanent marker pen compared to more expensive, specialty water-based paint marker pens). However, the self-report format of the Fitzpatrick Skin Type Questionnaire relies heavily on a subjective evaluation of oneself (e.g., does your skin tan?), so it is possible that some participants may have been falsely categorized (specifically in the dark skin pigmentation group) due to over-estimating their skin's reactivity to the sun, reducing the need for markers with enhanced contrast. Consequently, the validity of this questionnaire for categorizing skin pigmentations should be addressed if it is to be used to determine contrast requirements for soft tissue motion capture, as done in this study.

A vital assumption of using massless skin markers to quantify soft tissue movement following impact is that the superficial soft tissues (i.e., skin) move synchronously with the underlying deep soft tissues (i.e., muscle and fat), and thus, produce identical impact responses relative to bone (Brydges et al., 2015). Since this could not be tested in the current study, given the superficial and non-invasive nature of the approaches used, it could be viewed as a potential source of measurement error. Furthermore, the motion of the rigid tissue (i.e., bone) was not directly measured. As a result, the intra-segmental marker motion may have been influenced, to a certain extent, by the whole limb motion of the forearm (Pain & Challis, 2002). However, the impact of this limitation was minimised by carefully instructing participants to maintain proper upper extremity posture during data collection and inspecting the captured video footage after each impact trial. In addition, factors that have been shown to influence impact shock attenuation in the upper extremity, such as muscle activation levels (Pain & Challis, 2002; Burkhart & Andrews, 2010a) and joint angles (DeGoede, Ashton-Miller, Schultz & Alexander, 2002b), were not directly controlled for, as quantifying these measures without the use of devices which need to be externally affixed to the skin (e.g., electromyography, electrogoniometers, etc.) was a challenge that could not be met during the current study.

The generalizability of the results of this study is limited to a younger adult population (17–30 years of age). It is likely that the significant changes in body composition, such as sarcopenia (Baumgartner, 2000) and progressive declines of skin elasticity (Sumino et al., 2004; Luebberding, Krueger & Kerscher, 2014) that occur with age, would influence the forearm soft tissue impact responses of people older than the participants in this study. This will have implications for modelling segmental responses following impact events across different age groups. Considering that current wobbling mass biomechanical models include very simplified soft tissue components with respect to their shape and motion characteristics (Gruber, Ruder, Denoth & Schneider, 1998; Gittoes et al., 2006; Pain and Challis, 2006), further examination of the relative motions of soft tissue elements within individual segments of different aged participants will help improve the biofidelity and generalizability of future biomechanical modeling efforts.

CONCLUSIONS

In summary, as suggested by Pain and Challis (2002), ignoring the importance of soft tissue motion for attenuating impact shock in the body, and dismissing it as error (i.e., soft tissue artifact) that needs to be removed from biomechanical analyses (Peters, Galna, Sangeux, Morris & Baker, 2010), may limit our knowledge of the injury mechanisms at play during dynamic impact events. To the authors' knowledge, this is the first study to quantify the motion associated with the impact response of the forearm soft tissues following a forward fall onto the hands of outstretched arms. Consequently, this research provides novel insight into the shock attenuating characteristics of the soft tissues in the forearm, wherein peak soft tissue displacement and velocity were found to generally increase moving distally to proximally along the forearm, with the greatest impact responses occurring in the distal direction; females and males showed no significant differences for this body segment, on average. Future work should look to better comprehend how soft tissue responds both independently and in conjunction with other injury prevention strategies proven to help mitigate impact forces, such as wrist guards (Burkhart & Andrews 2010b) and energy-absorbing flooring systems (Laing & Robinovitch, 2009). Moreover, with multiple studies investigating both in- and out-of-plane motion of soft tissues (Manal, McClay Davis, Galinat & Stanhope, 2003; Stagni, Fantozzi, Cappello & Leardini, 2005; Akbarshahi et al., 2010; Mills, Scurr & Wood, 2011), 3D analysis utilizing either of the marker setups evaluated in the current study, would be a logical next step to advance the scope of this research, and to fully understand the effect that soft tissue motion has on the propagation and attenuation of impact forces in the forearm and body.

ACKNOWLEDGEMENTS

The financial support from NSERC is gratefully acknowledged as well as the efforts of Lauren Gyemi and Mary Birkner for their assistance with pilot data collection and data analysis.

REFERENCES

Akbarshahi, M., Schache, A., Fernandez, J., Baker, R., Banks, S., & Pandy, M. (2010). Non-invasive assessment of soft-tissue artifact and its effect on knee joint kinematics during functional activity. *Journal of Biomechanics*, 43(7), 1292-1301.

Baumgartner, R. N. (2000). Body composition in healthy aging. *Annals of the New York Academy of Sciences*, 904, 437-448.

Brydges, E. A., Burkhart, T. A., Altenhof, W. J., & Andrews, D. M. (2015). Leg soft tissue position and velocity data from skin markers can be obtained with good to acceptable reliability following heel impacts. *Journal of Sports Sciences*, 33(15), 1606-1613.

Burkhart, T. A., & Andrews, D. M. (2010a). Activation level of extensor carpi ulnaris affects wrist and elbow acceleration responses following simulated forward falls. *Journal of Electromyography and Kinesiology*, 20(6), 1203-1210.

Burkhart, T. A., & Andrews, D. M. (2010b). The effectiveness of wrist guards for reducing wrist and elbow accelerations resulting from simulated forward falls. *Journal of Applied Biomechanics*, 26(3), 281-292.

Burkhart, T. A., Andrews, D. M., & Dunning, C. E. (2012). Failure characteristics of the isolated distal radius in in response to dynamic impact loading. *Journal Orthopaedic Research*, 30(6), 885-892.

Burkhart, T. A., Quenneville, C. E., Dunning, C. E., & Andrews, D. M. (2014). Development and validation of a distal radius finite element model to simulate impact loading indicative of a forward fall. *Proceedings of the Institution of Mechanical Engineers. Part H, Journal of engineering in medicine*, 228(3), 258-271.

Choi W. J., & Robinovitch, S. N. (2011). Pressure distribution over the palm region during forward falls on the outstretched hands. *Journal of Biomechanics*, 44(3), 532-539.

Cole, G. K., Nigg, B. M., van den Bogert, A. J., & Gerritsen, K. G. M. (1996). Lower extremity joint loading during impact in running. *Clinical Biomechanics*, 11(4), 181-193.

Crammond, G., Boyd, S. W., & Dulieu-Barton, J. M. (2013). Speckle pattern quality assessment for digital image correlation. *Optics and Lasers in Engineering*, 51(12), 1368-1378.

DeGoede, K. M., & Ashton-Miller, J. A. (2002a). Fall arrest strategy affects peak hand impact force in a forward fall. *Journal of Biomechanics*, 35(6), 843-848.

DeGoede, K. M., Ashton-Miller, J. A., Schultz, A. B., & Alexander, N. B. (2002b). Biomechanical factors affecting the peak hand reaction force during the bimanual arrest of a moving mass. *Journal of Biomechanical Engineering*, 124(1), 107-112.

Fitzpatrick, T. B. (1988). The validity and practicality of sun reactive skin types I through VI. *Archives of Dermatology*, 124(6), 869-871.

Fuller, J., Liu, L., Murphy, M., & Mann, R. (1997). A comparison of lower-extremity skeletal kinematics measured using skin- and pin-mounted markers. *Human Movement Science*, 16(2-3), 219-242.

Gao, B., & Zheng, N. (2008). Investigation of soft tissue movement during level walking: translations and rotations of skin markers. *Journal of Biomechanics*, 41(15), 3189-3195.

Gittoes, M. J., Brewin, M. A., & Kerwin, D. G. (2006). Soft tissue contributions to impact forces simulated using a four-segment wobbling mass model of forefoot–heel landings. *Human Movement Science*, 25(6), 775-787.

Greenwald, R. M., Janes, P. C., Swanson, S. C., & McDonald, T. R. (1998). Dynamic impact response of human cadaveric forearms using a wrist brace. *American Journal of Sports Medicine*, 26(6), 825-830.

Gruber, K., Ruder, H., Denoth, J., & Schneider, K. (1998). A comparative study of impact dynamics: wobbling mass model versus rigid body models. *Journal of Biomechanics*, 31(5), 439-444.

Haddadi, H., & Belhabib, S. (2008). Use of rigid-body motion for the investigation and estimation of the measurement errors related to digital image correlation technique. *Optics and Lasers in Engineering*, 46(2), 185-196.

Hwang, I. K., Kim, K. J., Kaufman, K. R., Cooney, W. P., & An, K. N. (2006). Biomechanical efficiency of wrist guards as a shock isolator. *Journal of Biomechanical Engineering*, 128(2), 229-234.

Idzikowski, J. R., Janes, P. C., & Abbott, P. J. (2000). Upper extremity snowboarding injuries. Ten-year results from the Colorado snowboard injury survey. *American Journal of Sports Medicine*, 28(6), 825-832.

Kim, K. J., & Ashton-Miller, J. A. (2003). Biomechanics of fall arrest using the upper extremity: Age differences. *Clinical Biomechanics (Bristol, Avon)*, 18(4), 311-318.

Kuo, M. Y., Tsai, T. Y., Lin, C. C., Lu, T. W., Hsu, H. C., & Shen, W. C. (2011). Influence of soft tissue artifacts on the calculated kinematics and kinetics of total knee replacements during sit-to-stand. *Gait & Posture*, 33(3), 379-384.

Laing, A. C., & Robinovitch, S. N. (2009). Low stiffness floors can attenuate fall-related femoral impact forces by up to 50% without substantially impairing balance in older women. *Accident; Analysis and Prevention*, 41(3), 642-650.

Lattimer, L. J., Lanovaz, J. L., Farthing, J. P., Madill, S., Kim, S., & Arnold, C. (2016). Upper limb and trunk muscle activation during an unexpected descent on the outstretched hands in young and older women. *Journal of Electromyography and Kinesiology*, 30, 231-237.

Lattimer, L. J., Lanovaz, J. L., Farthing, J. P., Madill, S., Kim, S., Robinovitch, S., & Arnold, C. (2017). Female age-related differences in biomechanics and muscle activity during descents on the outstretched arms. *Journal of Aging and Physical Activity*, 25(3), 474-481.

Leardini, A., Chiari, L., Croce, U., & Cappozzo, A. (2005). Human movement analysis using stereophotogrammetry: Part 3. Soft tissue artifact assessment and compensation. *Gait & Posture*, 21(2), 212-225.

Luebberding, S., Krueger, N., & Kerscher, M. (2014). Mechanical properties of human skin in vivo: a comparative evaluation in 300 men and women. *Skin Research and Technology*, 20(2), 127-135.

Manal, K. K., McClay Davis, I. I., Galinat, B. B., & Stanhope, S. S. (2003). The accuracy of estimating proximal tibial translation during natural cadence walking: bone vs. skin mounted targets. *Clinical Biomechanics (Bristol, Avon)*, 18(2), 126-131.

Maughan, R. J., Abel, R. W., Watson, J. S., & Weir, J. (1986). Forearm composition and muscle function in trained and untrained limbs. *Clinical Physiology*, 6(4), 389-396.

Mazess, R. B., Barden, H. S., Bisek, J. P., & Hanson, J. (1990). Dual-energy x-ray absorptiometry for total-body and regional bone-mineral and soft-tissue composition. *American Journal of Clinical Nutrition*, 51(6), 1106-1112.

Mills, C., Scurr, J., & Wood, L. (2011). A protocol for monitoring soft tissue motion under compression garments during drop landings. *Journal Biomechanics*, 44(9), 1821-1823.

Mirhadi, S., Ashwood, N., & Karagkevrekis, B. (2015). Review of rollerblading injuries. *Trauma*, 17(1), 29-32.

Muller, M. E., Webber, C. E., & Bouxsein, M. L. (2003). Predicting the failure load of the distal radius. *Osteoporosis International*, 14(4), 345-352.

Myers, E., Sebeny, E., Hecker, A., Corcoran, T., Hipp, J., Greenspan, S., & Hayes, W. (1991). Correlations between photon absorption properties and failure load of the distal radius in vitro. *Calcified Tissue International*, 49(4), 292-297.

Nellans, K. W., Kowalski, E., & Chung, K. C. (2012). The epidemiology of distal radius fractures. *Hand Clinics*, 28(2), 113-125.

Nevitt, M. C., & Cummings, S. R. (1993). Type of fall and risk of hip and wrist fractures: The study of osteoporotic fractures. The Study of Osteoporotic Fractures Research Group. *Journal of the American Geriatrics Society*, 41(11), 1226-1234.

Pain, M. T., & Challis, J. H. (2002). Soft tissue motion during impacts: Their potential contributions to energy dissipation. *Journal of Applied Biomechanics*, 18(3), 231-242.

Pain, M. T., & Challis, J. H. (2006). The influence of soft tissue movement on ground reaction forces, joint torques and joint reaction forces in drop landings. *Journal of Biomechanics*, 39(1), 119-124.

Palvanen, M., Kannus, P., Parkkari, J., Pitkäjärvi, T., Pasanen, M., Vuori, I., & Järvinen, M. (2000). The injury mechanisms of osteoporotic upper extremity fractures among older adults: A controlled study of 287 consecutive patients and their 108 controls. *Osteoporosis International*, 11(10), 822-831.

Peters, A., Galna, B., Sangeux, M., Morris, M., & Baker, R. (2010). Quantification of soft tissue artifact in lower limb human motion analysis: A systematic review. *Gait & Posture*, 31(1), 1-8.

Prichasuk, S. (1994). The heel pad in plantar heel pain. *Journal of Bone and Joint Surgery. British Volume*, 76(1), 140-142.

Robinovitch, S. N., & Chiu, J. (1998). Surface stiffness affects impact force during a fall on the outstretched hand. *Journal of Orthopaedic Research*, 16(3), 309-313.

Sangeux, M. M., Marin, F. F., Charleux, F. F., Dürselen, L. L., & Ho Ba Tho, M. C. (2006). Quantification of the 3D relative movement of external marker sets vs. bones based on magnetic resonance imaging. *Clinical Biomechanics (Bristol, Avon)*, 21(9), 984-991.

Sati, M., de Guise, J. A., Larouche, S., & Drouin, G. (1996). Quantitative assessment of skin-bone movement at the knee. *The Knee*, 3(3), 121-138.

Stagni, R., Fantozzi, S., Cappello, A., & Leardini, A. (2005). Quantification of soft tissue artefact in motion analysis by combining 3D fluoroscopy and stereophotogrammetry: A study on two subjects. *Clinical Biomechanics (Bristol, Avon)*, 20(3), 320-329.

Stefanczyk, J. M., Brydges, E. A., Burkhart, T. A., Altenhof, W. J., & Andrews, D. M. (2013). Surface accelerometer fixation method affects leg soft tissue motion following heel impacts. *International Journal of Kinesiology and Sports Science*, 1(3), 1-8.

Südhoff, I., Van Driessche, S., Laporte, S., de Guise, J.A., & Skall, W. (2007). Comparing three attachment systems used to determine knee kinematics during gait. *Gait & Posture*, 25(4), 533-543.

Sumino, H., Ichikawa, S., Abe, M., Endo, Y., Ishikawa, O., & Kurabayashi, M. (2004). Effects of aging, menopause, and hormone replacement therapy on forearm skin elasticity in women. *Journal of the American Geriatrics Society*, 52(6), 945-949.

Winter, D. A. (2005). *Biomechanics and motor control of human movement* (2nd ed). Hoboken, NJ: John Wiley and Sons Inc.

Wolf, A., & Senesh, M. (2011). Estimating joint kinematics from skin motion observation: modelling and validation. *Computer Methods in Biomechanics and Biomedical Engineering*, 14(11), 939-946.

Wrbaškić, N. N., & Dowling, J. J. (2007). An investigation into the deformable characteristics of the human foot using fluoroscopic imaging. *Clinical Biomechanics (Bristol, Avon)*, 22(2), 230-238.

26

Demographic Characteristics Related to Motor Skills in Children Aged 5-7 Years Old

You Fu[1]*, Ryan D. Burns[2]

[1]*School of Community Health Sciences, University of Nevada, Reno, 1664 N Virginia Street, Reno, NV 89557*

[2]*Department of Health, Kinesiology, and Recreation, University of Utah, 250 S 1850 E, Salt Lake City, UT 84112*

Corresponding Author: You Fu, E-mail: youf@unr.edu

ARTICLE INFO

Conflicts of interest: None
Funding: None

ABSTRACT

Background: Motor skill is important to young children's overall well-being. However, there has been a paucity of work examining the demographic characteristics on young children' motor skill. **Objective:** The purpose of this study was to examine the differences in motor skills across socio-economic status (SES) and grade levels in elementary school children. **Method:** Participants were 651 kindergarten to 2nd grade children (mean age = 6.2 ± 0.9 years; 305 girls, 346 boys) recruited from two low SES schools and another two high SES schools. Selected motor skill items were measured using the Test for Gross Motor Development-3rd Edition (TGMD-3) instrument. Data were collected once at each school during physical education class and recess period. A $4 \times 3 \times 2 \times 2$ Multivariate Analysis of Variance (MANOVA) test was employed to examine the differences among grade, SES, ethnicity, and sex on TGMD-3 scores. **Results:** There were significant main effects for grade (Wilks' lambda = 0.34, $F (2, 1274) = 229.6, p < 0.001$) and SES (Wilks' lambda = 0.70, $F (2, 637) = 136.3, p < 0.001$). Follow-up tests revealed statistically significant differences between grades on locomotor, object control and overall TGMD-3, with the 2nd graders displaying highest mean scores, followed by 1st graders and kindergarteners. Follow-up tests suggested that high SES children displaying statistically significant higher mean scores than low SES students on all motor skill variables. **Conclusion:** Older children demonstrated higher motor competence levels, and those with high SES displayed higher motor skill levels than lower SES children.

Key words: Motor Skills, Exercise, Child, Social Class

INTRODUCTION

Motor skills are the basic human movements that are commonly identified by locomotor skills (e.g. running, jumping, sliding, etc.) and manipulative skills (e.g. kicking, throwing, or catching, etc.) (Burton & Miller, 1998; Pangrazi & Beighle, 2013; Barnett, Ridgers, & Salmon, 2015). The development of motor skills is a continuous and age-related process of change in movement. As age progresses, motor skills proceed from simple to complex locomotor and manipulative movements, which function as the building blocks for more advanced skills (Burton & Miller, 1998; Payne & Isaacs, 2011). According to Burton and Miller's (1998) movement skill assessment model, motor skills facilitate young aged individuals control bodies, adopt surrounding environments, achieve complex tasks that are involved in athletic and daily life activities (Davis & Burton, 1991). Therefore, an optimal development of young children's motor skills is of significant importance for their healthy physical and social conditions, sport performance, and general daily living activities (Deflandre, Lorant, Gavarry, & Falgairette, 2001; Williams et al., 2008; Trudeau & Shephard, 2008; Lai et al., 2014; Robinson et al., 2015; Burns, Brusseau, Fu, & Hannon, 2017).

Although an optimal development of these skills is important for the growing child, many children are still unable to achieve motor skill competence (Robinson et al., 2015). In fact, children who demonstrated low level of motor skills may also display low level of motivation, such as perceived physical competence and self-efficacy (Robinson, Rudisill, & Goodway, 2009; Barnett et al., 2015). The lack of motivation compromises physical activity participation and health-related fitness, and thus can exacerbate health risk if low levels of these constructs track through adolescence and into adulthood (Stodden, Goodway, & Langendorfer, 2008; Burns, Brusseau, Fu, & Hannon, 2015; Ali, Pigou, Clarke, & McLachlan, 2017).

Previous research has suggested that incompetency in motor skills was associated with lower levels of physical activity behaviors (Hardy, et al., 2012; Logan, Webster, Getchell, Pfeiffer, & Robinson, 2015). In addition, a recent research reported a significant correlation between children's motor skills and their cardio-metabolic risk that was mediated through aerobic fitness (Burns, Brusseau, Fu, & Hannon, 2017). Although it is beneficial for all students to develop motor skills in school settings, children with low socio-economic status (SES), or those from low-income families, may have low motor skill levels. This is because of fewer opportunities to participate in sports and recreational activities before and after school, and the limited physical education time during school (Lampard, Jurkowski, Lawson, & Davison, 2013). Particularly, it has been documented that low-income Hispanic and African American preschool children had a delayed proficiency in motor skills (Goodway & Branta, 2003; Goodway & Rudisill, 1997).

Compared to children from middle and high-income households, children from low-income families may be at risk for poor motor skill development due to the limited access to physical activity and sport participation outside of school settings. These children may also have limited resources to safe playground areas or equipment for motor skill competence (Kercood et al., 2015; Eime, et al., 2017). Despite these positive findings in disadvantaged preschool children, there has been a paucity of work examining the demographic factors relating to motor skill levels in young elementary school-aged children with the consideration that young individual's motor skill development is a continuous process and changes rapidly during the early years of age. Due to the importance of developing motor skills, the purpose of this study was to examine the differences in motor skills among SES and grades in a sample of young elementary school-aged children. It was hypothesized that older grade cohorts will display greater TGMD-3 scores compared to younger grade cohorts. We also hypothesized that high SES children will demonstrate higher levels on both locomotor and ball skills compared to children from lower income schools.

MATERIALS AND METHODS

Participants

A convenience sample of 651 kindergarten through 2nd grade children (mean age = 6.2 ± 0.9 years; 305 girls, 346 boys) were recruited from four urban elementary schools located in the Western U.S. There were two high SES schools in the middle and high-income household areas. All schools were within the same school district. In the high SES sample (141 girls, 172 boys), approximately 43.9% of the children were of Caucasian ethnicity, 24.4% were Hispanic/Latino, 16.3% were African American, 10.9% were Asian, and 4.5% were classified as other. In the low SES sample (164 girls, 174 boys), approximately 14.2% of the children were of Caucasian ethnicity, 45.0% were Hispanic/Latino, 27.5% were African American, 5.3% were Asian, 8.0% were classified as other. Children were recruited in this research only if they met the inclusion criteria: (1) aged 5 - 7 years; and (2) not diagnosed with physical and/or mental disability according to school records. Written assent was obtained from the children and consent was obtained from the parents prior to data collection. The University Institutional Review Board approved the study protocols.

Study Design

Children in the high SES schools were scheduled to have 2-3 physical education classes per week taught by certified

physical educators, in addition to recess opportunities for physical activity. The two low SES schools were both "Nevada Zoom" schools that received government financial assistance. "Nevada Zoom" schools are given supplemental government funding for tutoring, smaller class sizes, and extended learning opportunities. This additional funding has the purpose to accelerate learning for students where English is not the primary language. There was no physical education at these schools, but children participated into physical activities during multiple recesses in every school day.

Instrumentation and Tools

The Test for Gross Motor Development Edition-3 (TGMD-3) was used to assess children's motor skills (Webster & Ulrich, 2017). The TGMD-3, upgraded from TGMD-2 (Ulrich, 2000), is a validated assessment battery of gross motor skills for children 3-10 years old. The TGMD-3 assessed motor skills across 13 movement skills within locomotor and object control subtests, respectively. The locomotor sub-tests comprised run, skip, slide, gallop, hop, and horizontal jump. The object control sub-tests included the overhand throw, underhand throw, catch, dribble, kick, one-hand strike, and two-hand strike. The locomotor and object control subtest scores were 46 and 54 respectively, and the total TGMD-3 scores were 100. Each child in this study performed the test items across two trials that were individually scored using specific performance criteria (0 = did not perform correctly; 1 = performed.

Procedures

Gross motor skills were measured once at each school in the order of two low SES schools first, followed two high SES schools. Upon the entrance to the gym, a typical class of students was divided into two stations, which comprised of locomotor sub-tests and object control sub-tests with one research assistant supervised each station. Students switched over stations after completing all their sub-tests. For each sub-test, the research assistants demonstrated the movement before collecting data then scored using the protocols outlined in Webster & Ulrich (2017). Two trained research assistants scored all TGMD-3 data live in these four schools during physical education classes or recess in the spring semester. One research assistant scored locomotor sub-tests at all schools and the other research assistant scored object control sub-tests at all schools to maintain testing consistency. Throughout the entire data collection period, the two research assistants were not aware of the SES difference among schools, which may increase the internal validity of the results and reduces the potential for bias.

Research assistants were trained for one week prior to the commencement of data collection. Training included a seminar tutoring the TGMD-3 guideline and scoring protocol. Two research assistants also practiced coding TGMD-3 among a sample of elementary school-aged children from a difference school for two sessions, with the purpose to calculate inter- and intra-scorer agreement using live and video coding. Each research assistant scored both locomotor and object control sub-tests. The inter-observer agreement (the agreement of coefficient between different observers) was 0.90. The intra-observer agreement (the agreement of coefficient within the same observer over time) was 0.91 for the first observer and 0.93 for the second observer.

Statistical Analysis

Data were checked for Gaussian distributions using k-density plots and screened for outliers using z-scores (± 3.0 z-score cut-point). To determine the eligibility to use a multivariate model, bivariate associations among the observed variables were examined using Pearson product-moment correlations. All of the correlations among the dependent variables were statistically significant, being moderate-to-strong in magnitude. Therefore, a $4 \times 3 \times 2 \times 2$ Multivariate Analysis of Variance (MANOVA) test was used to examine the differences among ethnicity (White, Black, Asian, Other), grade level (Kindergarten, 1st grade, 2nd grade), sex (girl, boy), and SES (high, low) on the gross motor skill variables. Both main effects and interactions were examined within the multivariate model. The dependent variables were the locomotor subtest score, the ball skill subtest score, and the TGMD-3 total score. If a statistically significant omnibus multivariate model was found using Wilks' lambda, follow-up univariate tests were explored with Bonferroni post hoc tests. Pair-wise comparison effect sizes were calculated using Cohen's delta (d), in that d < 0.20 indicting a small effect size, d = 0.50 indicating a medium effect size, and a d > 0.80 indicating a large effect size (Cohen, 1988). Alpha level was set a $p \leq 0.05$ and the analysis was conducted using SPSS 25.0 statistical software package (IBM Inc., Armonk, NY, USA).

RESULTS

The descriptive data for the total sample and within sex groups was presented in Table 1. Pearson correlations among all motor skill observed variables (individual items and subtest scores) were presented in Table 2. There were statistically significant positive and weak-to-strong (r = 0.13 to 0.88) correlations among the TGMD-3 subtests scores and total scores ($p < 0.01$), warranting multi-variate analysis.

The omnibus MANOVA model yielded two statistically significant main effects for grade (Wilks' lambda = 0.34, F (2, 1274) = 229.6, $p < 0.001$) and SES (Wilks' lambda = 0.70, F (2, 637) = 136.3, $p < 0.001$). There is no other statistically significant multivariate main effects or interactions. Assumptions of MANOVA were confirmed via approximately univariate Gaussian distributions across all dependent variables (multivariate normality), no clustering within the data structure (independence of observations), adequate sample size achieving at least 80% power (a priori), a lack of extreme multicolinarity among the dependent variables (r < 0.90), and a non-significant Box's M test supporting homogeneity of variance-covariance matrices. Grade and SES mean differences on gross motor skill are presented in Figures 1 and 2, respectively. The follow-up Bonferroni post-hoc tests showed that there were statistically significant differences on locomotor sub-

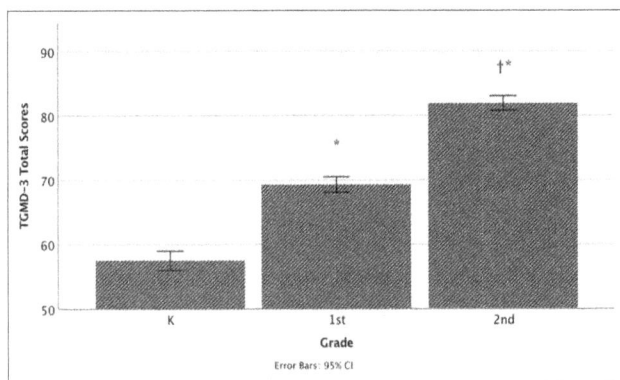

Figure 1. TGMD-3 scores across observed grades levels. * indicates statistical significance, p < 0.05; † indicates statistical significance, p < 0.01; Error bars are standard deviations

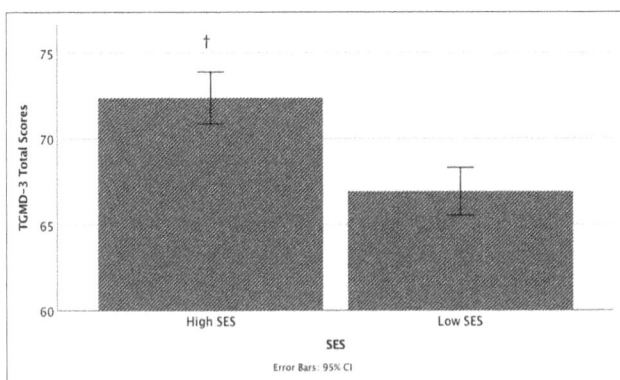

Figure 2. TGMD-3 scores between SES groups. † indicates statistical significance, p < 0.05; Error bars are standard deviations

test scores across grades. Specifically, the 2nd graders displayed higher mean scores compared to the 1st graders (mean difference = 4.4, $p < 0.001$, d = 0.91), the 1st graders displayed higher mean scores compared to the kindergarteners (mean differences = 4.30, $p < 0.001$, d = 0.68), and 2nd graders displaying higher mean scores compared to kindergateners (mean difference = 8.65, $p < 0.001$, d = 1.11). With respect to the ball skill subtest scores, the 2nd graders displayed higher mean scores than the 1st graders (mean differences = 8.19, $p < 0.001$, d = 1.23); the 1st graders displayed higher mean scores than the kindergarteners (mean difference = 7.55, $p < 0.001$, d = 1.14), and the 2nd graders displayed higher mean scores than the kindergarteners (mean difference = 15.74, $p < 0.001$, d = 2.38). In terms of the TGMD-3 total scores, the 2nd graders displayed higher mean scores as compared to 1st graders (mean difference = 12.57, p < 0.001, d = 1.14), 1st graders displayed higher mean scores as compared to kindergarteners (mean difference = 11.82, p < 0.001, d = 1.07), and 2nd graders displayed higher mean scores as compared to kindergarteners (mean difference = 24.38, $p < 0.001$, d = 2.22).

The follow-up Bonferroni post hoc tests also suggested that there were statistically significant differences between SES levels, with the high SES students displaying statistically significant higher mean scores compared to low SES students on locomotor sub-test scores (mean difference = 1.09, $p < 0.001$, d = 0.17), object control sub-test scores (mean difference = 2.56, $p < 0.001$, d = 0.31), and TGMD-3 total scores (mean difference = 5.45, $p < 0.001$, d = 0.42).

DISCUSSION

Although there is a growing body of evidence, the work examining the demographic characteristics on young children's motor skills has not yet been explored in depth. Accordingly, the purpose of this cross-sectional study was to investigate the demographic characteristics on motor skills in a sample of aged 5-7 years old children recruited from four rural schools. One of the salient findings was that the development of children's motor skills improved with the progression of age, as older children in the sample demonstrated statistically significant higher TGMD-3 sub-tests and overall scores than the younger participants. Another salient finding was that children with high SES had a significantly higher motor skill level compared to low SES children, or those from low-income families.

In the present study, the 2nd grade students achieved statistically higher mean scores than the 1st grade students on locomotor, object control, and overall TGMD-3, and a similar finding was further detected between the 1st grade students and kindergarteners. These results demonstrated that there was a positive relationship between the development of motor skill and gerontology. Based on the theoretical perspectives in motor development, maturational theory of child development (Gesell, 1928) explained young children's motor developmental changes as the function of maturational processes, particularly, through the central nervous systems, which control the motor development. The maturational theory of child development further claimed that children's motor development is an internal growth driven by biological development (Gesell, 1928). The theoretical

perspectives were soundly echoed by the findings of the present study, in that older students in the sample who characterized with higher level of biological and physiological development demonstrated higher levels of the motor skills development.

Present results were also in line with another research (Martinek et al., 1978) that aimed to compare the race and age differences on elementary school students' physical activity and motor skills. The study reported a progressive improvement in motor skill scores across grades, in specific, the motor skill mean scores for Grade 1, 2 and 3 were 27.30, 30.09, and 37.62, respectively. The findings of this study strengthened the contention that the process of maturation has a definite effect on motor performance in young children. It has also been suggested that motor skills and physical activity were significant associated with each other (Fisher at al., 2005; Stodden at el., 2008; Holfelder & Schott, 2014; Barnett et al., 2015). Therefore, a better understanding on the development of gross motor skills across various school grades may further lead to increased physical activity participation and health-related fitness levels, as this cohort tracks through adolescence and into adulthood (Stodden, Gao, Goodway, & Langendorfer, 2014).

We also found high SES sample in this study achieved statistically higher scores on locomotor, object control, and overall TGMD-3 as compared to the low SES children. This finding is in line with our hypothesis and is partially supported by theoretical perspectives as well as previous studies. Gesell (1928) claimed that children's social environment plays an important role in their motor skills development, and these external incentives were most effective when they were synchronized with the inner maturational timeline. Stodden et al. (2008) suggested that young children's different experiences might have attributed to the various lev-

Table 1. Descriptive statistics for the total sample and within each sex group (means and standard deviations)

	Total (N=651)	Girls (n=305)	Boys (n=346)
Run (Raw score 0-4)	3.2 (0.7)	3.2 (0.7)	3.2 (0.7)
Gallop (Raw score 0-4)	3.2 (0.8)	3.1 (0.8)	3.3 (0.8)
Hop (Raw score 0-4)	3.2 (0.8)	3.2 (0.8)	3.3 (0.8)
Horizontal jump (Raw score 0-3)	2.2 (0.8)	2.1 (0.8)	2.2 (0.8)
Skip (Raw score 0-4)	2.3 (0.8)	2.2 (0.8)	2.4 (0.8)
Slide (Raw score 0-4)	2.6 (0.9)	2.6 (1.0)	2.6 (0.9)
Locomotor sub-test (Raw score 0-46)	33.3 (7.2)	32.6 (7.4)	33.9 (7.0)
Two-hand strike (Raw score 0-5)	2.8 (1.2)	2.7 (1.2)	2.9 (1.1)
One-hand strike (Raw score 0-4)	2.9 (0.9)	2.9 (0.9)	2.9 (0.9)
One-hand dribble (Raw score 0-3)	1.8 (0.9)	1.8 (0.9)	1.8 (0.9)
Catch (Raw score 0-3)	2.1 (0.8)	2.1 (0.8)	2.1 (0.9)
Kick (Raw score 0-4)	2.7 (1.0)	2.6 (1.0)	2.8 (1.0)
Over-hand throw (Raw score 0-4)	2.9 (0.9)	2.9 (0.9)	2.9 (1.0)
Under-hand throw (Raw score 0-4)	3.0 (0.9)	3.0 (0.9)	3.0 (0.9)
Ball skill sub-test (Raw score 0-54)	36.3 (8.6)	36.0 (8.4)	36.5 (8.7)
TGMD-3 total score (Raw score 0-100)	69.5 (13.5)	68.6 (13.4)	70.4 (13.6)

TGMD-3 stands for the Test for Gross Motor Development-3rd Edition.

Table 2. Correlation matrix

	Run	Gallop	Hop	H-Jump	Skip	Slide	Loco subtest	Two-h strike	One-h strike	One-h dribble	Catch	Kick	Over-h throw	Under-h throw	Ball subtest	TGMD-3
Run	1															
Gallop	0.46**	1														
Hop	0.46**	0.46**	1													
H-Jump	0.43**	0.42**	0.81**	1												
Skip	0.73**	0.46**	0.37**	0.35**	1											
Slide	0.58**	0.38**	0.31**	0.25**	0.51**	1										
Loco subtest	0.82**	0.71**	0.75**	0.72**	0.77**	0.70**	1									
Two-h strike	0.20**	0.25**	0.14**	0.13**	0.21**	0.21**	0.26**	1								
One-h strike	0.23**	0.24**	0.15**	0.19**	0.28**	0.36**	0.33**	0.19**	1							
One-h dribble	0.25**	0.28**	0.17**	0.16**	0.36**	0.37**	0.36**	0.19**	0.39**	1						
Catch	0.22**	0.25**	0.16**	0.17**	0.29**	0.25**	0.30**	0.19**	0.35**	0.60**	1					
Kick	0.22**	0.19**	0.15**	0.13**	0.28**	0.34**	0.30**	0.17**	0.27**	0.41**	0.33**	1				
Over-h throw	0.17**	0.23**	0.12**	0.14**	0.28**	0.27**	0.28**	0.19**	0.27**	0.39**	0.25**	0.57**	1			
Under-h throw	0.19**	0.25**	0.21**	0.21**	0.24**	0.25**	0.30**	0.21**	0.26**	0.37**	0.30**	0.47**	0.64**	1		
Ball subtest	0.33**	0.37**	0.24**	0.25**	0.42**	0.45**	0.47**	0.51**	0.59**	0.71**	0.64**	0.60**	0.72**	0.71**	1	
TGMD-3	0.64**	0.62**	0.55**	0.54**	0.68**	0.66**	0.83**	0.46**	0.55**	0.65**	0.57**	0.60**	0.60**	0.61**	0.88**	1

TGMD-3 stands for the Test for Gross Motor Development-3rd Edition; H-Jump stands for horizontal jump; Loco stands for locomotor; Two-h stands for two-hand; One-h stands for one-hand; Over-h stands for over-head; Under-h stands for under-hand; * indicates a statistically significant bivariate correlation, $p \leq 0.05$; ** indicates a statistically significant bivariate correlation, $p \leq 0.01$.

els of motor skill competence. These experiences including environment, physical education, SES, parental support, etc. Additionally, Venetsanou and Kambas (2010) also reported that family SES affected children's motor development. In this review study, they found in majority of relevant studies children of lower socioeconomic classes seem to perform worse than those of the middle/high classes in motor development. Consequently, a number of plausible reasons may explain the lower-class children's in the present study had poorer motor competence. Low SES children's motor incompetence may be associated with poor pre-and post-natal nutrition supplementation, which may have affected the central nervous system. In the present study, Low SES children in "Nevada Zoom" schools may not be encouraged to develop motor skills during school day, as they did not have physical education classes in regular school schedule. In contrast, high SES children had 2-3 physical education classes taught by certified physical educators each week, plus recess opportunities for physical activity in every school day. Therefore, high SES sample in this study may have plenty of opportunities for perceptual-motor experiences, which are beneficial to their motor skill development. In terms of the out-of-school settings, low SES children living in disadvantage communities may suffer from the lack of facilities and space that prevents them from developing their motor skills (Eime et al., 2015; Kercood et al., 2015; Eime, et al., 2017). On the other hand, children from higher classes may have a greater number and variety of resources than children from lower classes.

There are a number of limitations to this study that must be considered before the results can be generalized. First, the sample consisted of children recruited across four schools from the Western U.S., specifically from a state characterized as having an arid climate; therefore the results are questionable if generalized to children belonging to other geographical regions. Second, the study design was observational and cross-sectional; therefore, no causal inferences can be made. Third, potential confounding not controlled for that may have influenced the results included physical activity behaviors and health-related fitness. Because of the bi-directional relationship between these constructs and gross motor competency, it is unknown whether the variability in TGMD-3 scores observed among grade levels and SES strata were partially because of variability in these behaviors and characteristics. Finally, as stated in the Methods, children from the high SES schools had physical education classes and children from lower SES schools did not; therefore, the differences in gross motor competency may have been due to the presence of physical education curricula, not the SES of the schools.

CONCLUSION

In conclusion, gross motor skill competency varied across grade levels and SES strata in a sample of young children from the Western U.S. The results of this study support previous work and clarify the potential relationship between gross motor competency and SES. Interestingly, sex did not modify any of the observed relationships. Given the importance of gross motor competency and its relationship with healthy physical activity behaviors and consequent health-related fitness levels, exploring the factors relating to gross motor competency, such as grade level and SES, is imperative to improve the health of at-risk youth.

Conflicts of Interest

The author declares no conflict of interest.

REFERENCES

Ali, A., Pigou, D., Clarke, L., & McLachlan, C. (2017). Literature review on motor skill and physical activity in preschool children in New Zealand. *Advances in Physical Education, 7,* 10-26.

Barnett, L. M., Ridgers, N. D., & Salmon, J. (2015). Associations between young children's perceived and actual ball skill competence and physical activity. *Journal of Science and Medicine in Sport, 18,* 167-171.

Burns, R. D., Brusseau, T. A., Fu, Y., & Hannon, J. C. (2015). Predictors and trends of motor skill performance in at-risk elementary school-aged children. *Perceptual and Motor Skills, 121,* 284-299.

Burns, R. D., Brusseau, T. A., Fu, Y., & Hannon, J. C. (2017). Gross motor skills and cardiometabolic risk in children: A mediation analysis. *Medicine & Science in Sports & Exercise, 49(4),* 746-751.

Burton, A. W., & Miller, D. E. (1998). Movement skill assessment. Champaign, IL: Human Kinetics.

Davis, W. E., & Burton, A. W. (1991). Ecological task analysis: Translating movement behavior theory into practice. *Adapted Physical Activity Quarterly, 8,* 154-177.

Deflandre, A., Lorant, J., Gavarry, O., & Falgairette, G. (2001). Determinants of physical activity and sports activities in French school children. *Perceptual and Motor Skills, 92,* 399-411.

Eime, R. M., Casey, M., Harvey, J. H., Sawyer, N. A., Symons, C. M., & Payne, W. R. (2015). Socioecological factors potentially associated with participation in physical activity and sport: A longitudinal study of adolescent girls. *Journal of Science and Medicine in Sport, 18,* 684-690.

Eime, R. M., Harvey, J. H., Charity, M. J., Casey, M., Westerbeek, H., & Payne, W. R. (2017). The relationship of sport participation to provision of sports facilities and socioeconomic status: a geographical analysis. *Australian and New Zealand Journal of Public Health, 41,* 248-255.

Fisher, A., Reilly, J. J., Kelly, L. A., Montgomery, C., Williamson, C., Paton, J. P., & Grant S. (2005). Fundamental movement skills and habitual physical activity in young children. *Medicine & Science in Sports & Exercise, 37,* 684-688.

Goodway, J. D., & Branta, C. F. (2003). Influence of a motor skill intervention on fundamental motor skill development of disadvantaged preschool children. *Research Quarterly for Exercise and Sport, 74,* 36-46.

Gesell, A. (1928). *Infancy and human growth.* New York: Macmillan.

Goodway, J. D., & Rudisill, M. E. (1997). Perceived physical competence and actual motor skill competence of African American preschool children. *Adapted Physical Activity Quarterly, 14,* 314-326.

Hardy, L. L., Reinten-Reynolds, T., Espinel, P., Zask, A., & Okely A, D. (2012). Prevalence and correlates of low fundamental movement skill competency in children. *Pediatrics, 130,* 390-398.

Holfelder, B., & Schott, N. (2014). Relationship of fundamental movement skills and physical activity in children and adolescents: A systematic review. *Psychology of Sport and Exercise, 15,* 382-391.

Kercood, S., Conway, T. L., Saelens, B. E., Frank, L. D., Cain, K. L., & Sallis, J. F. (2015). Parent rules, barriers, and places for youth physical activity vary by neighborhood walkability and income. *Children, Youth and Environments, 25,* 100-118.

Lai, S. K., Costigan, S. A., Morgan, P. J., Luban, D. R., Stodden, D. F., Salmon, J., & Barnett, L. M. (2014). Do school-based interventions focusing on physical activity, fitness, or fundamental movement skill competency produce a sustained impact in these outcomes in children and adolescents? A systematic review of follow-up studies. *Sports Medicine, 44,* 67-79.

Lampard, A. M., Jurkowski, J. M., Lawson, H. A., & Davison, K. K. (2013). Family ecological predictors of physical activity parenting in low-income families. *Behavioral Medicine, 39,* 97-103.

Logan, S, W., Webster, E. K., Getchell, N., Pfeiffer, K. A., & Robinson, L. E. (2015). Relationship between fundamental motor skill competence and physical activity during childhood and adolescence: a systematic review. *Kinesiology Review, 4,* 416-426.

Pangrazi, R. P., & Beighle, A. (2013). Dynamic physical education for elementary school children. 17th Ed. New York, NY: Pearson.

Payne, V.G., & Isaacs, L.D. (2011). Human motor development: A lifespan approach, 8th ed., McGraw-Hill, Boston, MA (2011)

Robinson, L. E., Rudsill, M. E., & Goodway, J. (2009). Instructional climates in preschool children who are at-risk. Part II: Perceived physical competence. *Research Quarterly for Exercise and Sport, 80,* 543-551.

Robinson, L. E., Stodden, D. F., Barnett, L. M., Lopes, V. P., Logan, S. W., Rodrigues, L. P., & D'Hondt, E. (2015). Motor competence and its effect on positive developmental trajectories of health. *Sports Medicine, 45,* 1273-1284.

Stodden, D. F., Gao, Z., Goodway, J. D., & Langendorfer, S. J. (2014). Dynamic relationships between motor skill competence and health-related fitness in youth. *Pediatric Exercise Science, 26,* 231-241.

Stodden, D. F., Goodway, J. D., & Langendorfer, S. J. (2008). A developmental perspective on the role of motor skill competence in physical activity: An emergent relationship. *Quest, 60,* 290-306.

Trudeau, F., & Shephard, R. J. (2008). Physical education, school physical activity, school sports and academic performance. *International Journal of Behavioral Nutrition and Physical Activity, 5,* 10. doi:10.1186/1479-5868-5-10

Ulrich, D.A. (2000). Test of Gross Motor Development. 2nd ed. Austin, TX: Pro-Ed, 1-5.

Venetsanou, F., & Kambas, A. (2010). Environmental factors affecting preschoolers' motor development. *Early Childhood Education Journal, 37,* 319-327.

Webster, E. K., & Ulrich, D. A. (2017). Evaluation of the psychometric properties of the test of gross motor development-third edition. *Journal of Motor Learning and Development, 5,* 45-58.

Williams, H. G., Pfeiffer, K. A., O'Neill, J. R., Dowda, M., Mclver, K. L., Brown, W. H., & Pate, R. R. (2008). Motor skill performance and physical activity in preschool children. *Obesity, 16,* 1421-1426.

27

Evaluation of Oxygen Uptake Kinetic Asymmetries in Patients with Multiple Sclerosis

Rebecca D. Larson[1]*, Monica Barton[1], John W Farrell III[1,2], Gregory S. Cantrell[1,3], David J. Lantis[1,4], Christopher D. Black[1], Carl J. Ade[1,5]

[1]*Department of Health and Exercise Science, University of Oklahoma, Norman, OK, USA*

[2]*Interdisciplinary School of Health Sciences, University of Ottawa, Ottawa, ON, CDN.*

[3]*Health and Physical Education Department, Northern State University, Aberdeen, SA, USA*

[4]*Department of Kinesiology, St. Ambrose University, Davenport, IA, USA*

[5]*Department of Kinesiology, Kansas State University, Manhattan KS, USA*

Corresponding Author: Rebecca D Larson, E-mail: rdlarson@ou.edu

ARTICLE INFO

Conflicts of interest: None
Funding: None

ABSTRACT

Background of Study: Observations of limb to limb differences (bilateral asymmetry) in leg strength, power, peak oxygen uptake (VO_2) and bone mineral density has been reported in individuals with Multiple Sclerosis (MS). **Objetives:** The purpose of this study was to quantify the magnitude of bilateral asymmetries in oxygen uptake (VO_2) kinetics response to single leg cycling (SLC) in relapsing-remitting multiple sclerosis (MS) patients. **Methods:** Five MS patients (2 men, 3 women; age 43±7 yrs) performed constant work rate SLC trials to determine VO_2 kinetics in each leg. Asymmetry scores were used to quantify the magnitude of the bilateral asymmetries. **Results:** Significant asymmetries were seen in VO_{2peak} and parameters of VO_2 kinetics. VO_{2peak} asymmetry score was significantly different than 0% (p=0.015). Similarly, significant asymmetry for VO_2 kinetic response to exercise as mean response time was observed (p=0.03). In addition the VO_2 response to exercise resulted in a significant asymmetry in VO_2 deficit between legs (p=0.03). No correlation between EDSS scores and any asymmetry scores existed. **Conclusions:** These findings provide insight into the potential differences in metabolic perturbation and limb specific symptomatic fatigue within the MS population.

Key words: Multiple Sclerosis, Exercise, Oxygen, Asymmetry

INTRODUCTION

Pulmonary oxygen uptake (VO_2) kinetics is generally described as the time where oxygen consumption (VO_2) is elevated to meet the demands of the cardiovascular, pulmonary, and muscular systems until the attainment of steady state VO_2 during the beginning of moderate-intensity, aerobic exercise (Poole et al., 2012). Typically VO_2 kinetics occurs within the first 2-3 minutes of aerobic exercise where energy production (ATP) meets energy demands. Prior to reaching steady state, phosphocreatine (PCr) and anaerobic glycolysis compensate for the energy needs (oxygen deficit) created by the delay in skeletal muscle mitochondria production of ATP (energy) until the occurrence of aerobic metabolism (Whipp et al., 1982). A clinical population of interest to examine pulmonary VO_2 kinetics is multiple sclerosis (MS). MS is a chronic, autoimmune disease of the central nervous system (CNS) characterized by the destruction of the myelin that surrounds and insulates nerve fibers. This demyelination results in scarring which slows nerve signal transmission from the brain to the working muscles, resulting in neural

and muscular impairments. These impairments can have a negative impact on exercise tolerance and on quality of life (Compston et al., 2008). To date, only a few researchers have studied pulmonary VO_2 kinetics in individuals with MS and observed that the individuals with MS have significantly slower oxygen uptake at the onset of exercise than healthy individuals (Hansen et al., 2013; Ponichtera-Mulcare et al., 1993). These researchers suggest that slowed pulmonary VO_2 kinetics might play a role in exercise intolerance. One interesting aspect of MS is that it can affect one side of the body more than the other (bilateral asymmetry) which has the potential to create an imbalance in function and performance. Bilateral asymmetry also contributes to fatigue, reported to be the most problematic symptom of MS, leading to reductions in strength and impairments in mobility (Ponichtera-Mulcare, 1993). Although there has been little research quantifying bilateral asymmetries in skeletal muscle function and performance in individuals with MS, the research that has been done has observed significant differences in aerobic capacity, balance, and muscular differences between the lower limbs in a MS group compared to a matched control group by approximately 30% (Larson et al., 2013). The degree to which pulmonary VO_2 kinetics affects those with MS has not been well observed. Hansen et al. (2014) observed that pVO_2 kinetics was slowed in the MS population by approximately 30% of the mean response time (MRT) during double leg cycling when compared to healthy controls (Hansen et al., 2014). However, pulmonary VO_2 kinetics for a single limb of an MS individual has yet to be studied. If a limb is unable to produce the required force as well as incapable of adequately delivering oxygen quickly enough to the exercising muscle, an imbalance could reduce the body's ability to metabolically synchronize the legs, compromising bilateral movements (Sandroff et al., 2013). Since fatigue is reported in the multiple sclerosis (MS) population and is a primary disabling symptom (Romani et al., 2004) and MS bilateral asymmetries in muscular strength are associated with fatigue and exercise performance, highlighting the importance of exercise related asymmetries in this population (Chung et al., 2008). The rate of increase of pulmonary oxygen uptake (VO_2) at the transition from rest to exercise depends on the coordinated muscular and cardiorespiratory responses to meet the increased VO_2 demand of the activity. If this rate of change in VO_2 (i.e. VO_2 kinetics) at exercise onset is decreased a greater VO_2 deficit and metabolic perturbation will occur, which is associated with the onset of fatigue and exercise intolerance (Poole et al., 2008). Here, we provide a pilot investigation of the single-leg VO_2 kinetic response and bilateral asymmetries in a group of MS patients. We hypothesized that asymmetries in would exist in our sample of MS patients.

METHODS

Subjects and Design

This pilot study included 5 relapsing-remitting MS patients (2 men, 3 women; age 43 ± 7 yrs; stature 170.5 ± 7.4 cm; weight 90.2 ± 18.5 kg). The inclusion criteria for patients included age (18-65 years), relapsing-remitting progression, stable for at least 3 months, and Expanded Disability Statistics Scale (EDSS) of 6.0 or less. Exclusion criteria were past or present prednisone medication, past or present lower-body orthopedic injury, and history of cardiovascular disease. Informed consent was obtained per the University of Oklahoma Institutional Review Board for Research Involving Human Subjects requirements.

Protocols

A single-leg ramp exercise test (15W/min) to exhaustion was performed on a cycle ergometer to evaluate each participant's leg specific peak VO_2 (VO_{2peak}) and gas exchange threshold (GET). Each leg was tested on a separate day with 48 hrs between days. Following the ramp tests, over a period of 2-4 weeks, all participants performed 5-7 moderate-intensity constant work rate exercise tests in each leg corresponding to the leg specific 90% GET. These tests were performed over a minimum of 4 visits with 48 hrs between visits. At

each visit at least 3 individual constant work rate tests were performed with 10-minutes between tests. Metabolic and ventilatory data were measured via a gas exchange system (True One 2400, Parvo Medics, Sandy, UT).

Data Analysis and Statistics

For modeling the VO_2 response the 5-second averaged VO_2 from each constant work rate test were time aligned and ensemble-averaged to provide a single response for each participant's individual leg. The mean response time (MRT) of the overall VO_2 response in the transition from rest to end exercise was fit with a monoexponential model after removal of the cardiodynamic phase I (Whipp et al., 1982). The VO_2 deficit was calculated as MRT × the change in VO_2 from baseline. The functional "gain" of the VO_2 response was calculated as the change in VO_2 from baseline divided by the change in work rate. An absolute asymmetry (Chung et al., 2008) was calculated for each variable as

$$asymmetry\ score = 1 - \left(\frac{low\ performance\ leg}{high\ performance\ leg} \right) 100$$

Where the ratio was the value for the lesser performing leg divide by the value for the better performing leg for each tested variable. A value of 0% indicated and 100% indicated maximal asymmetry between legs. A one sample t-test was used to determine if the asymmetry scores were significantly different than 0% (i.e., determine if asymmetry in the limbs existed) for each tested variable (SigmaPlot/SigmaStat 12.5, Systat Software, Point Richmond, CA). Linear correlation analyses were used to determine the association between asymmetry scores and EDSS values. Statistical significance was declared when $P<0.05$ (mean ± SD).

RESULTS

Patients had a mean Expanded Disability Status Scale (EDSS) score of 3.0 ± 1.0 (range: 2-4.5) indicating mild to moderate impairment. On average our sample performed 24.0 ± 20.12 minutes of physical activity for 4.0 ± 2.45 days per week. The VO_{2peak}, GET, MRT, SEE for the modeling, and O_2 deficit for each patient's left and right legs along with individual asymmetry scores are displayed in Table 1. The asymmetry score for VO_{2peak} was significantly different than 0% (p=0.015). Similarly, significant asymmetry for VO_2 kinetic response to exercise, described as the MRT, was observed (p=0.03). This difference in VO_2 response to exercise resulted in a significant asymmetry in VO_2 deficit between legs (p=0.03).

A representative subject's VO_2 kinetic response is illustrated in Figure 1. Note the different MRTs between legs and the associated differences in VO_2 deficit. There was no correlation between EDSS scores and any asymmetry scores.

DISCUSSION

This pilot study suggests that significant asymmetries in the VO_2 response at exercise onset was present in relapsing-remitting MS patients. These findings support our hypothesis and provide insight into the potential differences in the met-

Table 1. Individual data during single leg cycling

Patient #	Leg	VO_{2peak}, ml kg^{-1} min^{-1}	GET, W	MRT, s	SEE	O_2 deficit, ml
1	Right	12.1	58	78.3	0.042	50.3
	Left	12.6	63	76.3	0.053	52.4
	Asymmetry score	3.97	7.94	2.63		4.2
2	Right	21.2	67	40.4	0.072	27.2
	Left	22.1	66	48.8	0.077	30.7
	Asymmetry score	4.07	1.49	20.7		11.3
3	Right	23.2	70	51.9	0.049	38.6
	Left	21.3	64	37.7	0.041	23.8
	Asymmetry score	8.19	8.57	37.7		62.3
4	Right	14.1	43	36.2	0.048	13.4
	Left	13.9	43	44.9	0.056	17.5
	Asymmetry score	1.44	0.00	23.9		23.4
5	Right	30.1	55	76.2	0.104	53.6
	Left	27.9	53	74.2	0.039	39.0
	Asymmetry score	7.31	3.64	2.6		27.2

Abbreviations and symbols are as follows: VO_{2peak}, peak oxygen uptake; GET, gas exchange threshold; MRT, mean response time; SEE, standard error of the estimate.

abolic perturbation and limb specific symptomatic fatigue previously reported in this population (Romani et al., 2008; Larson et al., 2013). Hansen et al. (2013) previously evaluated VO_2 kinetics during bipedal cycling in MS patients with an EDSS score of ~3.1 and demonstrated that MS patients have a significantly slower MRT compared to healthy participants (Hansen et al., 2013). Our work expands on this data by demonstrating differences in MRT between legs of a given MS patient. The primary component of the VO_2 kinetics provides an accurate analog of muscle VO_2 and therefore provides unique insight into muscle energetics beyond that obtained with traditional measurements of aerobic exercise capacity (Poole et al., 2008; Poole et al., 1991). The speed of VO_2 kinetics can be VO_2 delivery independent and dependent, with the latter occurring in situations in which muscle O_2 availability are compromised. Given the high ratio of cardiac capacity to skeletal muscle recruitment during single leg cycling it is likely that the asymmetries in VO_2 kinetics are due to difference within the muscle, not bulk O_2 transport. Given the MS is primarily a neurodegenerative disorder it is possible that these asymmetries are a secondary consequence of the disease and dependent on neurodegenerative dependent differences in limb training status. However, mitochondrial myopathy has been reported in some MS patients (Mao et al., 2010). It has been shown that individuals with MS exhibit bilateral asymmetry and elevated muscle fatigue, especially in the lower limbs compared to healthy controls. This study focused on possible lower leg asymmetry in VO_2 kinetics as a potential mechanism for muscle fatigue in individuals with MS. A majority of MS studies on muscle function and fatigue do not specify the leg used during the study or conduct experimentation on the same leg for each participant, whether or not this leg is the weaker or stronger leg. This study utilized assessment of both limbs and calculating an asymmetry score.

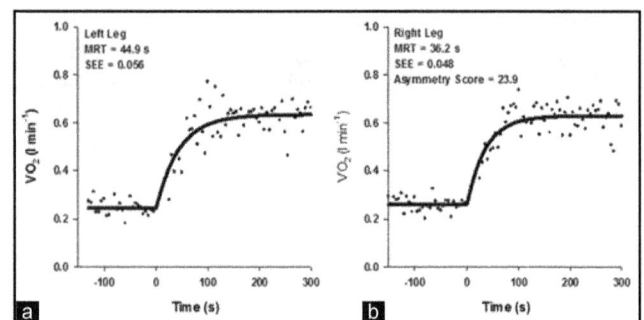

Figure 1. Representative subject's O_2 kinetic response

This is one of the first studies of its kind that Should be accessed and quantified pulmonary VO_2 kinetics during single leg cycling in individuals with MS. A similar study by Hansen et al. (2013) quantified pulmonary VO_2 kinetics during double leg cycling in individuals with MS (Hansen et al., 2013). Due to the effect of MS on bilateral symmetry in the lower limbs in individuals with MS, it is important to access pulmonary VO_2 kinetics of each limb independently to eliminate any compensation from the other leg in exercise performance. This study accurately quantified pulmonary VO_2 kinetics by having each subject perform at least 5 pulmonary VO_2 kinetics trials on each leg at a submaximal workload taken from 90% of GET (Poole et al., 2012). Hansen et al. (2013) had participants perform only two pulmonary VO_2 kinetics trials at 25% peak power output (Hansen et al., 2013). The present study corrected for the age of each subject by eliminating phase I from pulmonary VO_2 kinetics analysis, which Hansen et al. (2013) did not take into consideration. Therefore, this study is the first stepping stone in developing proper exercise prescriptions for individuals with MS to help them to prosper in everyday life. This study is limited by the small sample size, and no control group. Likewise, no evaluation of the mechanistic determinates of the VO_2 kinetic response occurred, which limits our interpretation of the data. However, the data reinforces the potential cardiorespiratory changes in the MS population that by association may contribute to symptoms of fatigue and exercise intolerance.

CONCLUSION

The findings from this study of significant asymmetries in VO_2 peak and parameters of VO_2 kinetics provide valuable insight into the potential metabolic perturbations associated with asymmetries in individuals with MS. However, further research is needed due to the small sample size and lack of control group.

ACKNOWLEDGMENTS

No external funding was used to support the current study. The authors have no relationships with any companies who will benefit from the results of the present study. In addition there was no conflict of interest with this project or manuscript.

REFERENCES

Abbiss, C. R., & Laursen, P. B. (2005). Models to explain fatigue during prolonged endurance cycling. *Sports Medicine, 35*(10), 865-898.

Compston, A., & Coles, A. (2008). Multiple Sclerosis. *Multiple Sclerosis, 372*(9648), 1502–17.

Chung, L.H., Remelius, J.G., Van Emmerik, R.E. & Kent-Braun, J.A. (2008). Leg power asymmetry and postural control in women with multiple sclerosis. *Medicine and science in sports and exercise, 40*(10), 1717-24.

Hansen, D., Wens, I., Kosten, L., Verboven, K. & Eijnde, B.O. (2013). Slowed exercise-onset Vo2 kinetics during submaximal endurance exercise in subjects with multiple sclerosis. *Neurorehabilitation and neural repair, 27*(1), 87-95.

Larson, R.D., McCully, K.K., Larson, D.J., Pryor, W.M. & White LJ. (2013). Bilateral differences in lower-limb performance in individuals with multiple sclerosis. *Journal of rehabilitation research and development, 50*(2), 215-22.

Mao, P., & Reddy, P.H. (2010). Is multiple sclerosis a mitochondrial disease? *Biochimica et biophysica acta, 1802*(1), 66-79.

Ponichtera-Mulcare, J. A. (1993). Exercise and multiple sclerosis. *Medicine & Science in Sports & Exercise, 25*(4), 451–465.

Poole, D.C., Barstow, T.J., McDonough, P., & Jones, A.M. (2008). Control of oxygen uptake during exercise. *Medicine and science in sports and exercise, 40*(3), 462-74.

Poole, D. C., & Jones, A. M. (2012). Oxygen uptake kinetics. *Comprehensive Physiology, 2*(2), 933–996.

Poole, D.C., Schaffartzik, W., Knight, D.R., Derion, T., Kennedy, B., Guy, H.J., Prediletto, R., & Wagner, P.D. (1991). Contribution of exercising legs to the slow component of oxygen uptake kinetics in humans. *Journal of applied physiology, 71*(4), 1245-60.

Romani, A., Bergamaschi,R., Candeloro, E., Alfonsi, E., Callieco, R., & Cosi, V. (2004). Fatigue in multiple sclerosis: multidimensional assessment and response to symptomatic treatment. *Multiple sclerosis, 10*(4), 462-8.

Sandroff, B. M., Sosnoff, J. J., & Motl, R. W. (2013). Physical fitness, walking performance, and gait in multiples sclerosis. *Journal of the Neurological sciences, 328*(1-2), 70–76.

Whipp, B. J., Ward, S. A., Lamarra, N., Davis, J. A., & Wasserman, K. (1982). Parameters of ventilatory and gas-exchange dynamics during exercise. *Journal of Applied Physiology, 52*(6), 1506–1513.

PERMISSIONS

LIST OF CONTRIBUTORS

Cordial M. Gillette
Exercise and Sport Science, University of Wisconsin – La Crosse, 1725 State Street, 148 Mitchell Hall, La Crosse, Wisconsin, 54601, USA

Scott T. Doberstein
Exercise and Sport Science, University of Wisconsin – La Crosse, 1725 State Street, 144 Mitchell Hall, La Crosse, Wisconsin, 54601, USA

Danielle L. DeSerano
UW-Health Sports Medicine, 621 Research Drive, Madison, Wisconsin, 53711, USA

Eric J. Linnell
Athletics, University of Wisconsin – Madison, 1440 Monroe Street, Madison, Wisconsin, 53711, USA

Ciro Agnelli and John A. Mercer
Department of Kinesiology & Nutrition Sciences, University of Nevada, Las Vegas, 4505 Maryland Parkway, Las Vegas, NV 89154-3034, USA

Athanasios Tsiokanos
Department of Physical Education and Sports Science, Laboratory of Biomechanics, University of Thessaly, Trikala 42100, Greece

Dimitrios Tsaopoulos
Institute for Research and Technology Thessaly (IRETETH), Kinesiology Sector, Center for Research and Technology Hellas (CERTH), 51 Papanastasiou St, 41222, Larissa, Greece

Arsenis Giavroglou and Eleftherios Tsarouchas
Hellenic Sports Research Institute, OAKA, Kifisias 37, Maroussi 15123, Athens, Greece

Melissa M. Montgomery and Andrew J. Galpin
Center for Sport Performance, Department of Kinesiology, California State University, Fullerton, 800 N. State College Blvd., Fullerton, CA 92831 USA

Risto H. Marttinen
Department of Kinesiology, California State University, Fullerton, 800 N. State College Blvd., Fullerton, CA 92831 USA

Nicole M. Sauls and Nicole C. Dabbs
Department of Kinesiology, California State University, San Bernardino, 5500 University Parkway, San Bernardino, CA 92407

Megan M. Adkins, Matthew R. Bice and John P. Rech
Kinesiology and Sport Science, University of Nebraska-Kearney, 2504 9th Ave, Kearney, NE 68849, United States

Danae Dinkel
Health and Physical Education, University of Nebraska-Omaha 6001 Dodge Street, Omaha, NE 68182, United States

Martin Weigert, Nico Nitzsche, Felix Kunert, Christiane Lösch, Lutz Baumgärtel and Henry Schulz
Institute of Human Movement Science and Health, Chemnitz University of Technology, Thüringer Weg 11, 09126 Chemnitz, Germany

Darien T. Pyka, Pablo B. Costa, Jared W. Coburn and Lee E. Brown
Department of Kinesiology, California State University, Fullerton, 800 N. State College Blvd. USA

John Porcari, Abigail Ryskey and Carl Foster
Department of Exercise and Sport Science, University of Wisconsin- La Crosse, La Crosse, WI USA

Kaitlin M. Jackson and David M. Andrews
Department of Kinesiology, University of Windsor, 401 Sunset Avenue, Windsor, ON, Canada N9B 3P4

Tyson A. C. Beach
Faculty of Kinesiology & Physical Education, University of Toronto, 55 Harbord St, Toronto, ON, Canada M5S 2W6

Joel Jackson, Alex Game, Pierre Gervais and Gordon Bell
Faculty of Physical Education and Recreation, University of Alberta, Edmonton, Alberta Canada, T6G2H9

Gary Snydmiller
Augustana Faculty, University of Alberta, Camrose, Alberta Canada, T4V2R3

Cale Bechtel, Joshua A. Cotter and Evan E. Schick
Physiology of Exercise and Sport (PEXS) Laboratory, Department of Kinesiology, Long Beach State University, 1250 Bellflower Blvd., Long Beach, CA, 90840-4901

John W. Farrell III, David J. Lantis, Debra A. Bemben and Rebecca D. Larson
Department of Health and Exercise Science, University of Oklahoma, 1401 Asp Ave, Norman, OK, 73019, USA

Carl J. Ade
Department of Kinesiology, Kansas State University, 920 Denison Ave, Manhattan, KS, 66506, USA

Oladipo Eddo, Bryndan Lindsey, Shane V. Caswell and Nelson Cortes
Sports Medicine Assessment, Research & Testing Laboratory, George Mason University, 10900 University Blvd., Manassas, 20110, United States

Christopher F. Kelly, Adam M. Gonzalez, Robert W. Spitz, Katie M. Sell and Jamie J. Ghigiarelli
Department of Health Professions, Hofstra University, 110 Hofstra Dome, 220 Hofstra University, Hempstead, NY 11549, USA

Godefroid K. Mabele, Constant N. Ekisawa, Teddy B.Linkoko and Nicaise K. Ngasa
Department of Physical Medicine and Rehabilitation, University of Kinshasa Faculty of Medicine, Democratic Republic of Congo (DRC) Kinesiology service

Christophe DELECLUSE
Faculty of movement and Rehabilitation sciences Departement of movement science K.U. Leuven, Belgique

Francois L. Bompeka
Department of Internal Medicine, University of Kinshasa Faculty of Medicine, Democratic Republic of Congo (DRC) Nephrology service

Jongil Lim
Department of Counseling, Health and Kinesiology, Texas A&M University - San Antonio, One University Way, San Antonio, TX, USA

Seung Ho Chang and Adriane Cris Tomimbang
Department of Kinesiology, San Jose State University, 1 Washington Square, San Jose, CA, USA

Jacob R. Gdovin
Department of Kinesiology; Missouri State University 901 S. National Ave., Springfield, MO 65897 USA

Charles C. Williams
Department of of Exercise Science; LaGrange College, 601 Broad Street, LaGrange, GA 30240 USA
Department of Health, Exercise Science and Recreation Management; The University of Mississippi 215 Turner Center, University, MS 38677 USA

Lauren A. Luginsland
Department of Health, Exercise Science and Recreation Management; The University of Mississippi 215 Turner Center, University, MS 38677 USA

Samuel J. Wilson
Department of Health, Exercise Science and Recreation Management; The University of Mississippi 215 Turner Center, University, MS 38677 USA
Department of Health Sciences and Kinesiology; Georgia Southern University Statesboro, GA 30460 USA

Vanessa L. Cazas-Moreno
Department of Human Performance and Sport Sciences; Tennessee State University 3500 John A. Merritt Blvd., Nashville, TN 37209 USA

Charles R. Allen
Department of Exercise Science; Florida Southern College 111 Lake Hollingsworth Dr., Lakeland, FL 33801 USA

Harish Chander
Neuromechanics Laboratory, Department of Kinesiology; Mississippi State University Mississippi State, MS 39762 USA

Chip Wade
Department of Industrial and Systems Engineering; Auburn University Auburn, AL 36849 USA

John C. Garner III
Department of Kinesiology and Health Promotion; Troy University 112G Wright Hall, Troy, AL 36082 USA

Amanda Gier MS, Shelley Kirk, Christopher Kist and Robert Siegel
Center for Better Health and Nutrition, Cincinnati Children's 3333 Burnet Ave., MLC 5016, Cincinnati, OH, 45229, USA

Nicholas M. Edwards
Orthopaedics, University of Minnesota Medical Center 2450 Riverside Ave. South, Suite R200, Minneapolis, MN, 55454, USA

Philip R. Khoury
Heart Institute, Cincinnati Children's, 3333 Burnet Ave., MLC 7002, Cincinnati, OH 45229, USA

John W. Farrell and Daniel J. Blackwood
Department of Health and Exercise Science, University of Oklahoma 1401 Asp Ave, Norman, OK 73019, USA

George M. Dallam, Steve R. McClaran and Carol P. Foust
Department of Exercise Science, Health Promotion and Recreation, Colorado State University – Pueblo; Pueblo.2200 Bonforte Boulevard, Pueblo, CO, USA 81001-4901

Daniel G. Cox
Staff TherapistArizona Orthopedic Physical Therapy 9980 W. Glendale Rd ste 110 Glendale, AZ 85307

Jordan M. Glenn
Neurotrack Technologies Inc.399 Bradford St #101, Redwood City, CA 94063

Michelle Gray
Exercise Science Research Center, University of Arkansas HPER 321-E, University of Arkansas, Fayetteville, AR 72701

Nicole E. Moyen
Hopkins Marine Station of Stanford University Pacific Grove, CA 93950

Jennifer L. Vincenzo
Department of Physical Therapy, University of Arkansas for Medical Sciences Fayetteville, Arkansas 72703

Kylie K. Harmon
Neuromuscular Physiology Lab, University of Central Florida 12354 Research Pkwy, St #221, Orlando, FL 32826

Lee E. Brown
University of West Florida 7178 Loysburg St., Navarre, FL 32566

Thiago F. Lourenço, Fernando O. C. da Silva, Lucas S. Tessutti and Carlos E. da Silva
Biochemistry Department, State University of Campinas, Cidade Universitária Zeferino Vaz, Campinas, SP, 13083-970, Brazil

Cesar C. C. Abad
Department of Phyical Education, SENAC University, Av. Eng.Eusébio Stevaux São Paulo, SP 04696-000, Brazil

Yang Song
The Division of Liberal Studies and Education, Lane College, Jackson, Tennessee, United States

Stephen Harvey
Patton College of Education, Department of Recreation and Sport Pedagogy, Ohio University Athens, Ohio, United States

James Hannon
College of Education, Health and Human Services, Kent State University Kent, Ohio, United States

Karen Rambo-Hernandez
College of Education and Human Services, West Virginia University Morgantown, West Virginia, United States

Emily Jones
College of Applied Science and Technology, Illinois State University Normal, Illinois, United States

Sean Bulger
College of Physical Activity and Sport Sciences, West Virginia University Morgantown, West Virginia, United States

Danielle L. Gyemi, Don Clarke and Paula M. van Wyk
Department of Kinesiology, University of Windsor, 401 Sunset Avenue, Windsor, ON, Canada, N9B 3P4

William J. Altenhof
Department of Mechanical, Automotive and Materials Engineering, University of Windsor, 401 Sunset Avenue, Windsor, ON Canada, N9B 3P4

You Fu
School of Community Health Sciences, University of Nevada, Reno, 1664 N Virginia Street, Reno, NV 89557

Ryan D. Burns
Department of Health, Kinesiology and Recreation, University of Utah, 250 S 1850 E, Salt Lake City, UT 84112

Rebecca D. Larson, Monica Barton and Christopher D. Black
Department of Health and Exercise Science, University of Oklahoma, Norman, OK, USA

John W Farrell III
Department of Health and Exercise Science, University of Oklahoma, Norman, OK, USA
Interdisciplinary School of Health Sciences, University of Ottawa, Ottawa, ON, CDN.

Gregory S. Cantrell
Department of Health and Exercise Science, University of Oklahoma, Norman, OK, USA
Health and Physical Education Department, Northern State University, Aberdeen, SA, USA

David J. Lantis
Department of Health and Exercise Science, University of Oklahoma, Norman, OK, USA
Department of Kinesiology, St. Ambrose University, Davenport, IA, USA

Carl J. Ade
Department of Health and Exercise Science, University of Oklahoma, Norman, OK, USA
Department of Kinesiology, Kansas State University, Manhattan KS, USA

Index